Sexualized Children

Sexualized Children

Assessment and Treatment of Sexualized Children and Children Who Molest

Eliana Gil & Toni Cavanagh Johnson

Launch Press

Printed in the United States of America

03 02 01 00   12 11 10 9 8

Library of Congress Cataloging-in-Publicaton Data

Gil, Eliana.

Sexualized children : assessment and treatment of sexualized children and children who molest / by Eliana Gil & Toni Cavanagh Johnson.

p. cm.

ISBN 1-877872-07-5 : pbk. 1-877872-05-9

1. Psychosocial disorders in children. 2. Children and sex.

3. Children—Sexual behavior. 4. Teenage child molesting.

I. Johnson, Toni Cavanagh. II. Title.

[DNLM: 1. Child Behavior Disorders—therapy. 2. Psychosexual Development—in infancy & childhood. 3. Sex Behavior—in infancy & childhood. WS 105.5.S4 G463s]

RJ506.P72G55 1992

618.92'8583—dc20

DNLM/DLC

for Library of Congress   92-49422
                                                                         CIP

In loving memory of my godmother, Irene Valero, a guiding light, a shelter in the storm, and a source of joy.

E. G.

To my husband Bill, and children Matthew, Taj, and Alexis.

T. C. J.

Contents

Foreword

William N. Friedrich, Ph.D.

Although I now realize that I had probably worked with a number of sexually abused children prior to 1976, that year marks the beginning of my "knowing" involvement with child sexual abuse. I wasn't very successful with the incestuous family that presented itself to me, and moved on as if they had been a rare aberration in my clinical career. I had no reason to think otherwise, since my clinical supervisor had also had no experience in the area.

But something serious happened. I now had an awareness that sexual abuse occurred, and in the same way that once a new word is learned you begin to hear it, once an awareness happens, information and data about the awareness have a way of finding you.

I began to meet many victims, and before I left graduate school, my experiences as a psychologist with a county social services agency and as a foster parent/group home house parent had left me with the realization that many children, particularly female, were molested. Being an empirically grounded person, I wasn't yet convinced that many males had been abused.

But by the end of the 1970's, I was regularly treating male victims, and in 1982, I received a referral to evaluate and treat a young boy who looked surprisingly like some of the adolescent and adult sex offenders I had worked with to that point. Always the skeptic, a true realization of the extent of sexual abuse and its range of impact in children was only now complete.

As Toni Johnson mentions in Chapter 5 of this book, my paper on sexually aggressive young children was published almost simultaneously with her paper on child perpetrators. I had never met Dr. Johnson prior to these papers being published, and the simultaneity added to the validity of our findings. At conferences when I talk about sexually aggressive children, I still see in fellow clinicians the same look of disbelief that I had at one time. It's as if each of us have a level of tolerance for the abhorrent, and the thought of children as sexually aggressive exceeds this level for many.

And now, the National Center on Child Abuse and Neglect (NCCAN) has funded two separate grants to study sexually aggressive children, one a collaborative project involving Barbara Bonner in Oklahoma City and Lucy Berliner in Seattle, and the other a Vermont-wide study involving Bill Pithers and Alison Stickrod-Gray. This speaks to the urgency that sexually aggressive children instill in the practitioner, and the need to know more about them and how to treat them.

I am pleased to have had the chance to read this book which distills, for the first time in a full-length volume, the range of pertinent theory, practice and networking that is required to best serve these children. I had read Eliana Gil's *The Healing Power of Play*, a warmly compassionate and clinically rich book, and I have since had the opportunity to get to know Toni Johnson, who brings a developmental perspective that is central to these children, and I believe that this book reflects some of the best of what each has to offer.

For example, sexually aggressive children, despite their acts, need to be viewed compassionately and hopefully, and this is best done by thinking about them as developing organisms who are also victims of some form of maltreatment, most often sexual. I think it is poor clinical practice to not see the victim part as primary in young, sexually aggressive children. While sexual abuse as the etiologic agent is not always clearly evident, these children have had more than their share of experiences in which they were rejected, discounted and not treated empathically.

Rather than lumping them together in a homogenous group, another contribution of this book is Johnson's preliminary typology of sexually aggressive children. Only when we see accurately the full range of behavior and its context, can we then develop treatment plans that do these children service. One of the seminal papers in the adolescent offender treatment literature is a paper on typology by Michael O'Brien and Walter Bera (1986), and the typology offered in this book, while not validated, is a welcome beginning.

Along the same lines is the chapter on assessment, which in addition to discussing various techniques, is another avenue to help the clinician not only accurately perceive these children, but also document any treatment progress that is made.

Another critical piece is the emphasis on community involvement, including working with foster parents and networking with legal and other treatment professionals. The amount of extra-therapy telephoning and conferencing I do in regards to abusive families is enormous, but must be done if all of the players are to be helpful to the treatment process.

I agree with Drs. Gil and Johnson's contention about the primacy of group therapy for sexual abuse victims, but I want to remind the reader of two things. The first is the fact that we don't know what works with these children. The longer this lack of empirical knowledge exists, the longer we operate in the dark. We need to evaluate our treatment effectiveness if we are to be able to lobby for the services that children need. The second is the fact that sexually reactive children are also behaviorally more reactive in group settings, and we owe it to them not to retraumatize them in treatment.

I have been using pair therapy (Selman & Schultz, 1990) with several sexually aggressive boys, and this combination of two children, in a carefully structured setting, has been more useful than a larger group, which would have been both overwhelming and invited rejection. Attachment failure is something that is discussed with some of the most traumatized children, and expecting remotely appropriate group behavior is premature for some of the children that get placed in group. This is even more so the case when one thinks of sexually aggressive children, who by their very definition, have failed peer experiences.

The sensitive practicing clinician also is fully aware of the impact working with traumatized children has on one's world view. Victims who have become victimizers will often leave a therapist feeling invaded, literally and figuratively. I very much appreciated their final chapter on transference and countertransference issues with these children and their families. Only by labelling the feelings we get in the therapy office can we master them. This is a technique we teach children and one that works for us as well.

Finally, I have found it enormously useful to think about the following theoretical perspectives when working with sexually aggressive children: developmental, attachment, emotional/behavioral regulation, and development of self. Sexual abuse stems from and affects attachment to parents and peers, creates disregulation in behavior and affect, and disturbs the child's developing sense of self. These perspectives are discussed throughout this text.

I encourage the reader to keep these perspectives in mind as another way to integrate the material presented here. For example, I was pleased to see Gil's focus on dissociative processes, which are manifestations of disregulation. The longer I work with victims, either as children or adults, the more I realize that dissociation exists, in a variety of presentations, and while very rare, this includes multiplicity in children.

Read the extensive therapy material presented here with the question of how this furthers and corrects attachment. The therapy described is designed to be corrective of the insecure and insufficient attachments present in these children. The chapters on group and family therapy list a number of strategies to engage difficult children and families in the therapeutic process. The more corrective the attachment experience, the more children can develop the "internal working model" of relatedness that enables them to view other children accurately, and not as victims. This directly and indirectly affects the end result, which is the emergence of a more coherent self that can do the "love and work" of mature life.

O'Brien, M. & Bera, W. (1986). Adolescent sexual offenders: A descriptive typology. *Preventing Sexual Abuse*, 1, 1-4.

Belman, R. L. & Schultz, L. H. (1990). *Making a friend in youth*. Chicago: University of Chicago Press.

Preface

Sexuality is seldom treated as a strong or healthy force in the positive development of a child's personality in the United States. We are not inclined to believe that our children are sexual or that they should be sexual in any of their behaviors. Although it is difficult to generalize in our pluralistic society, there is typically no permission for normal child sexual experiences. Children are not taught to understand their sexual experiences nor to anticipate sexual experiences as enjoyable. Rather, they are taught to be wary of most sexual experiences, both interpersonally and intrapsychically.

Floyd M. Martinson

This book was written out of a concern that parents and professionals too often minimize harmful or dangerous molesting behaviors between children, or identify children's age-appropriate sexual behaviors as something alarming, deviant, or warranting punishment.

In our experience, parents and/or professionals often ignore, dismiss, or underreact to situations in which children engage in aggressive or hurtful sexual play. When children's molesting behaviors are ignored, child victims are negatively affected, children's molesting behaviors can increase, and neither children who molest nor child-victims receive needed therapeutic services.

On the other hand, many professionals and parents struggle with situations such as children kissing, children who disrobe together, children showing their genitals, children masturbating, or children who are "caught" playing doctor. These children may be engaged in age-appropriate, joyful, and spontaneous sexual interest and experimentation. Overreacting to children's age-appropriate sexual interest or play can be alarming and confusing to children. This book clarifies issues regarding child sexuality.

There has been a gradual increase of reports of suspected sexual abuse involving children who molest other children or children with problematic sexual activity. A well-publicized California case caused a furor when a ten-year-old child allegedly sodomized approximately four or five children in the neighborhood. Child abuse agencies received numerous phone calls from individuals asking if a ten-year-old could get and maintain an erection that could penetrate another child. This is not an isolated case; similar referrals have been made to authorities across the country. A Texas court for example, recently (1992) awarded the child-victim molested by a five-year-old classmate over $11 million, citing the daycare's negligence in protecting the child.

In this book, we provide preliminary information based on our combined experience working with children twelve and under who molest, and who exhibit problematic sexual behaviors. We discuss age-appropriate childhood sexuality; provide a way to distinguish "normal sex play" from problematic sexual behaviors including sexual abuse; and offer ideas for evaluation, individual and group treatment for children who molest, and family treatment.

We made some choices in presenting the material. First, we are using the term "sexualized children" to refer to children who engage in sexual behaviors that seem problematic and elicit adult concern. We use this phrase to avoid the word "seductive," which has been used often to describe observed sexual behaviors in children. The word seduction implies intent, and we believe that many children with problematic sexual behaviors are children who have been conditioned to respond in specific ways. A sexually abused boy who is taken into a shelter and grabs the genitals of personnel in the facility is not "coming on" to staff: the child is doing what he has been taught to do, and what he expects others want from him.

The use of the word "sexualized" should not be taken to mean that we believe some children are sexual and some children are not. We believe that all children are sexual beings, and sexual development includes a gradual progression of interest, curiosity, and activity. We have also tried to avoid the use of words such as "normal" or "abnormal" sexual behaviors, choosing instead to use phrases such as "natural and expectable," "age-appropriate," or "problematic sexual behaviors."

The literature uses many terms to refer to children who act out sexually. We use the term sexualized children for children who exhibit a range of problematic sexual behaviors such as sexual language, excessive masturbation, or sexual preoccupation. We reserve the term children who molest for children who force, coerce, bribe, or trick other children into engaging in a range of sexual behaviors. We are not using the phrase "abuse reactive" because we believe this may inadvertently confuse readers into believing that all children who molest have a documented history of overt sexual or physical abuse. Some children who molest come from environments in which there is covert sexual abuse, and we devote some time to discussing the importance of this variable. Last, we simply prefer to use the descriptive term "children who molest" rather than "sex offenders" due to the often negative associations evoked by the term sex offenders, particularly regarding the possibility of rehabilitation. We feel optimistic about the likelihood of reversing the molesting behaviors of young children who have not solidified patterns of arousal and behavior, and have not yet had the opportunity to develop their own sexual maturity and choice.

We recognize the difficulty of working with this population, and we are impressed by the similarities between young children's sexually abusive behaviors and those of their adolescent counterparts. At the same time, dissimilarities exist between children who molest and older offenders: children who molest, and their parents, across the board, have more highly disturbed interpersonal relationships, levels of family disruption, sexual confusion, and victimization. In contrast to adolescent sex offenders, most children who molest have severe oppositional disorder, frequently diagnosed Conduct Disorder; have significant disruptions in development of their core self, as well as their capacity to make meaningful attachments. In addition, the thrust of sexual behaviors in young children is less frequently toward obtaining sexual pleasure, and more frequently toward expressing internalized anger or tension. The relationship between masturbation and deviant fantasies is less evident in children who molest, and patterns of sexual arousal are not yet well-established. Finally, cognitive treatment approaches that are very helpful for older offenders, should be imbedded in experiential and process-oriented interventions, helpful to young children who often exhibit Attention Deficit Disorder and severe learning problems.

We believe that the clinical response with children who molest should rigorously provide limits, education, accountability, and supervision. The therapy must be abuse-specific and individually tailored to each child's unique pattern of molesting. The therapeutic outcomes for children who molest are strongly correlated to a successful treatment outcome for their parents. Family treatment is critical in helping the child reverse his or her molesting behaviors; the younger the child, the more influence the family has, and the more we must rely on the family's ability and willingness to change dysfunctional patterns, provide support and supervision to their children, and cooperate with treatment.

In closing, we want to make clear that in assessing children who molest children, we do not consider the issue of intent or consent to be relevant. We raise this at the outset, because we have noted that many professionals who evaluate these cases may rely on issues of intent and/or consent to draw conclusions. Although the issues of consent may be relevant when investigating potential child abuse cases among adolescents, it cannot be used to draw conclusions about young children and possible sexual abuse. Young children are clearly not capable of giving informed consent, and assessing whether or not a victimization has occurred based on this variable seems totally unacceptable. Gail Ryan (1990) has pinpointed important elements of consent including understanding what is being proposed without confusion, misconception, or misattribution and having an awareness of possible consequences. Clearly, young children cannot meet these demands for consent.

We have been fortunate to write this book at a time when many professionals are making contributions to our understanding of this problem. In particular we would like to acknowledge the work of Sandra Ballester, Lucy Berliner, Jan Ellen Burton, Henrika Cantwell, Barbara Christopherson, Carolyn Cunningham, David Finkelhor, William Friedrich, Alison Stickrod Gray, Fern Grunberger, Sandra Hewitt, Connie Isaacs, Fay Honey Knopp, Sandra Lane, Kee MacFarlane, Floyd Martinson, John Money, Michael O'Brien, Frederique Pierre, Lucinda Rasmussen, Les Rawlings, Gail Ryan, and Alayne Yates.

One of the advantages of coauthoring, is that we can offer a broad perspective based on our individual experiences, and we can emphasize slightly different approaches—we believe this strengthens our collective effort. We present our thoughts with humility and a clear understanding that work in this field is in its earliest stages. Nothing we say is intended to be the final word on this topic.

References

Martinson, F. M. (1991). Normal sexual development in infancy and early child-hood. In G. D. Ryan & S. L. Lane (Eds.), *Juvenile sexual offending: Causes, consequences, and correction.* Lexington, MA: Lexington.

Ryan, G. (1990). Sexual behavior in childhood. In J. McNamara & B. H. McNamara (Eds.), *Adoption and the sexually abused child.* Human Services Development Institute, University of Southern Maine.

Acknowledgments

I would like to acknowledge the ongoing love and support of my family: Eillen and Norm, Jim, Renee and Char; my children Eric, Teresa and Christy; my mother Eugenia, my brothers Peter and Tony; my sister Monica, brother-in-law Juan, step-mother Fanny, wonderful niece Geovanna and my godson Xavier Antonio; my beloved nephew John Brady; my special cousin Tere; and my newest god-daughter, Sarah Fox Hansen. Also, a warm thanks to my closest friends Teresa & Toni Davi, Melissa and Melinda Brown, Don Wilson, Uncle Hal, Mary Herget, Robert Green, Steve Santini, Sue Scoff, Kathy Baxter, Lorraine Heath, Lou Fox Hansen and Ken Miller. I also thank my friend and colleague Jeff Bodmer-Turner for being available night or day to help me sort things out or give me help with reference materials. I thank Toni Cavanagh Johnson for making my first coauthoring experience as painless as possible and for her generosity in talking things out with me, giving and taking constructive feedback, negotiating, and offering many helpful insights. My gratitude to Laura Miller and Beatrice Sussman for their skillful editing. Laura edited early drafts with great care, and Beatrice tackled the final manuscript, ensuring clarity and continuity, and offering countless suggestions which strengthened the final product. My assistant Lisa Metro maintains my general chaos organized, helped research the topic, and typed and retyped drafts with patience and efficiency. My thanks to my husband, John, for being helpful, supportive, and understanding the nature of writing and writing spurts. Last but not least, thanks to the parents and children with whom I've worked for helping me gain insight and always delighting me with their resiliency.

Eliana Gil

I am extremely grateful to Eliana Gil for inviting me to co-author this book with her. Eliana guided me through the process with kindness, editorial assistance, and fairness. I hope that I would be so helpful and gracious to someone with comparatively little experience.

Without the assistance of my wonderful husband, there is no way I could have completed this work. He is generous with his time, keeping all the electronic equipment working, and giving emotional support when it seemed as though I would never finish. My thanks to my children, who never complained while remarking that they always knew where to find me, in front of the computer.

I am very grateful to all the people who gave large amounts of time to read and comment on my material: Bill Breer, Connie Bohan, Conrad Bowden, Colleen Friend, Fern Grunberger, Dorothy Haverbush, the clinical staff at Intermountain Children's Home, Floyd Martinson, Mary Beth Olender, Michael Perry, Gail Ryan, John Stoner, John Taylor, Michele Winterstein, Kathy Wood, and Alayne Yates. Without their comments, the chapters I wrote would not be as complete.

My deep gratitude and respect goes to the children who molest and their families who taught me all I know about them. I stand in awe at their ability to work through the tremendous pain of their lives, to survive, and often flourish.

Toni Cavanagh Johnson

Client identity has been rigorously protected in presenting "case histories," by altering some combination of age, gender, circumstances, and often by combining the stories of several individuals into one presentation. When actual dialogue is presented it is reconstructed from memory using a variety of conversations with children, and therefore, does not violate children's actual confidences.

1

Childhood Sexuality

Toni Cavanagh Johnson, Ph.D.

Child development proceeds along many lines. Most textbooks separate child development into biological, cognitive, and social and personality headings. Sexual development is generally discussed under the biological and social and personality areas.

Childhood sexuality is generally discussed as a single entity. This chapter examines separate developmental lines within child sexuality, allowing a more thorough understanding and a greater possibility of the assessment of problems that can occur in children's sexual development. Seven different lines of development are discussed: biological, sensual/erotic, behavioral, gender, cognitive, relationship, and socialization.

Starting in utero, the *biological* substrates of sexuality begin to develop. After children are born, *sensuality* in relation to touch and skin contact is experienced and is later expressed in the *eroticism* of adult sexuality. In utero, erections and orgasms occur. As children develop manual dexterity and physical coordination, they begin to engage in *sexual behaviors*. Children grow in cognitive awareness of the world, accumulate sexual knowledge, and consolidate *gender* identity through interaction with the environment. As children experience others in relation to their own sexuality, the *relational* aspects of sexuality develop and mature. *Sexual socialization* is a powerful force in aligning all aspects of sexuality in developing children.

After birth, the lines of childhood sexual development occur simultaneously, but at different rates and with different emphases at different times. Although the lines can be delineated separately, they overlap in many respects. If disruption or acceleration occurs in one line, other lines may be disrupted or accelerated. There may be "critical periods" in sexual development as in other aspects of children's development.

Biological

Natural and Expectable Development

At conception, all embryos are female. As the fetus develops, if there is an influx of gonadal androgens during the sixth to twelfth week of fetal development, the child will be born with male sexual apparatus. As the fetus grows in utero, the sexual apparatus of males and females develops and begins to function. Involuntary penile erections have been observed in the womb (Reinisch & Beasley, 1990).

Lubrication and orgasm, which are normally associated with adult sexual responses, have been observed during infancy. These are physiological responses of the organism and are reflexive in nature (Martinson, 1982).

During childhood and latency, children's bodies, including their sexual apparatus, grow and develop. Both sexes at about the age of seven experience an increase in adrenal androgens, although gonadotropin levels remain low (Yates, 1991).

Between eleven and fourteen years of age most children experience a substantial increase in their hormonal levels, accounting for the vast physical changes of puberty. Pubescent males experience an increase in testosterone and other hormone levels from age eleven until age seventeen. The physical changes for males include hair growth, increases in height and weight, growth of the penis and pubic hair, a deepening of the voice, development of sperm, and ejaculation. With the increase in hormones, girls increase in height and weight, develop breasts, pubic hair, and begin to menstruate. The influx of serum androgenic hormones at puberty is a precursor to the surge in sexuality seen in adolescents. Although the mechanism by which androgens cause the motivation for engaging in sexual behaviors is unknown, their influence has been established (Udry et al., 1985). After the physiological changes of puberty, the individual has the physical capability to procreate.

Disruptions in Development

There are no reported cases of biological abnormalities in children who molest known to me. Children whose prenatal hormones contradict their sex of assignment, children born with the genitalia of both sexes, children with highly disfigured genitalia in need of surgery during infancy, or other physical abnormalities of the genitalia are unknown among children who molest.

It has been speculated that there may be an excessive or pathogenic influx of hormones in some sexualized children and children who molest (Johnson, 1988). Prepubertal children engage in more sexual behaviors than other children, possibly a result of an excess or deficiency of certain hormones—a topic worthy of research.

Children who molest are a heterogeneous group. It is possible that hormonal excesses account for some subsets of the children. One of the subsets to which this may apply is sexually preoccupied children (see Preliminary Findings, Chapter five). These children who bribe, cajole, and threaten other children into the sexual interactions describe their behavior as striving for pleasurable feelings. They often have more highly developed fantasies than other children who molest, and their fantasies do not seem to have the aggressive component, but mainly sexual and pleasurable aims. If they were molested, they often describe it as having been pleasurable. They do not want to stop the sexual behaviors and are frequently very difficult to supervise.

Money (Money & Lamacz, 1989) discusses the use of sex hormone suppressants or antagonists as a treatment for adult paraphilias. These suppressants lower the level of circulating androgen in the bloodstream to the level of prepuberty. Medroxyprogesterone acetate (Depo-Provera) is used most commonly in the United States and lowers the secretion of androgen and testosterone from the testicles. Depo-Provera also has a calming effect on the sex-regulating brain cells of the preoptic area of the hypothalamus. Future research may determine whether differing levels of hormones exist between sexualized children, children who molest, and children with natural and healthy sexual interest and behaviors. Although it is not well understood, hormonal levels may increase in some children who experience abuse.

Children who live in unstable, unpredictable environments frequently experience different states of physiological arousal. Unsure of what is going to happen when someone gets angry, sobs, slams the door while fleeing the house, curses and hits them, or caresses their genitals, children feel various types of physiological arousal that generally are incomprehensible to them. Many children seek to discharge the arousal as quickly as possible. Children who molest also describe heightened physiological arousal to different emotions. For example, when they fear for their bodily safety, are extremely lonely, feel hopeless or helpless, or when they feel jealous, angry, or rageful, they describe feeling anxious or tense, which are both states of physiological arousal. The environmental factors and the feelings are often paired so that children who feel sad, and recall a violent scene, feel aroused and seek to discharge the arousal immediately. The arousal is sometimes sexual and other times a more complex arousal with both sexual and aggressive elements; at other times the arousal may simply feel rageful and explosive. Erections and lubrication can occur with any of these physiological states. Because the pairing with high arousal has multiple elements, children may seek to discharge the arousal by acting in physically, sexually, or emotionally aggressive ways. Although some children seek to discharge high arousal by acting inwardly, children who molest have no models for doing so. Arousal is discharged against the environment, and most frequently against people, through physically, verbally, or sexually aggressive means.

Although most children feel uncomfortable with this high state of arousal and seek to discharge it, some may seek the arousal. One subset of the children, the violent children who molest (see Preliminary Findings, Chapter five), may be seeking to increase their level of physiological arousal. They may feel readier to act and defend themselves and hurt others in this higher state of arousal and more vulnerable when not aroused. Many of these children have been victims of extreme physical abuse. When not keyed up, they are at risk of experiencing their unending sadness and feelings of loss and abandonment. They prefer rage and aggression, which they can direct outward.

Studies indicate that, at least in animals, once a physiological response has been established (e.g., a hormonal response to sexual or aggressive stimuli) it is more easily reevoked when exposed to similar stimuli. When children who feel overwhelmed or highly aroused in threatening situations reexperience a similar situation, it can reevoke the physiological response.

Future research may indicate that some children, based on their history, temperament, brain anatomy, and hormonal patterns develop a physiological response pattern that relates to sexually aggressive behavior patterns.

Sensual/Erotic

Natural and Expectable Development

Beginning in earliest childhood, infants respond to kissing, rubbing, patting, and caressing by caretakers. Infants have a sensual and gratified response to closeness. They are soothed and nourished while sucking at the breast. Thumbsucking and toesucking are sensual experiences that bring pleasure. Children may get a positive sensual experience from the withholding of urine and feces. Sensuality in children is evidenced by their pleasure in manipulating objects. Stroking the fur of stuffed animals or the edge of a blanket calms children. Masturbation provides physical pleasure. Although some young children may actively seek orgasm from self-stimulation, masturbation generally provides a soothing sensual pleasure and may act as a method of tension reduction and distraction (Yates, 1990).

Latency-aged and older prepubescent children describe fascination with genitalia. Because of the external nature of the penis, boys have greater access to and knowledge of their genitalia. Boys participate in fanciful games of childhood: making exciting designs with their urine, measuring their penises, seeing whose penis can stand up higher, or seeing how many rubber bands can be balanced on an erect penis. During prepubescence, children experience feelings that awaken the erotic components of their sexuality. The genitalia begin to take on a new meaning. Pleasure is experienced as the genitalia become associated with desire.

> Wild and confused dreams made me feel funny—just as if I had to urinate. The dreams included boys and girls kissing, and the funny feeling I got was both distressing and exciting. I had no idea as to what the dreams meant, but I definitely realized they pertained to sex (Martinson, 1973). When I touch myself, it feels weird. I kind of like it but I kind of don't. (Personal communication from an eleven-year-old boy)

Preliminary results of a retrospective study indicate that approximately 18 percent of adults surveyed describe feeling "sexually stimulated as an adult might feel" while engaging in sexual experiences when they were twelve years old or younger. Most adults surveyed described feeling "excited [not sexually]" during childhood sexual experiences (Johnson, 1992).

Eroticism and sexual desire focused on sexual arousal and orgasm generally accompany pubertal and postpubertal sexual experiences. Sensuality remains, but in addition is a sexual and erotic pleasure that comes from kissing, looking, fantasizing, genital touching, self-stimulation, sexual intercourse, and other sexual experiences.

Disruptions in Development

In equatorial Africa, southern Asia, and the South Pacific are cultures in which infants' genitals are intentionally stimulated by adults if children are cross or restless (Yates, 1991). This may not create any confusion or disturbed feelings in children because the sensual pleasure derived is for the children's benefit and continues only as long as it takes for the soothing to occur. Confusion and anxiety can result when children's genitalia and other parts of their bodies are used by others for their erotic satisfaction. Adult sexual desire and erotic pleasure seeking is foreign to children. Faced with the need to satisfy the erotic desires of an older person, some children become overwhelmed by feelings of helplessness, confusion, inadequacy, and fear.

If children's genitalia become the focus of another's attention, children begin to organize their lives around their own genitalia. As Yates states, "The child's genitals may function as a central, organizing principle in their development" (Yates, 1990). Children may begin to seek out other opportunities for sexual experiences. Some begin to confuse all touch with sexual touch (Finkelhor, 1984). When another person is using them as a sexual object, children may feel highly aroused. Whether this arousal in children is similar to sexual arousal of adults is unclear. Differences exist between children in the sensations they feel. Some postpubertal children report sexual arousal while being molested including vaginal lubrication, sexual pleasure, and orgasm. Reports by some prepubertal children appear to indicate pleasure and arousal; however, whether this is similar or identical to postpubertal sexuality is unclear. In some children who describe pleasurable feelings during sexual encounters, this may be related to feeling wanted, loved, and cared for. These feelings, which are more emotional than genital, are similar to those many females strive for in a sexual relationship.

Research through the National Institute of Mental Health (NIMH) is studying the effects of trauma and sexual abuse on the onset of puberty. Early data indicate that girls who have been sexually abused appear to have an early onset of the hormonal changes associated with puberty (Trickett & Putnam, 1990). Studies of girls raised in families in which persistent family conflict occurred indicate an earlier onset of puberty, which may be related to stress (Sapolsky, 1992).

An example using a therapy group of young boys who molest illustrates sexual behavior that focuses on aggression. The shift to sexual pleasure is noted in the final stages of therapy as children enter puberty.

Tom, a nine-year-old boy, abused five girls and two boys in a residential setting. In each case he exposed himself, snuck up on a child, and yelled profanities or sidled up to a child and talked about sexual urges and needs using slang phrases. He had an extremely angry demeanor when engaging in sexual acts. He identified that before doing the sexually aggressive behaviors he felt angry, and sometimes he would wonder where his mother and father were. (Tom had not seen his parents, who had physically abused and neglected him, since he entered the residential facility five years earlier.) During the first two years of treatment, he could identify high arousal before sexually aggressive behaviors, but did not identify anything that sounded like sexual arousal. (See previous section.) Toward the end of therapy, as Tom entered the middle half of his eleventh year, he began to speak about sexual arousal. He said that he had started putting his pillow a certain way so that he could rub his penis on it. He was reticent to speak about it, but wanted to know if any of the other children in the group were doing the same thing and felt the same feelings.

Sexual Behaviors

Natural and Expectable Development

Erections, lubrication, and pelvic thrusting occur in infants. These are the body's responses to the internal experiences of children and are mainly reflexive in nature. Although they may eventuate in orgasm, they are not consciously oriented toward that goal, as is generally found in adults (Martinson, 1982).

Genital exploration begins in infancy and brings pleasurable and soothing feelings. Masturbation is more orchestrated than genital play. When masturbating, children rhythmically thrust the genitals rubbing them on something to produce soothing and pleasurable stimulation. Many children use their hands, others use stuffed animals, blankets, arms of chairs, other children, etc.

Other sexual behaviors of children include showing their genitals to others or being embarrassed and covering themselves up. Peeking to catch others in sexual behaviors is frequently observed in children. Sex play between children that includes exploring or touching other children's genitals is common. Some sexual behaviors include kissing, using dirty words, and telling "dirty" jokes. As children get older and try to understand the social and interpersonal aspects of sexuality, games such as spin the bottle and strip poker gain prominence. Sexual rehearsal play, including rehearsal of coital motions and positioning, is common among children and primates according to Money (Money & Lamacz, 1989). It should be noted that there is very little research on sexual behaviors among children in different races, ethnic groups, socioeconomic levels, and religious groups. Finkelhor (1983), Haugaard and Tilly (1988), Goldman and Goldman (1988), and Johnson (1992) indicate that when adults respond to questions about their childhood sexual experiences, approximately forty percent (Haugaard & Tilly, 1988) to seventy percent (Finkelhor, 1983; Goldman and Goldman, 1988; Johnson, 1992) of adults recall sexual activity before age thirteen. Friedrich surveyed mothers regarding their children's sexual behaviors (Friedrich et al., 1992) and sixty percent of them were aware of their children's sexual activity.

Disruption in Development

Studies of sexually abused children frequently cite increased sexual behaviors in these children (Friedrich et al., 1987; Friedrich et al., 1988). Disturbed sexuality between the child and others may increase the child's interest in the behaviors, and perhaps stimulate the child into wishing to repeat the sensation. Some children may possibly engage in the behavior, as a form of repetition compulsion; others may be trying to understand or master the traumatic aspects of the experience by repeating it. (See Chapter four.)

Friedrich (Friedrich et al., 1992) asked 880 mothers of children who were not sexually abused and 276 mothers of children who were sexually abused to indicate the sexual behaviors they observed in their children. The boys and girls were two to twelve years of age, with a mean age of 6.3 for the normative sample and 7.1 for the clinical sample. On the thirty-five sexual behavior items of the Child Sexual Behavior Inventory (CSBI) (Appendix C), twenty-five of the behaviors were observed statistically more frequently in sexually abused children than in non-sexually abused children. A higher frequency of sexual behaviors in the clinical sample was directly related to more severe abuse, a greater number of perpetrators, and the use of force or threats. It was also found that sexual abuse itself does not occur in isolation, but is associated with greater levels of family distress and fewer educational and financial resources. The greater the amount of nudity in the home, the higher the mean frequency of sexual behaviors in both samples. For the frequency of sexual behaviors in both samples and the items that discriminated between them see Appendix A.

Friedrich's data indicate that sexual behaviors observed in children by mothers decline with age; however, due to the difficulty in collecting data on children's sexual behaviors, this may be erroneous. Finkelhor asked college students to recall their sexual behaviors when they were age twelve and younger. Of the 796 students surveyed, 63 percent of the males and 59 percent of the females who engaged in sexual behaviors reported that only 12 percent of behaviors between siblings were disclosed to anyone else (Finkelhor, 1980) and for sexual experiences with siblings, friends, and relatives, 30 percent were disclosed (Finkelhor, 1983).

Children who molest engage in sexual behaviors that go beyond those of the sexually abused children in Friedrich's work. Children who molest engage with a higher frequency in the more advanced behaviors of sexually abused children, while also engaging in oral sex, sodomy, and sexual intercourse (Friedrich & Luecke, 1988; Johnson, 1988; Johnson, 1989).

Gender Development

Natural and Expectable Development

Infants are born with an inclination toward a particular gender identity, which usually conforms to the individual's anatomic sex. There is a question as to what extent the prenatal hormonal environment influences sexual preference or gender role. The hormonally determined maleness or femaleness of the brain may predispose persons toward one sexual preference or another. Prenatal hormones most likely contribute to, but do not determine, object choice (Yates, 1991). Recent research by neurobiologist Levay, at the Salk Institute in San Diego, may shed light on the biological derivatives of sexual object choice (Hoffman,1992).

Children develop an awareness of their gender early in their lives. Parents overtly and covertly reinforce the child's gender. "What a nice little boy." "Little girls don't do those kinds of things." "Boys are brave." Not only do these types of statements underline gender, but also gender role. Children learn which gender they are and how that gender is to act . During this period, children are aware of their genitals and develop a boy-self or girl-self; gender identity is defined in the first few years of life.

Children learn their gender role through interaction with parents, friends, and the social milieu. Before latency most children have defined themselves by their behaviors and mannerisms into gender-specific roles. Although sexual orientation awaits further elaboration and development, homosexuals and heterosexuals indicate that during their early elementary years many had an awareness of their sexual preference. Little is known about the development of bisexual preference. By adolescence, sexual orientation becomes fixed, and there is movement away from the parents toward peers as love objects and partners.

Disruption in Development

Presently no empirical evidence exists of a disturbance related to gender identity among children who molest. There is a congruence between the children's biological sex and their gender identification. Rarely are cases of cross-dressing seen within this population.

Many children exaggerate their gender roles: boys may over-emphasize their maleness, claiming to be tough, strong, and invincible. In some boys this appears to be in direct relation to their feelings of insecurity and inability to control their destinies. This is also seen in relationship to having been a victim of a male, and not infrequently, children (and their parents) fear they may become homosexual. This does not appear to be as salient for girls who were molested by females. There does not appear to be as much exaggeration of being female among children who molest as among sexually victimized children. Some sexually victimized girls have been found to walk, talk, and dress more like adult females than young girls.

Available research indicates that boys who molest other children, molest girls more frequently than boys (Johnson, 1988). Girls molest boys two times more frequently than girls (Johnson, 1989). This may be related to sexual preference, but it may be more related to availability or a victim targeted due to jealousy. In cases in which boys molested younger siblings, the sibling-victim was the favored child in the family, and the sex of the child was seemingly not of major significance (Johnson, 1990).

Most children who molest, especially those over seven years old, have inculcated the negative stereotypes in this culture and are strongly homophobic. This is true, even though they may have had many same-gender sexual encounters; both boys and girls often appear to be oblivious to the incongruity of their statements. This may be understood in some cases by the children focusing on the sexual activity as an expression of anger or anxiety reduction and not sexuality.

One seven-year-old boy had bribed eighteen classmates into having oral sex with him in the school bathroom. When asked if he preferred to do touching things with boys, he retorted, "No that's sick, I want to do it with girls, but I would get caught if I took them in the boys' bathroom."

Sexual Knowledge

Natural and Expectable Development

Children learn about sex and sexuality from their parents, friends, and the world around them. Much of their knowledge is gained through self-exploration; their natural curiosity stimulates this exploration. Toddlers generally discover that there are different anatomical parts on different people. Children may explore the genitalia of other-gender children and same-gender children to discover the similarities and differences. Trying to peek at the genitalia of their parents may become a quest. As children continue to explore the differences and similarities between males and females, they notice the different positions for urination. Older children attach words to the various parts of their universe, including the genitalia, and hopefully, parents supply the correct words.

As children grow and develop, they question adults about what the genitalia are for, where babies come from, and how they are born. They become more aware of the universe around them and interested in male-female relationships, dating, courtship, and marriage, and often play dress up and simulate adult roles. Based on their developing knowledge of sexuality, children have make-believe weddings and play house. Gender identity and sex roles become a focus of play. All of these play activities are in the service of attempting to understand the meaning of the world around them.

During latency and preadolescence, children begin to use slang terms such as fuck, faggot, cunt, queer, bitch, etc. Understanding of the terms lags far behind acquisition: substantial misinformation often arises during childhood through the process of language acquisition without meaning acquisition. Not infrequently, children attach a meaning to words not only from the context, but also from the affect associated with the word when they heard it. Gaps in knowledge are also filled by peers, print and visual media, and society at large.

Schools encourage students at preadolescence and adolescence to study the physiology of sexuality including menstruation, conception, pregnancy, and contraception. In the era of AIDS, addressing sexually transmitted diseases has become prevalent.

Parents have an important role in teaching their children about sex and sexuality. Unfortunately, parents take on this responsibility to different degrees. Some parents provide children with absolutely no information regarding sex and sexuality.

Disruption in Development

Is the sexual knowledge gained by children through visual and print media contributing to the development of accurate knowledge, or is it creating confusion? Although the answer to this has not been reliably researched, this is an area that could use serious scrutiny. Daytime talk shows discuss every area of sexuality from sex-enhancing techniques to transvestite makeup to transsexual lovemaking. Michael Jackson and Madonna have raised music and dance to an erotic height to which children can only aspire. Does the sexual information, and perhaps misinformation, acquired through the media facilitate age-appropriate sexual knowledge, exploration, and expression?

When sexualized children and children who molest are questioned about what in their immediate environment stimulates their desire to act in a sexual way, they invariably mention television soap operas. They also mention watching movies such as *Dirty Dancing* and videos made by

Michael Jackson. Particularly stimulating to children who molest are movies that have the dual themes of sex and violence.

Children who have been oversexualized or children who molest other children have more and less sexual information than other children. Although these children may know more about the mechanics of sexual behavior, they often have less understanding of the human body. Often latency-aged children have some idea of conception and birth, but sexualized children may not. Frequently, these children have focused to such an extent on the sexual body parts and sexual behaviors that they have not expressed their natural curiosity about childbirth.

The parents of sexualized children are generally less apt to provide positive and healthy sexual information to their children. In some cases, the parents themselves have been sexually misused, and may be reticent to talk about sex and sexuality.

More than other children, sexualized children and children who molest tend to have skewed values and perceptions about sexuality. Overexposure to sexuality has generally overwhelmed their ability to assimilate the information in an orderly fashion. Many incorrectly surmise the connections between fragments of sexual information gleaned while in emotionally heightened states.

Relationship Aspects of Sexuality

Natural and Expectable Development

Children's first sexual experience may be the pleasure derived from nursing at their mother's breast (Yates, 1991). The sensuous infant moves from the warm comfort of the nursing mother to the soothing and pleasurable aspects of self-stimulation. As children grow and develop, there is a transition from the symbiosis with the mothering figure and a gradual transition to separation and individuation. During this process infants learn to create their own pleasure.

The gentle physical contact when being bathed, dried, and diapered are all part of children's growing experience of a relationship to another. These circumstances combine physical, and often verbal contact between young children and the parent around the children's genitals. Children learn to enjoy and expect the parents' caring and warmth.

As young children develop in the context of the family, there are frequently strivings for the affection of the parents. Freudian theory posits that preschool children, especially females, strive for the sexual affection of the parent of the opposite sex. This remains without substantial empirical backing. It is more likely that children are aware of the special relationship between their parents, feel jealous due to their exclusion, and seek special attention from the parents. Miller (1986) cautions against overemphasizing the Freudian theory of the sexual attraction of the female child for the father, which may lead to a conjecture that a male parent would be seduced by a female child who is seeking sexual satisfaction.

As children go through the latency period, they focus on developing peer relationships while still remaining closely tied to their parents. They learn about male-female sexual relationships through observation of their home life. Children become even more aware of gender roles and relationship roles between family members. They internalize concepts of father and mother, husband and wife, girlfriend and boyfriend roles from their observations, which will strongly influence the way they relate to others in sexual relationships in the future. As they perceive their role in relation to the other persons in their home, they define their family role.

Disruption in Development

Families in which children who molest are raised have extreme difficulties in their relationships. The emotional and sexual nature of the adult-child relationship and relationships between adults show vast disturbances. Healthy adult sexual relationships are virtually absent; positive male or female role models are almost nonexistent. Negative relationship models, including role reversals, are the standard for children.

During infancy, the parents of these children are often unable to attend to the children's emotional and physical needs due to their own unmet dependency and sexual needs. Many of these children are found wandering alone in parks or are left unattended for extended periods. This type of early deprivation of adequate touch and healthy physical intimacy can affect adult sexual functioning (Yates, 1991). Lack of physical affection has also been associated with higher levels of violence in cultures (Broude, 1976; Prescott, 1975).

Some mothers of children who molest are unable to tolerate nursing their children or become overly stimulated by the child sucking on their breasts. Mothers have described becoming confused due to their sexual and orgasmic reactions or intolerant attitudes toward the infants sucking or touching their breasts. Mothers have described hitting their infants when the infants bit them, feeling the children were being hostile toward them. The nature of the parent's response may be anxiety or tension producing in infants. Trust in physical touching, eating, and closeness with a caring individual is not furthered.

Toilet training can become a battlefield, with the parents trying to force children to conform to urinating and evacuating their bowels. Focus on the genital area can persist, with children continuing to be enueretic and encopretic late into latency. This becomes a battleground used by the children to oppose their parents' wishes in an area that the parents cannot control. Some sexualized children and children who molest have intense issues around toileting, leading them to soil their clothes, urinate in the parent's favorite chair, outdoors, in sinks, pans, or other nonconventional areas. Some children smear their feces on walls or on the parents' clothes. The struggle with parents around toileting has led children to use feces and urine as weapons.

Parents of sexualized children or children who molest may use their children to fulfill their own needs, frequently trying to disguise this as fulfilling the children's needs. Parents' needs for sexual and emotional comfort may be fulfilled by having children sleep in their bed. Children may be told that sleeping there is to provide them comfort and prevent bad dreams. This is inherently confusing to children, who become unable to separate their needs from the sexual and dependency needs of their parents. Parents often project their own needs onto children and insist and believe that it is, in reality, the children's expressed need. This merging of need states can have serious sequelae for the mental health of children and their ability to develop mutually satisfying intimate relationships.

The confusion in their understanding about relationships becomes more intense when the parent has a sexual partner. Instead of inviting the child into his or her bed, the parent may throw the child out of the bed. The child is unconsciously aware that he or she is being used, but this cannot be articulated. Parental rejection and the ephemeral nature of relationships is underscored.

As children observe their parents' volatile relationships to each other or to other partners, the impermanence and unreliability of male-female relationships becomes the norm.

Sexual Socialization

Natural and Expectable Development

Parents, parents' friends, teachers, relatives, siblings, television, published materials, and videos contribute to the sexual socialization of children.

Sexual socialization starts immediately after birth with the closeness and comfort infants receive. From holding and soothing, children learn about closeness, soothing touch, and emotional caring. Infants and children learn to expect that their parents' warm feelings and appreciation of them are accompanied by kisses and hugs.

Children's genital awareness and self-touching, when accepted by parents, leads children to accept their bodies. Positive toilet training does not center children on urination and defecation, but allows children to feel competent and to gain mastery of a body function.

Parents teach their children how to use emotional and physical space by how close they sit and stand to people, whether they require or allow privacy for themselves and their children, and the topics they discuss with their children and with others in their children's presence. When and where to express sexuality, and what to discuss with whom about sexuality, is transmitted to children via their parents' actions.

Children learn about when sexual behaviors between people can begin by their parents' example. The age at which parents began their intimate sexual interactions with others is a guideline frequently followed by children for their own behaviors.

Parents teach values and morals regarding sex and sexuality to their children as they grow. As children begin to experiment with nudity, touching and exploring other's genitals, sexual games, and sexual jokes, the guidelines set by parents teaches them the balance for these activities in their lives. Exaggerated, angry, or horrified reactions by parents send messages to children about themselves, sexuality, and sexual expression. If parents openly engage in these behaviors, their actions provide a stronger message than their words.

Parents express attitudes about sex and sexuality by the words they use when describing sexual behaviors. The choice of expressions used in the heat of anger, if including sexual reference, will teach attitudes and values to their children. Parents' personal choices of television shows, movies, videos, and magazines teach values. Which television shows, movies, videos, and magazines the parents allow their children will teach sexual values. Parents' choice of attire, the sexual behaviors in which they engage in front of children, the friends they choose, how they define their gender role and the gender role of the opposite sex send messages to their children.

Disruption in Development

Sex and sexuality are issues in all homes. The home environment is of crucial importance in the sexual socialization of children. The manner in which sex and sexuality are expressed, and how parents relate to one another, varies from family to family. Unspoken messages are often as potent or more potent than spoken messages: actions speak louder than words.

There is a range of sexual environments in families (Bolton et al., 1989). They range from supportive of or destructive to healthy and natural sexuality: on the one end of the continuum are natural and healthy homes and on the other end are multigenerational sexually abusive homes. In between are sexually neutral homes, open or communal living homes, sexually repressed homes, sex is dirty homes, homes with overt values and covert norms, sexually overwhelming homes, sexually and emotionally needy homes, homes where sex is an exchange commodity, sexually abusive homes, and multigenerational sexually abusive homes (Johnson, In press).

Adolescent perpetrators may come from *sexually repressed, sex is dirty*, and *homes with overt values and covert norms*. Children who molest other children generally come from sexually and emotionally needy homes, homes where sex is an exchange commodity, sexually abusive homes or multi-generational sexually abusive homes. Frequently, these children are raised in a sexually abusive home for a time and then live with a single parent who is sexually and emotionally needy (Johnson, 1989).

In *sexually and emotionally needy homes*, sex is used as a way to meet the unsatisfied longing of the adults. Generally, coming from an abusive and neglectful background, the parents in these families are constantly in search of love, caring, and companionship to fill their inner void. Because genuine love is difficult for them to find among the people they attract, sex is the substitute. Sex is often confused with love, and the parents engage in sex trying to compensate for their emptiness. If a parent is without a partner, a child may be used as a substitute partner. Although parents are generally unaware of using children as a substitute, children may feel the pull to fulfill the parent's emotional and sexual needs. Substitution of children in this role lasts only until adult partners are found and then children are put aside. Parents using their children as substitutes may have them sleep in their bed, go out to the movies with them, walk hand in hand with them, or invite them to snuggle while watching television together. The emotional, physical, and sexual boundaries in these families are very poorly managed.

Because adult relationships in these families are generally based on a desperate attempt to fulfill intense emotional and sexual neediness and not love, aggressive interchanges between the adults are common. Adults may hit one another as the children look on helplessly. Aggressive interchanges between adults and children are frequent as the children compete with the abusive adult for the attention of the abused adult, while trying to protect the abused adult and seek emotional comfort for themselves.

In homes where *sex is an exchange commodity*, the parents engage in sex for money, drugs, and other things that they want or need. Children may or may not be used as vehicles for this exchange. Observation of the sexual activities by the children may occur because the parents are not generally focused on the children's needs, but their own. Physical aggression is frequently part of the environment. If the mother is a prostitute, the children may see her beaten by her pimp. The children may engage in incestuous behaviors, forced or mutual. Alcohol, drug abuse, and other illegal activities are frequent.

In *sexually abusive homes,* incest by one or both of the parents occurs. In some cases, one of the parents does not know that the other is molesting their child. In other cases, one parent knows and is unwilling or unable to step in to end the abuse. If extended family members live in the home or visit, abuse may be by relatives. Children who are abused may be unsure of getting the full support of the nonabusive parent and so endure the abuse. In families in which children believe they will get the support of the nonabusive parent if they tell, the abuser uses threats to keep the child quiet or abuses a young child whose disclosures will be suspect. Abusive parents may use threats of aggression to keep children quiet. In sexually abusive homes, there may be alcohol or drug abuse.

In *multigenerational sexually abusive homes,* there is concurrent incestuous activity between grandparents, parents, siblings, and perhaps aunts, uncles, and cousins. Sexual abuse and misuse is by the more powerful to the less powerful. Although some of the relationships appear to be mutual, consent is impossible because both covert and overt sexual messages are so pervasive that family members and relatives are totally confused about sexual expression and its limits and boundaries. Family members use physical punishment and physical and emotional bullying as techniques to gain compliance. Rules for sex and aggression between family members have never been formulated or discussed.

Children who molest generally come from one of the home environments listed above. They are socialized to sex and aggression occurring in tandem. The language about sexuality is often violent and debasing. The naked body is used as a weapon or as a commodity. Children's bodies are used as vehicles for the pleasure of adults. Touching is not for the child's comfort, but for someone else's pleasure. Anxiety, tension, anger, rage, and cruelty become intimately associated with sex. The meaning of love is contorted. Relationships are based on sex and need, not love and caring. Sex and love are destructive. The way to stop emotional emptiness and pain is through sex, which is often accompanied by hitting and violence and quick exits and loss. Men are seen as aggressive, often violent, and free to come and go. By and large, they are not expected to take responsibility for their actions or to care for their children. Women are generally victims who are angry and needy and search for men to fill them up and save them.

The type of people to trust, and with whom it is mutually beneficial to develop relationships, is not modeled. The places to frequent are not taught to the children. Many children, not knowing who to trust, get molested outside their homes as they seek emotional sustenance from their friends' parents or from others on their street.

Children who molest are not adequately socialized about emotional and physical boundaries. As they observe their parents and learn from how they are treated, they gain no sense of when they are intruded upon and when they are intruding on someone else. Parents may share the intimate details of their sexual encounters, discuss their contraceptives, or lament the loss of a sexual partner with the children. Adequate physical space boundaries are not taught; parents invade children's bed, or bathe the children far beyond what is necessary, or do not allow privacy for toileting or changing clothes. Often there are no doors on rooms, even bathrooms. Parents may be overly interested in children's genitals and require the children to undress for inspection. Mothers of children who molest have described being fascinated with their children's erections. Children have described their genitals being played with or overly valued by their parents, and in some cases having their genitals mocked.

Children whose sexuality is beyond natural and healthy expression may come from any of these families; very few come from natural and healthy homes, sexually neutral homes, or open or communal living homes.

Summary

Sexualized children and children who molest experience a disruption in their sexual development. This chapter discusses separate lines of sexual development, which helps us understand the types of disturbances in children. Seven different lines of development are discussed: biological, sensual/erotic, behavioral, gender, cognitive, relationship, and socialization. Natural and disturbed development within each developmental line are delineated.

References

Bolton, F., Morris, L., & MacEachron, A. (1989). *Males at risk*. Newbury Park, CA: Sage.

Broude, G. (1976). Cross-cultural patterning of some sexual attitudes and practices. *Behavioral Science Research* 11:227-262.

Finkelhor, D. (1980). Sex among siblings: A survey on prevalence, variety, and effects. *Archives of Sexual Behavior* 9(3): 171-194.

Finkelhor, D. (1983). Childhood sexual experiences: a retrospective survey. Durham, NH: University of NH.

Finkelhor, D. (1984). *Child Sexual Abuse*. New York: Free Press.

Friedrich, W., Beilke, R., & Urquiza, A. (1987). Children from sexually abusive families. *Journal of Interpersonal Violence* 2(4): 391-402.

Friedrich, W., Beilke, R., & Urquiza, A. (1988). Behavior problems in young sexually abused boys. *Journal of Interpersonal Violence* 3(1): 21-27.

Friedrich, W., Grambsch, P., Damon, L., Koverola, C.,Wolfe, V., Hewitt, S., Lang, R., & Broughton, D. (1992). The child sexual behavior inventory: Normative and clinical comparisons. *Psychological Assessment* 4(3): 303-311.

Friedrich, W., & Luecke, W. (1988). Young school-age sexually aggressive children. *Professional Psychology Research and Practice* 19(2): 155-164.

Goldman, R., & Goldman, J. (1988). *Show me yours: Understanding children's sexuality*. New York: Penguin.

Haugaard, J., & Tilly, C. (1988). Characteristics predicting children's responses to sexual encounters with other children. *Child Abuse and Neglect* 12:209-218.

Hoffman, P. (1992). The science of sex. *Discover*, 13(6): 4.

Johnson, T. C. (1988). Child perpetrators—children who molest other children: Preliminary findings. *Child Abuse and Neglect* 12:219-229.

Johnson, T. C. (1989). Female child perpetrators: Children who molest other children. *Child Abuse and Neglect* 13(4): 571-585.

Johnson, T. C. (1990). (Manuscript). Commonalities in sibling incest cases when the perprtrators are boys younger than thirteen.

Johnson, T. C. (1992). Cross-cultural study of childhood sexual behaviors: Preliminary data. Unpublished manuscript.

Johnson, T. C. (In press). Assessment of sexual behavior problems in preschool and latency-aged children. In A. Yates (Ed.), *Child and adolescent psychiatric clinics of North America*. Philadelphia, PA: Saunders.

Martinson, F. (1973). *Infant and child sexuality: A sociological perspective*. St. Peter, MN: The Book Mark.

Martinson, F. (1982). Sensory/erotic development: Embryo, fetus, infant, child. In *Sixth World Congress of Sexology*, Washington, DC.

Miller, A. (1986). *Thou shalt not be aware: Society's betrayal of the child*. New York: Meridian.

Money, J., & Lamacz, M. (1989). *Vandalized lovemaps*. Buffalo, NY: Prometheus.

Prescott, J. (1975). Body pleasure and the origins of violence. *Futurist* 9(64).

Reinisch, J., & Beasley, R. (1990). *The Kinsey Institute new report on sex*. New York: St. Martin's Press.

Sapolsky, R. (1992). Growing up in a hurry. *Discover* 13(6):40–45.

Trickett, P. K., and Putnam, F.(1990). The psychobiological effects of sexual abuse. American Psychiatric Association annual meeting, New Orleans.

Udry, J., Billy, J., Morris, N., Groff, T., & Raj, M. (1985). Serum androgenic hormones motivate sexual behavior in adolescent boys. *Fertility and Sterility* 43(1): 90–94.

Yates, A. (1990). Eroticized children. In M. E. Perry (Ed.), *Handbook of sexology: Childhood and adolescent sexology*. New York, NY: Elsevier Science Publishers.

Yates, A. (1991). Sexual and gender development. In P. Wilner (Ed.), *Psychiatry*. Philadelphia: J. B. Lippincott.

2

Age-Appropriate Sex Play Versus Problematic Sexual Behaviors

Eliana Gil, Ph.D.

Two things about childhood sexuality can be said with certainty: (1) sexual curiosity, interest, experimentation, and behavior is progressive over time and (2) sexual development is affected by a number of variables.

The Progressive Nature of Child Sexuality

Those who have studied and discussed age-appropriate sexual behaviors in children (Martinson, 1976, 1991; Rutter, 1971, 1980; Green 1988; Sgroi, Bunk & Wabrek,1988, among others) have agreed on the progressive nature of childhood sexual behaviors. Whether assessing these behaviors based on Freud's theory of psychosexual development or any current adaptations of this framework, it is clear that there is an upward movement in the development of childhood sexual behaviors. Martinson (1991) reminds us that "Each child's development will be markedly influenced by the cultural norms and expectations, familial interactions and values, and the interpersonal experiences encountered." He goes on to say that "Organic capacities, cognitive development and integration, and intrapsychic influences further determine the rate and extent of development of the sexual capacity" (p. 58).

Preschoolers

Children from birth to age four share common experiences: They have limited peer contact (i.e., they usually don't attend school with a classroom full of other children); they tend to be mostly involved in self-exploration or self-stimulation that is random and sporadic; and they tend toward disinhibition.

It is common for children in this age group to "discover" that when certain parts of the body are touched, poked, rubbed, or otherwise stimulated, pleasant sensations occur. When something pleasurable occurs, children may seek to repeat the event; the younger the child the more likely the repetition occurs by accident. Children may learn that during diapering there is an opportunity to reach over and touch their genitals. Parents or caretakers provide a positive or negative reinforcement by how they react to children's self-exploration. If the caretaker hits the child's hands or genitals when self-exploration occurs, it is less likely to reoccur. The child will make a negative association between self-touching and pain. If the parent allows the self-exploration while continuing to change the diaper and does not punish the child, a positive or neutral association is made between self-exploration and the diapering circumstance. From birth children have occasional erections or vaginal secretions (Martinson, 1976); masturbation has been observed in the first year of life, and by the age of five any child is capable of autoerotic experiences. Martinson (1991) distinguishes between genital play and masturbation in infancy, stating that infants in the first year of life are not capable of the direct volitional behavior required to masturbate. Levine (1957) notes that rhythmic manipulation with the hand does not appear to occur until children are approximately two and a half to three years of age, likely because small muscle control is not sufficiently developed.

Young children may observe and take notice of all the different parts of the bodies around them. Young children who sit on women's laps may poke or squeeze what they call "boobies." When they do this, they may laugh or run away with delight.

Preschoolers may show their genitals to others from an early age. Again, this depends on the guidance and limits set by parents or caretakers. If children are punished for running around without diapers or underwear, they may learn that being nude elicits a specific response. Children who are then trying to get a rise out of their parents or caretakers, or who want to cause a little commotion, may "streak" at regular intervals.

Children around the age of two may increase their interest in genitals. Many preschoolers engage in sex play or genital handling. By the age of four, children engage in exhibitionistic and voyeuristic behaviors with other children and adults (Gallo, 1979), and they typically initiate or become involved in games in which there is undressing or sexual exploration. Bathroom activities are of interest to children and are frequently associated with sex (Rutter, 1971). Children's attention is first focused on bathroom activities during toilet training. Around this time (two to four years of age) children may want to follow adults into the bathroom and watch as adults use the toilet. They may use an inordinate number of bathroom words. There are few children who engage in the "poo-poo, caca, diarrhea" monologue without great amusement. They may also learn slang words for body parts and use these words relentlessly, to the dismay of concerned parents or caretakers. Often, adults make the mistake of assuming that the child is using the word with a correct understanding of what it means. Children simply repeat what they hear and then sit back and watch the responses they can produce.

A three-year-old child may "play house" and orchestrate the mother and father dolls into situations in which they kiss, lay in bed together, make babies, and have arguments. Playing house is a normal childhood activity, and many children enjoy role-playing "mommy" or "daddy." This is mostly imitative behavior, and it is remarkable to notice the amount of detail children can absorb through observation. The specificity of children's play is likely based on what they have observed. For example, children with little knowledge of adult sexuality may lay the mom and dad dolls in the same bed, cover them up, and say they are making a baby. Children with more knowledge about adult sexuality may undress the dolls, put the male on top of the female, and rub them together while making guttural sounds. Both children are showing what they know about adult sexuality. Money and Ehrhardt (1972) have found that young children from the age of three can impersonate mannerisms of parents, siblings, or television actors, and can look "outrageously flirtatious and seductive."

The same is true of playing doctor. This is an age-old activity for children, probably because every child visits a physician. Toy companies have produced many medical toys that children like to play with; usually they assume the role of physician or nurse and examine a chosen doll patient. On occasion, children may give each other a medical once-over. Observation of this play shows how children are capable of storing information in memory and retrieving that information for play. Children examine each other the way a physician does: ears, nose, throat, chest, back. They poke here and there, asking if there is pain. They may dispense shots, splints, medicines, etc.

It is unlikely that doctor play will progress beyond what the children have experienced. It would be highly unlikely, for example, for doctor play to include a pelvic examination. It would not be unlikely, however, for one child to attempt to take another child's temperature by inserting a toy thermometer, or by creating something that looks like a toy thermometer (a pencil or popsicle stick). This can inadvertently hurt a child, however, and can precipitate a referral to child protective services by a concerned parent or caretaker. This is why it is very important that assessments be made on a case-by-case basis, taking child development issues into account.

Last, children in this age group can experiment with sticking fingers or other small objects inside any and all of their openings. Young children poke their nostrils, ears, bellybutton, eyes, mouth, or genitals just because they are there. Initially everything goes into the mouth. Later, children may like putting things in their nose or ears. Children may discover a vaginal or anal opening and may want to see if something goes in. Usually, this causes pain or discomfort and the behavior tends to stop. If children persist with the behavior, it's helpful to assess. Children who are sexually abused tend to insert objects into their vaginal or anal openings more than nonabused children (Friedrich et al, 1992). It is also possible that a child who makes excessive contact with the genitals is indicating a medical problem.

Young School-Age Children

School-age children have increased peer contact, go through periods of inhibition, and have a broad range of experimental interactive behaviors. Lewis (1965) states that children begin to be socialized away from body contact by age four.

Although younger children are more self-exploratory as a result of spending more time with adults and being more egocentric, school-age children have more contact with same-gender and opposite-gender children, and the possibility of exposure to new sexual behaviors increases.

Young school-age children may begin to masturbate in a less random way. They may have discovered creative ways of masturbating and may repeat them. Young girls often stumble on the fact that if they lift their vagina to the water spout in the bathtub, the water stimulation feels good. This information may then be shared between girlfriends. Similarly, young boys may discover that climbing or shimmying poles feels good on their penis, and they may do it frequently.

Children in this age group watch and ask questions. The infamous "Where did I come from?" question tends to pop up around this time. They may want to see pictures of the human body, and may giggle a great deal when they see people kissing on TV. They may be repulsed by and drawn to overt sexual behaviors. In public, children this age may say they are "grossed out" by displays of affection; in private, they may be fascinated by similar scenes.

Feelings of sacred privacy emerge at this age. Children may unexpectedly drape towels around their bodies and demand that parents, siblings, or caretakers knock on their doors before entering. One young girl yelled at the top of her lungs, "Mother, please, I'm dressing in here and I'd like my privacy." Just the day before, the child had dressed in the living room in front of her parents.

Young school-age children are notorious for telling "dirty jokes." They repeat them endlessly and they revel in testing limits. They may or may not fully understand the punch lines.

Depending on regional and cultural differences, some children this age begin to "date," although this is usually done in groups. Some young children may hold hands and kiss. Most parents do not allow this activity, and others may think it cute. Children of all ages may mimic or practice behaviors they have seen or experienced.

Latency-Aged Children

Latency-aged children (approximately seven to twelve) engage in a range of sexual interests. They continue to have peer contact in school, they may begin to experiment with sexual behaviors, and they may have alternating periods of disinhibition and inhibition.

Children in this age group vary greatly. During this time frame most children enter puberty. Boys may develop pubic hair and the ability to masturbate to ejaculation. Girls may develop pubic hair, breasts, and begin their menses. Both boys and girls can have a growth spurt during this period, and it is certain that physiological changes are imminent.

These children have active hormonal changes that create a range of physical and emotional sensations. They may give more time to masturbatory activities. They may or may not become exhibitionistic.

Young boys develop a certain locker room behavior in which they are often nude, and they may slap each other on the buttocks and tell dirty jokes. Some youngsters have confided their participation in ejaculation contests to see who can ejaculate first or most. Girls in locker rooms can also behave in a disinhibited manner, comparing breast sizes, and experimenting with varying degrees of nudity.

Children of this age range may begin dating, and some parents allow their children to go on unsupervised dates. Children may experiment with kissing, "french" kissing, petting over and under clothes, touching each other's genitals, dry humping, or having digital or vaginal intercourse. Older children are subject to nonfamilial socialization experiences according to Friedrich (1990), and they are likely to assume cultural norms and restraints. Because of all the moral, religious, and health restrictions on sexuality, many children avoid penile/genital contact and engage in cunnilingus and fellatio. Other children fear and/or avoid sexual contact until much later.

Pre-School	Young School-Age	Latency/Preadolescence
0–4	5–7	8–12
Limited peer contact	Increased peer contact	Increased peer contact
Self-exploration	Experimental interactions	Experimental interactions
Self-stimulation	Inhibition	Disinhibition/inhibition
Disinhibition		
• Touches/rubs own genitals (random)	• Touches self (specific)	• Touches self/others
• Watches, pokes	• Watches, asks	• Mooning
• Shows genitals	• Inhibited (privacy)	• Exhibitionistic
• Interested/ask about bathroom functions	• Repulsed by/drawn to opposite sex	• Kissing/dating
• Uses dirty language	• Tells dirty jokes	• Petting
• Plays house— mom/dad	• Plays house	• Touches others' genitals
• Plays doctor (imitative)	• Kissing, holding hands	• Dry humping
• May insert/stops with pain	• May mimic/practice	• Digital or vaginal intercourse or oral sex in preadolescents or adolescents

Table 2-1   Summary of Sexual Development in Children

Parental Guidance

Probably one of the most critical factors in child sexual development is the level of parental guidance. Parents play an important part in instilling values about sexuality in their children. When parents view sex as dirty, inappropriate, or secretive they may set rigid and restrictive limits on self-exploration, language, questions, or curiosity considered healthy in children. When children are punished, chastised, or humiliated for their sexuality, they may associate sex with shame or guilt.

Children need an open environment in which they can ask questions and learn about sexuality. If they can't find that at home, they frequently designate their peers as educators.

Family Dynamics

It is clear that in some families there is an inordinate amount of sexual agitation and activity that can give rise to sexual acting-out in children. (See Chapter seven for a review of family dynamics.)

Parents can be either over- or undersexualized, creating a sexualized environment or one in which sex is taboo. Either polarity affects the child's sexual development.

Nudity may also influence a child's sexual development. Family members are almost always exposed to a certain amount of nudity. Going to and from the bathroom, changing or trying on clothes in front of each other— family members have more or less relaxed standards regarding nudity. Occasional glimpses of family nudity certainly is not damaging to children. However, when parents are nude in front of their children because they want adult sexual gratification, children are exposed to eroticization of nudity that can influence sexual interest and behavior.

Relaxed television-watching standards can also influence children's interest in sexuality. If young children are allowed to watch X-rated movies with explicit sexual information, they obtain knowledge that may influence their fantasies and arousal mechanisms. In other words, in expectable sexual development children gradually learn and experiment. At any given age, children may not be able to imagine beyond their own experience level. When explicit sexuality is available, children who may be in the kissing stage of sexual experimentation may now seek additional gratification, and the developmental process is therefore accelerated.

Traumatic events obviously have an impact on child sexual development. Sexually abused children are exposed to focused and excessive sexual stimulation, interrupting their normal sexual development. They are denied the opportunity to learn about sexuality at their own pace. Rather, attention to sexuality is refocused within the context of a "relationship" with an older person in which an inherent power imbalance exists. Sexually abused children experience sexual responses in tandem with feelings of helplessness and instinctual arousal. Sexual arousal is paired with feelings of fear or confusion or pain. Given the traumatic nature of the event, children may fixate on the traumatic event and develop resultant behavioral problems.

Examples of Questions Regarding Child Sexuality

1. A mother walks into her thirteen-year-old son's bedroom and finds that he is having sexual intercourse with his eight-year-old sister. In a panic, she rushes the young girl into the car and speeds to the pediatrician's office,

where she asks about the activity. Is the child all right? Is this normal for kids their age?

2. A preschool teacher becomes very frustrated and concerned when one of the children refuses to take a nap and instead quietly proceeds to put his hand inside the diapers of other sleeping children. He becomes surprised and annoyed when the teacher places him back in his cot, and after several attempts to repeat this behavior, he masturbates himself to sleep.

3. A six-year-old boy who plays unsupervised in his apartment complex after school is observed taking smaller children behind bushes, pulling them to the ground, turning them over, and attempting to insert a stick or finger in the children's anuses.

4. A nine-year-old girl causes great alarm when several of her girlfriends report that when they go to the bathroom with her, she shows them her breasts and wants everyone to show theirs. Sometimes she offers one or two dollars if friends will let her touch their breasts.

5. Two four-year-olds are "playing doctor," and when mother enters the room they yell at her to leave, saying they are doing "private things." The mother notices both children have disrobed down to their underwear.

6. A fourteen-year-old boy masturbates to orgasm in the presence of a six-year-old boy he is baby-sitting. The six-year-old is scared and talks to his mother when the teenager insists that the boy watch him ejaculate.

These are typical examples of the kinds of questions that are brought to the attention of police, social workers, physicians, nurses, and mental health professionals. The questions are posed by parents, teachers, daycare providers, concerned neighbors, and others who become alarmed after observing apparently unusual sexual behaviors in young children.

Probably never before have children's sexual behaviors been so disturbing and caused so much reflection among professionals, who are often at a loss to understand, let alone differentiate, between age-appropriate and problematic sexual activity in children. It's difficult to know why these behaviors have become so widespread. Is it a new phenomenon? Has it always occurred, but people ignored it or chose to keep quiet about it? How did parents cope with children's sexual behaviors in the past? Did parents and caretakers punish children, or simply wait for them to outgrow the activity? Are parents and others more willing to ask questions now? Is there a more relaxed climate about sexual issues in general that permits or encourages more open interest or conjecture about sexuality in childhood?

Although the "sexual revolution" has opened up a range of options including more relaxed standards about virginity, premarital sex, and consensual sex between adults, a certain amount of discomfort persists for many adults who consider the topic of child sexuality. The obvious lack of scientific study in this area has created a gap in reliable and comprehensive information about children and sexuality, and this gap makes it difficult to decipher what might be considered problematic sexuality in children. This book attempts to summarize some basic information about childhood sexuality and offers some preliminary ways of understanding how to approach the subject.

We have learned a lot about problematic sexuality in the last two decades, in particular about adult sex offenders. In addition, much information has emerged about adolescent sex offenders, and some of these data are helpful in analyzing sexualized behaviors in children, and in particular molesting behaviors among children.

Groth and Laredo (1981) studied adolescent sex offenders and offered eight basic criteria that could be used to distinguish "normative sexual behavior that is situational," from "what may be inappropriate, solitary sexual activity of a non-aggressive nature," from "what may be sexually assaultive behavior that poses some risk to another person"(p. 32). Although some of Groth and Laredo's determinants pertain primarily to adolescents, they also serve as a framework for later consideration of age-appropriate sex play versus sexual abuse in younger children, as follows:

- Age relationship of persons involved
- Social relationship between persons involved
- Type of sexual activity
- How sexual contact takes place
- How persistent it is
- Evidence of progression in regard to nature or frequency of sexual activity
- Nature of fantasies that accompany or precede sexual behavior
- Distinguishing characteristics of persons targeted for sexual activities

Sgroi and colleagues (1988) developed the following assessment criteria:

- Complaint status
- Behavioral indicators of sexual abuse
- Developmental perspective

- Relative power position
- Fear or intimidation
- Ritualistic or sadistic behaviors, and
- Secrecy

Using these frameworks as a foundation, I propose the following set of criteria that can be used to assess whether a situation is one of age-appropriate sex play between young children, or if the situation can be considered problematic or potentially dangerous. When making assessments, the professional cannot consider a single criterion, but must appraise the situation along several criteria before reaching a conclusion. Using a single criterion to establish a professional opinion is erroneous and can lead to over- or under-reacting.

Age Difference Between Children Engaged in Sex Play

When the age discrepancy between two children involved in sexual play is greater than three years, the situation warrants exploration. It can be considered age-appropriate for children of similar ages to have mutual sex play. If two nine-year-olds pull down their pants, look at each other, and run away giggling, chances are the situation is one of mutual exploration. If a nine-year-old and a five-year-old are engaged in sex play that consists of inserting a foreign object in the child's rectum, this signals a dangerous situation given both the age discrepancy and type of sexual activity. The most obvious concerns arise when adolescents initiate sexual exploration with latency-aged or preschool children; yet, due to the vast developmental differences in younger children, a three-year-old being approached for sex play by a seven-year-old would also be a high-risk situation given the cognitive and emotional disparity between the youngsters. Disparity in children's ages cannot and should not be used as the only criterion, since it could cause dangerous situations to be overlooked or minimized.

Size Difference Between Children

Another important distinction between problematic sexual play and age-appropriate sex play is disparity in size. Children mature physically at highly individualized rates, and when one child towers over another, underlying dynamics of dominance or threat can become relevant.

One pediatrician minimized the worry of an attentive mother when she asked how normal it was for her five-year-old to be found unrobed, playing doctor with another five-year-old child of the same sex. The pediatrician laughingly asked the mother, "Don't you remember doing that at her age?"

and then told the mother that her child's behavior was developmentally appropriate. Although it is certainly possible that the situation of two same-age children playing doctor can be age-appropriate, a proper assessment is also warranted. In this case, it turned out that one of the five-year-old children was a good foot and a half taller and ten pounds heavier than the other, and this larger child was clearly bullying the smaller child into undressing. The smaller child eventually refused to go and visit her friend's house, even with her mother, and developed regressed behavior and nightmares shortly after that. The mother brought the child to therapy after feeling that something was wrong. The clinician discovered that the child had experienced trauma in her "play sessions" with her peer, and the subsequent trauma could have been prevented if the pediatrician who was originally consulted had looked into the situation further.

Difference in Status

Another factor that can help decide the mutuality in sexual activity is the status of the children vis à vis one another. An older child can be delegated as baby-sitter. Older siblings may be assigned the role of temporary caretakers. In either case, one child has more authority and compromises the other child's ability to make choices, even when there is no apparent use of threat or force. A child with higher status or authority can use the inequality to coerce cooperation in another child. This may be a factor independent of chronological age.

One eleven-year-old male baby-sitter took off his clothes and ran around the house nude with an erection. The six-year-old boy in his care eventually took off his clothes and they then wrestled on the floor. The mother came home early one day and was shocked to find the two boys on the floor wrestling, with the baby-sitter erect. The eleven-year-old insisted that he had done nothing wrong, and he had never asked the younger child to take off his clothes. He didn't understand that his modeling the behavior, coupled with his elevated status, could create a situation in which the young child simply followed his lead. The young child's mother also failed to understand the situation properly and became infuriated with her six-year-old for not telling her what had been happening, and for taking off his own clothes. The younger child was left feeling much shame, yet didn't understand exactly what he had done wrong.

Type of Sexual Activity

Children become interested in, ask about, and obtain sexual information progressively over a period. They appear to become interested in their bodies first, and later develop an interest in experimentation with others. Sexual interests therefore range from self-stimulation, to exhibitionism, to periods of inhibition, to touching others, and finally, to experimenting with kissing, fondling, oral sex, and penetration. Types of sexual interest and activity vary depending on several social and familial factors, as societies and families provide or restrict sexual information based on cultural, moral, or religious values and beliefs. Development of sexualized behaviors may be accelerated by explicit sexual information available from family or peers, pictures or videos, observation of sexual activity between parents or among siblings or others, and direct sexual experience.

Although data about normative sexual behavior among children are minimal, a rule of thumb is to consider the progression of curiosity and activity on a continuum. For example, a six-year-old who wants to penetrate other children vaginally or anally with his fingers, penis or a foreign object is depicting unusual and potentially harmful behavior and should be evaluated carefully. A four-year-old girl who wants to orally copulate younger children is showing an unusual knowledge of sexuality.

Dynamics of Sexual Play vs. Problematic Sexual Behaviors

The dynamics of age-appropriate, exploratory sex play between young children usually include spontaneity, joy, laughter, embarrassment, and sporadic levels of inhibition and disinhibition.

On the other hand, problematic sexual behaviors have themes of dominance, coercion, threats, and force. Children seem agitated, anxious, fearful, or intense. They have higher levels of arousal, and the sexual activity may be habitual. It is as though no other activity gives the same degree of pleasure, comfort, or reassurance, and it becomes the focus of the child's life. This behavior is usually extremely unresponsive to any parental or caretaker limits or distractions.

The following section reviews the examples on pages 27–28, using my set of five criteria. In some situations, all the information may not be available, but the criteria provide direction about the types of information to obtain.

> Example 1: A mother walks into her thirteen-year-old son's bedroom and finds he is having sexual intercourse with his eight-year-old sister. In a panic, she rushes the young girl into the car and speeds to the pediatrician's office where she asks about the activity. Is the child all right? Is this normal for kids their age?

Age difference: The five-year age difference is a red flag. The disparity in developmental phases is great, and one would presume increased knowledge, maturity, and potential for force or persuasion in the thirteen-year-old. Developmentally, the thirteen-year-old has a more developed cognitive and physical interest in sexuality.

Size difference: In this particular case, the children are similar in size as the thirteen-year-old is very small for his age. This fact may have some impact on the situation, since the thirteen-year-old may feel like an outcast in his peer group due to his small size. This feeling may have contributed to his lack of adequate social contact (and opportunity for experimentation) with youngsters his own age.

Status difference: There is obvious inequality between the siblings, and the thirteen-year-old is often called on to baby-sit his sister. In addition, the eight-year-old girl has always been told to "do just what her brother says."

Type of sexual activity: Predicting with certainty when youngsters begin to engage in sexual intercourse is problematic, since there are so many variables that have an impact. Some youngsters claim that all their junior high school friends have had sexual intercourse. Self-report is not necessarily reliable. Some youngsters may want to be seen by others as sexually active in order to be "cool."

Most adolescents in small towns and rural settings begin to have sexual intercourse between the ages of sixteen and eighteen. It is likely that the average age drops for adolescents in big cities or more sophisticated communities. Still, many adolescents continue to wait until marriage to have sexual intercourse because of ingrained family values or religious dictates. In addition, the AIDS epidemic may be having some impact on adolescent sexual activity, with more adolescents regarding abstinence as the safest sex to have.

As mentioned above, it is difficult to say for certain when most adolescents begin to have sexual intercourse, but most people would not be as surprised today to find a sexually active teenager as twenty or thirty years ago. A recent study (Flax, 1992) found more than half of all high-school students in the ninth to twelfth grades had sex. Black students were more likely than Caucasian or Hispanic students to have had sex, and boys were more likely than girls to have done so. By the time they graduate from high school, nearly three-quarters of all students have had sexual intercourse.

When youngsters exhibit persistent or unusual sexual activity, several questions can be posed. Are children mimicking behavior they have seen or experienced? Have children been prematurely exposed to explicit sexual information? Why is the youngster in this example compelled to have (what was later discovered to be) forced sexual activity with his sister?

Dynamics: When the situation was assessed, the mother discovered that the young girl was frightened and ashamed of what occurred with her brother. She reported feeling trapped because he told her that if she told anyone he would never speak to her again. She idolized her brother and the thought of being rejected by him was intolerable to her. The thirteen-year-old viewed his sister as consenting because she did not resist him; she never said no to him—she also never said yes. The eight-year-old also viewed herself as consenting because she did not fight him off or tell her mother. Yet a sexual assault occurred, and the issue of consent between children is moot, since children cannot consent given their limited cognitive development. Children cannot consent to things they don't know about and don't fully understand. The absence of resistance is not consent.

In this situation, the outcome is noteworthy: The pediatrician told the mother that the sexual activity was developmentally appropriate. He later called to consult with me about the situation, and I was frankly happy that he chose to call. When I asked which developmental theory he was referring to when he had assessed the situation as normal, he said it had been a long time since he had reviewed child development material. I was very impressed with his calling because I recognized some uncertainty that he was willing to explore further. Obviously, the question the mother had posed perplexed him long after mother and child left his office.

After we talked, he realized that what troubled him was his unconscious knowledge that these two children were siblings and that sexual intercourse between siblings was probably not normal. I insisted that in fact this was incest and was reportable to the authorities. The report generated an investigation that revealed that the thirteen-year-old had been sexually abused by his own female baby-sitter when he was about ten years old. The mother then brought both children into therapy that consisted of individual therapy, parent-child sessions, and eventually family sessions.

> Example 2: A preschool teacher becomes very frustrated and concerned when one of the children refuses to take a nap and instead quietly proceeds to put his hand inside the diapers of other sleeping children. He becomes surprised and annoyed when the teacher places him back in his cot, and after several attempts to repeat this behavior he masturbates himself to sleep.

Age difference: In this example, the children are all the same age, and it bears repeating that age alone cannot be used as the differentiating criterion. Regardless of chronological age, many factors create a disparity between children.

Size difference: Not noteworthy.

Status difference: Although there is no formal difference in status, this situation involves children with a <u>compromised ability to participate or resist</u>. Children may be compromised in this way when they are asleep, physically ill, physically or emotionally disabled, etc.

Type of sexual activity: Preschoolers can be interested in looking or touching themselves and others, participating in bathroom activities alone or with others, and using language they regard as "bad," particularly about bathroom activities. Still, it is more common for preschoolers to engage in this behavior sporadically, and to be responsive to limits from caretakers. It is also possible that children three to five develop a sense of privacy about sexual matters, and may not feel comfortable with public displays. So although it may be somewhat common for a preschooler to spontaneously attempt to touch another child's private parts, it is not common for a preschooler to persist in touching other children's genitals while they sleep, particularly when the child is reprimanded and instructed to stop the behavior.

Dynamics: Two factors are worth consideration: The child was approaching other children while they were sleeping, making the circumstances unique. The child was approaching children who were in a vulnerable state, so the power dynamics were definitely an issue. In addition, the child could go to sleep only while masturbating, and although this may not be unusual for a child this age, it is a little less usual in a public setting, and may warrant exploration.

Outcome: The child was referred for a medical examination to rule out any organic reason for excessive masturbation and was found to have chlamydial infection, which is sexually transmitted. As a result of this medical finding, an investigation ensued and incest by an older brother was uncovered.

> <u>Example 3:</u> A six-year-old boy who plays unsupervised in his apartment complex after school is observed taking smaller children behind bushes, pulling them to the ground, turning them over, and attempting to insert a stick or a finger in the children's anuses.

Age difference: The child was approaching smaller children, although some of these children were his age.

Size difference: As stated previously, this six-year-old was particularly interested in smaller children.

Status difference: No specific status difference existed between the children except that inherent in the occasional age dissimilarity.

Type of sexual activity: For a six-year-old child, the sexual activity appeared sophisticated and extreme. Attempting to penetrate other children's anuses is definitely an alarming behavior for a child his age.

Dynamics: One of the most distinctive features of this case was the child's aggression. He wanted to dominate younger children, and he physically secluded them and forced them to the ground. The child merged aggression and sexuality and presented an unequivocal danger to other children.

Outcome: The child was placed in a residential treatment center because his behavior could not be curtailed otherwise. He required twenty-four-hour supervision and an in-depth therapy program. His treatment revealed a severe history of child sexual abuse beginning when he was three years old. His treatment plan necessitated long-term and comprehensive therapy, with a focus on child sexual abuse.

> Example 4: A nine-year-old girl causes great alarm when several of her girlfriends report that when they go to the bathroom with her, she shows them her breasts and wants everyone to show theirs. Sometimes she offers one or two dollars if friends will let her touch their breasts.

Age difference: She approached peers.

Size difference: She approached friends of all sizes.

Status difference: None.

Type of sexual activity: Wanting to see or touch genitals is not unusual for children this age. Depending on the child, there may be more or less inhibition about nudity.

Dynamics: There are a couple of factors to consider. First is that the child approached children in the school bathroom as opposed to in more public settings. The child probably had some sense that her behavior was not appropriate, and she may even have felt ashamed of herself. The second factor is the child's attempt to coerce other children to engage in this behavior by bribing them to do so. Her preoccupation with sexuality was excessive, and from reports, had not decreased as a result of rejection from peers. Further exploration would be appropriate.

Outcome: This nine-year-old child had been exposed to explicit sexual information by an older sister who had engaged in sexual intercourse on the bottom bunk bed they shared. She had done this many times and paid her younger sister to keep quiet. The nine-year-old eventually stated that her sister's boyfriend had fondled her breasts several times while her older sister slept.

> Example 5: Two four-year-olds are playing doctor, and when mother enters the room they yell at her to leave, saying they are doing "private things." The mother notices both children have disrobed down to their underwear.

Age difference: None.

Size difference: None.

Status difference: None. The children were friends and neighbors.

Type of sexual activity: Children customarily play doctor. They may mimic physical examinations and practice with peers. For example, young children may initiate a game in which they are the doctor and another child is the patient. Children may take turns doing examinations and usually are having fun while they play together.

When children report they are playing doctor or when parents observe this type of play, it is useful to pay attention and make sure that both children are safe, and that the play has not escalated into something harmful or painful to either child.

Outcome: In this situation the parent simply asked the children to keep playing while she picked up some things in the room. She observed the children using the medical toys to listen to each other's heart beat, giving each other pretend shots, and "prescribing" M&M medicine. Obviously, this was age-appropriate doctor play and the parent responded in a most suitable way.

It would be of concern if children who were playing doctor were inserting fingers or objects into genitals or if they were using the game as a way to encourage or coerce unwilling friends into compliance.

> Example 6: A fourteen-year-old boy masturbates to orgasm in the presence of a six-year-old boy he is baby-sitting. The scared six-year-old talks to his mother when the teenager insists that the boy watch him ejaculate.

Age difference: Significant. There is both a chronological difference and a developmental one. Even though these two children may be at the same emotional maturity level, the teenager was obviously more knowledgeable about sexuality and was more physically mature.

Size difference: Significant.

Status difference: There was an inherent disparity in power between these two children. The teenager was in a position of authority over the youngster in his care. The six-year-old child had been told to "obey" the baby-sitter. There is an implicit delegation of power from parent to baby-sitter.

Type of sexual activity: It is not unusual for a fourteen-year-old to masturbate to ejaculation. What is unusual is that the adolescent chose to masturbate in front of a much younger child for whom he was baby-sitting. This was highly inappropriate behavior for the adolescent and would certainly require further scrutiny.

Dynamics: There are certain disconcerting dynamics in this case. The adolescent chose to engage in sexual activity while baby-sitting. He used his position of authority to have a younger child observe him while he masturbated. The adolescent might have been aroused by the younger child, or by having the younger child's compliant observation. In either case, the dynamics suggest an adolescent with a problem around abusive sexuality.

Outcome: The adolescent had been reported to the authorities for molesting younger children when he was twelve. He had been in therapy for six months and claimed he would not fondle other children again. When the police investigated, the adolescent was outraged that the six-year-old had told his mother and appeared angry and potentially violent. He claimed that he had not molested the child in any way. When confronted with his masturbatory behavior, he stated, "The kid shouldn't have been watching me," and did not recognize his behavior as unusual or abusive in any way. The adolescent was referred back into treatment, this time with a therapist who specialized in the treatment of adolescent sex offenders.

Summary

We can say few things about childhood sexuality with certainty. First, normal sexual development follows suit with physical, emotional, psychological, cognitive, and moral development in that it is progressive over time.

Second, a large number of variables affects the child's ability to follow along the developmental path, and when assessing whether childhood sexual behavior is age-appropriate, those variables must be assessed.

Third, children seem to be having sexual experiences at earlier ages, and age-appropriate sexual play and experimentation between peers is neither harmful nor traumatic to children.

When evaluating the sexual behaviors of children, clinicians must neither under- nor overreact. Instead, clinicians and investigators are advised to proceed by making careful and sensitive assessments using the knowledge base available to them.

In order to fully comprehend the sexual behaviors of children that might be referred for evaluation, it is important to assert that children are sexual beings, capable of demonstrating a positive, healthy, creative, and spirited interest in sexuality. For too long, childhood sexuality has been stymied by adults seeking to curtail children's developing interest, curiosity, and experimentation.

At the same time, sexual interest or experimentation that is excessive and/or compulsive, devoid of the usual spontaneity and frolic of childhood, and that contains the dynamics of threat, force, or coercion, must be evaluated with a certainty that excessive interest or sophisticated sexual behaviors in children do not occur in a vacuum. Many of the problematic sexual behaviors that elicit adult concern can surface as a result of (1) inappropriate exposure to explicit sexual material in or out of the home; (2) a child's premature involvement in sexuality, often initiated by an older child or adult; or (3) as a result of living with a family that fails to provide the needed guidance, limits, or nurturance to children. Chapter three discusses a way to view children's sexual behaviors by offering a categorization system along a continuum, including age-appropriate childhood sexuality to child-molesting behaviors. To differentiate between age-appropriate sex play and sexual contact between children that could be considered problematic or symptomatic, professionals must distinguish on a broad base of criteria. A number of examples of children's sexual behaviors that caused concern or alarm were presented to provide specific assessment criteria.

References

Flax, E. (1992). Most high school students sexually active, CDC finds. *Education Week* XI (17): 10.

Friedrich, W., Grambsch, P., Damon, L., Koverola, C.,Wolfe, V., Hewitt, S., Lang, R., & Broughton, D. (1992). The child sexual behavior inventory: Normative and clinical comparisons. *Psychological Assessment* 4(3): 303–311.

Friedrich, W. N. (1990). Developmental considerations. In W. N. Friedrich, *Psychotherapy of sexually abused children and their families*. New York: W. W. Norton.

Gallo, A. M. (1979). Early childhood masturbation: A developmental approach. *Pediatric Nursing* 12:47–49.

Green, A. H. (1988). Overview of normal psychosexual development. In D. H. Schetky, & A. H. Green, *A handbook for health care and legal professionals*. New York: Brunner/Mazel.

Groth, N. A. & Laredo, C. M. (1981). Juvenile sexual offenders: Guidelines for assessment. *International Journal of Offender Treatment and Comparative Criminology* 25(1): 31–39.

Levine, M. I. (1957). Pediatric observations on masturbation in children. *Psychoanalytic Study of the Child* 6:117–124.

Lewis, W. C. (1965). Coital movements in the first year of life: Earliest anlage of genital love? *International Journal of Psychoanalysis* 46:372–374.

Martinson, F. (1976). Eroticism in infancy and childhood. *Journal of Sex Research* 12:251–262.

Martinson, F. M. (1991). Normal sexual development in infancy and childhood. In G. D. Ryan, & S. L. Lane, *Juvenile sexual offending*. New York: Lexington.

Money, J., & Ehrhardt, A. A. (1972) *Man and woman, boy and girl*. Baltimore, MD: Johns Hopkins University Press.

Rutter, M. (1971). Normal psychosexual development. *Journal of Child Psychology and Psychiatry* 2:259–283.

Rutter, M. (1980). Psychosexual development. *Scientific Foundations of Developmental Psychiatry* 16:322–339.

Sgroi, S., Bunk, B., & Wabrek, C. (1988). Children's sexual behaviors and their relationship to sexual abuse. In S. Sgroi (Ed.), *Vulnerable populations*, Vol. 1. New York: Lexington.

3

Sexual Behaviors: A Continuum

Toni Cavanagh Johnson, Ph.D.
with Joanne Ross Feldmeth

After extensive evaluations of children and their families who were referred as a result of the child's sexual behaviors, definable groups or clusters emerge. If there were a continuum based on the level of sexual disturbance, these children could be divided into four groups. Group I includes children engaged in natural childhood sexual exploration, group II is composed of sexually reactive children, group III includes children mutually engaged in the full range of adult sexual behaviors, and group IV includes children who molest other children.

This model applies to boys and girls ages twelve and under who have intact reality testing and are not developmentally delayed. Each group includes a very wide range of children. Some are on the borderline between groups, or move between groups over a period of time.

Normal Sexual Exploration	Sexually Reactive	Extensive Mutual Sexual Behaviors	Children Who Molest
Group I	Group II	Group III	Group IV

Table 3-1   A Continuum of Sexual Behaviors

Group I - Normal Sexual Exploration

Normal childhood sex play is an information-gathering process. Children explore each other's bodies visually and tactilely (e.g., playing doctor), or try out gender roles and behaviors (e.g., playing house). Children involved in age-appropriate exploration are of similar age and size, generally of mixed sex, and more often friends than siblings. (Finkelhor, 1973). They participate on a voluntary basis ("I'll show you mine if you show me yours!"). The relationship of these children outside the sexual interaction is amicable.

Another aspect of typical childhood curiosity is a delight in bathroom humor and games, an interest that sometimes flusters adults. Three ten-year-old boys threw the staff at one elementary school into conflict when they were discovered playing in the bathroom. The children were attempting to identify which boy could stand farthest from the toilet bowl and still "hit" it. The principal was convinced the behavior was "perverted" and suggested the children be removed from school (Morgan, 1984).

Despite the principal's alarm, the boys provide an excellent example of healthy—if, perhaps, mischievous—childhood behavior. The typical affect of children regarding normal behaviors related to sexuality is lighthearted and spontaneous. These boys were trying out something fun. They were exploring the capabilities of their bodies. In age-appropriate sex play or exploration, children are excited and feel silly and "giggly." Although they may also feel confused and guilty, they do not experience feelings of deep shame, fear, or anxiety.

The sexual behavior of children engaged in the natural process of childhood exploration is balanced by curiosity about other parts of their universe. They want to know how babies are made and why the sun disappears. They want to explore the physical differences between males and females, as well as figure out how to get their homework done quickly so they can play outside.

If children are discovered in normal sex play and instructed to stop, the sexual behaviors generally diminishes or ceases, at least within sight of adults, to arise again during another period of the child's development. Children engage in a wide range of sexual behaviors. Not all children engage in all behaviors; some may engage in none, whereas others engage in only a few (Finkelhor, 1973; Goldman & Goldman, 1988; Haugaard & Tilly, 1988). These behaviors include autostimulation and self-exploration, kissing, hugging, peeking, touching and/or exposing of genitals to other children, and perhaps simulating intercourse (Goldman & Goldman, 1988). Only 2 to 3 percent of children twelve and younger engage in intercourse (Haugaard & Tilly, 1988).

Because of this range, diagnosing a child based on sexual behavior alone can be misleading. Children with sexual behavior problems usually show many more sexual behaviors, but in some cases, they may vary only in degree from the behaviors of some group I children.

The need for careful evaluation of children referred for problematic sexual behaviors is evident in the case of eight-year-old Eddie, who was brought in for evaluation after a long and traumatic day. Eddie had been taken from his apartment in handcuffs and put into a squad car as the neighbors watched. Phoned by the police, Eddie's parents met him at the police station. The allegation against the third-grader was sexual assault.

Earlier that day, the apartment manager's two young daughters (ages four and five) came to their mother and announced that Eddie had pulled their pants down and tried to put his finger in their private parts. The manager immediately telephoned the police, who responded by transporting Eddie to the police station in handcuffs. After questioning Eddie and his parents, instead of filing charges, the police referred the family for evaluation at a center with expertise in treating children who molest other children. The family followed up by scheduling an appointment immediately.

As soon as the Smiths arrived, they presented an immediate contrast to the fragmented and dysfunctional families of most sexually troubled children (particularly children in group IV). Mr. and Mrs. Smith both attended the session with Eddie, and instead of being hostile or denying the allegations, made it clear they took the incident seriously and were very concerned about their son. Their intake information revealed a stable family history. The Smiths had been married for 18 years and had an older daughter, a sixteen-year-old who regularly attended the local high school. Both parents had worked for the same company for over a dozen years. There was no history of drugs, alcohol, physical or sexual abuse, or major family disruption.

Until his arrest, Eddie's history showed the same kind of positive stability and achievement. He was doing fine academically, was a Little League player, and had many friends. Assessment instruments filled out by Eddie's parents and teacher indicated no significant behavior problems. His parents filled out the Child Sexual Behavior Checklist (Johnson, 1992), which indicated sexual behaviors within normal limits. All questions related to abuse, abandonment, neglect, or a highly sexually charged family atmosphere were met with negative responses.

In the interview with Eddie alone, the eight-year-old quietly told the therapist that he knew what he had done was wrong and he was sorry. He explained that his motive in approaching the children was curiosity. Alone in the apartment all day during summer vacation, there was little to do. "And I really did wonder," Eddie said, "what girls look like." Then he added, "I hope I didn't scare them."

The two little girls were interviewed the following day, and the therapist asked them if they were afraid of Eddie. "No way!" they insisted, giggling. Further questioning revealed that Eddie did not play with them regularly and had never tried anything sexual with them before. The only time they were together was in the apartment's swimming pool; their interactions at those times were nonthreatening.

On the other hand, Eddie's sexual behavior with the children had clearly been inappropriate. He had not only asked to "look," but had pulled down both the children's pants and touched and poked their private parts. His behavior caused special concern because the little girls were considerably younger than he and not regular playmates who engaged in other mutually enjoyable activities. The girls indicated, however, that Eddie stopped immediately when they said no.

After assessing Eddie, the evaluator felt that he was a group I child who had engaged in behaviors that were inappropriate and needed to stop. Eddie and his parents were provided with materials regarding sexuality and encouraged to discuss sexual issues openly in the family. The evaluator also pointed out that Eddie needed a more structured schedule and planned activities. Eight-year-olds are not self-sufficient enough to be left alone all day in an apartment complex without same-aged playmates and supervision. His parents agreed and enrolled him in a local camp for summer and an afternoon daycare program for the school year.

Finally, the interviewing therapist gave Mr. and Mrs. Smith a list of sexual behaviors of children and other behaviors that occur in children who have sexual problems. "Call me if Eddie starts doing things on this list," the evaluator urged. "Let's set an appointment for two months from now to see how things are going for Eddie."

Group II - Sexually Reactive

Group II children display more sexual behaviors than same-age children in group I, and their focus on sexuality is out of balance in relation to their peer group. In general, sexual curiosity is one aspect of many in a child's life. There is a balance between sexual curiosity and expression, learning, running, jumping, reading, etc. As in each of the other groups, there is a wide range of children in group II. In the more distressed children in group II, the children's genitals may function as the central organizing principle in their development (Yates, 1990).

Many children in group II have been sexually abused. Other children in this group have been exposed to pornography, or live in households where there is too much sexual stimulation. Young children who watch soap operas, cable television, or videos excessively and who live in sexually explicit environments may display a multitude of sexual behaviors. Children who have been reared in a commune, in crowded quarters, on the streets, in a holistic life-style, in sexually permissive cultures or subcultures, or who have engaged in a good deal of normative sex play may exhibit more sexual behaviors than children raised in "a conventionally inhibited family" (Yates, 1987).

Many children who have been overstimulated sexually cannot integrate these experiences in a meaningful way. This can result in children acting out the confusion in the form of more advanced or frequent sexual behaviors, heightened interest and/or knowledge beyond what would be expected of that age. Sexually reactive children often feel deep shame, intense guilt, and pervasive anxiety about sexuality. Often the sexual behaviors of children in group II involve only their own bodies—that is, masturbation, exposing or inserting objects in themselves, etc. If they do engage in sexual behaviors with other children, the difference in age is usually not great, and they do not force other children into sexual behaviors. Group II children are not seeking out children to coerce and victimize and do not threaten other children into silence.

Tommy is a nine-year-old boy who fits into group II. Tommy was sexually abused by a man he called "Uncle Frank," who lived down the street. Ever since the abuse, he has shown an intense and anxious interest in anything sexual, and his teacher reports some behavior and attention problems in the classroom. He has initiated oral sex and other behaviors with an eight-year-old cousin on several occasions. He has not tried to force the boy or threaten him into silence. The activities Tommy engaged in with his cousin were the ones Uncle Frank had done to him or he saw while watching pornographic videos with his "uncle."

In Tommy's case, it would be valuable to explore with him whether the sexual behaviors may be part of Post-traumatic Stress Disorder caused by his own victimization. Since the behaviors in which he is engaging are almost identical to those done to him, he may be trying to play out or reenact the traumatic experience, using sexually explicit behavior. Like the post-traumatic play described by Terr (1981), sexualized post-traumatic reenactment is stereotyped, literal, and it follows the same format time after time. Engaging in this type of play does not relieve the child's anxiety, no matter how frequent the play behavior (Yates, 1991).

The sexual behaviors of these children often represent a repetition compulsion or a recapitulation (often unconscious) of previously overstimulated sexuality. The sexualized behavior can be seen in some cases as working through the confusion around sexuality. After being told their sexual behaviors need to be altered, group II children generally acknowledge the need to stop the behaviors and welcome help. Interventions with these children must be consistent, nonjudgmental, and proactive. They need help in identifying circumstances that may increase sexualized behaviors and in substituting other behaviors. (See Chapter eleven.)

The time between sexual overstimulation and sexual acting out is close, often overlapping or contiguous. In some instances, these sexual behaviors are an unconscious attempt by children to alert adults to the abuse (Yates, 1991). The sexual behaviors of many of the children in this group are relatively easy to stop, because they do not represent a long pattern of secret, manipulative, and highly charged behaviors as seen in children who molest (group IV).

Four-year-old Jenna is also a sexually reactive child, but unlike Tommy, she has never been molested. When Jenna's mother brought her in for an evaluation, the child's behavior was unusually sexualized. When Jenna met a man—even a complete stranger—she climbed into his lap, stroked his face, or put her arms around his neck and snuggled up against him. She often tried to stick her tongue into the mouths of people who kissed her and made sexual sounds. She spent hours sitting on the couch in front of the television, masturbating while humping her stuffed animals.

Jenna was brought in by her mother, a pretty eighteen-year-old named Jackie. Jackie told the evaluator she thought her child had been molested. After several interviews, there was no evidence of sexual abuse. What emerged, however, was a picture of a home that was sexually overstimulating, with virtually no developmentally appropriate activities. The little girl and her teenage mother lived in a one-room apartment with Jackie's boyfriend, Bob. There were no children in the complex, and Jenna did not have a single child friend. Every day, the four-year-old and her mother spent hours watching soap operas. Before Bob returned from work, Jackie and Jenna did their hair and dressed up to "look pretty for Bob." Frequently, Jackie let Jenna wear her makeup. At night, Jenna watched cable movies and slept on the sofabed where Bob and Jackie made love ("only after Jenna is asleep" Jackie told the psychologist).

Like most group II children, Tommy and Jenna were very responsive to treatment. In Tommy's case, treatment focused on his sexual confusion and victimization. Being in group therapy with other boys who had been molested was especially helpful. Within a period of months, his sexual behaviors decreased to normal levels.

For Jenna, recovery was even faster and primarily involved working with her mother. Jackie put up a curtained sleeping corner for Jenna, which created a little more privacy for the adults in the evening. She and her daughter enrolled in a "Mommy and Me" class that provided Jackie with knowledge of a four-year-old's needs and practice in interacting appropriately with Jenna. Jenna started attending nursery school, and Jackie took a parenting course at the local community center. Trips to the park, zoo, and library took the place of soap operas. As the overstimulating environment decreased, and age-appropriate activities increased, the sexualized behaviors disappeared.

Yates (1991) describes children who are sexually compulsive. These children appear driven to continue sexual behavior—usually masturbation, even when it interferes with their daily lives—which brings the wrath of adults on them and appears to bring no gratification. These children would be an extreme example of group II, or perhaps group III children. Compulsive masturbation is usually regarded as a sign of tension or intrapsychic disturbance (Lewis & Volkmar, 1990).

Group III - Extensive Mutual Sexual Behaviors

Todd and Joey are nine-year-old boys who have been in the foster system as long as they can remember. When their group home leader talks about them, he throws up his hands in frustration. "I literally cannot leave Todd or Joey alone in a room for ten minutes or they will try to have sex with one another or some other kid. Todd is always behind a tree or in bed with one of several girls, whereas Joey seems to be pretty available to girls or boys. So far, Joey has had sex—lots of it—with both roommates I've assigned to him. Neither of the boys told me—I found out from the other kids. At the moment, he is spending nights in the nurse's office until I can come up with a better plan. When I try to talk to either of them, I get nowhere. They don't seem to understand why I should care about this. The other day, Joey just looked at me, shrugged and said, 'Hey, this is just the way we play!'"

Children like Todd and Joey fall into group III. They have a far more pervasive and focused sexual behavior pattern than group II children, and they are much less responsive to treatment. They participate in the full spectrum of adult sexual behaviors (oral copulation, vaginal and anal intercourse, etc.), generally with other children in the same age range, and conspire to keep the behaviors secret. Although these children use persuasion, they usually do not use force or physical or emotional coercion to gain other children's participation in sexual acts. Some of these children, however, move between groups III and IV—that is, between mutually engaging in sexual behaviors, and forcing or coercing another child into sexual behaviors of their choice.

One of the striking differences between these children and the children in other groups is their affect—or more precisely, the lack of affect—around sexuality. Group III children do not have the lighthearted spontaneity of normal children, the shame and anxiety of sexually reactive children, or the anger and aggression typical of children who molest. Instead, they display a blasé, matter-of-fact attitude toward sexual behaviors with other children.

This attitude is reflected in Joey's explanation: "This is just the way we play." It might be more accurate to say that sex is one way group III children try to relate to their peers. As for grown-ups, most group III children expect only abuse and abandonment. On Todd's few remembered trips home, his mother beat him and left him locked in a room. Joey does not remember ever living with his parents, but he has "failed placement" in ten foster homes. In one of them, he was sexually molested by an older boy. Like Todd and Joey, a high percentage of group III children are in the care of the state and live in foster, group, or residential settings.

Other group III children have been sexually abused in a group by an adult and they continue or increase the sexual behaviors with one another after the abuse stops. Some group III children are siblings who mutually engage in extensive sexual behaviors as a way of coping in a highly dysfunctional family life.

All group III children have been emotionally and sexually and/or physically abused and/or have lived in highly chaotic and sexually charged environments. Through these experiences, their understanding of relationships has been skewed. Distrustful of adults, chronically hurt and abandoned, lacking in academic or social success, these boys and girls use sex as a way to make a "friend," even briefly. Some of these children are focused on the sexually arousing aspects of the behavior, for others the behavior functions as a coping mechanism. While their "what's the big deal?" attitude has a sophisticated appearance, it conceals significant emotional vulnerability. Their sexual activity appears to be an attempt to make some kind of human connection in a world that has been chaotic, dangerous, and unfriendly.

Group IV - Children who Molest

The sexual behaviors of group IV children go far beyond developmentally appropriate childhood exploration or sex play. Like the children in group III, their thoughts and actions are often pervaded with sexuality. Typical behaviors of these children may include (but are not limited to) oral copulation, vaginal intercourse, anal intercourse, and/or forcibly penetrating the vagina or anus of another child with fingers, sticks, and/or other objects. These behaviors continue and increase over time and are part of a consistent pattern rather than isolated incidents. Even if their activities are discovered, they do not and cannot stop without intensive and specialized treatment.

A distinctive aspect of group IV children is their feelings about sex and sexuality. The shared decision making and lighthearted curiosity in the sex play of group I children is absent. Instead, there is an impulsive, compulsive, and aggressive quality to the behavior. These children often link sexual acting-out to feelings of anger (or even rage), loneliness, or fear. In one case, four girls held a frightened, fighting, and crying eighteen-month-old child while another child orally copulated him. The other girls (all aged six to eight) each took a turn. The little boy required extensive medical attention as a result of penile injuries.

Although most of the case studies in this group are less physically violent, coercion is always a factor. Children who molest seek out children who are easy to fool and bribe or force them into sexual activity. The victim-child does not get to choose what the sexual behaviors are or when they will end. Often the victim is younger, and sometimes the age difference is as great as twelve years, since some of these children molest infants. On the other hand, some sexually aggressive children molest children who are age-mates or even older. In sibling incest with boys who molest, the victim is typically the favorite child of the parents. In other cases, the child is selected because of special vulnerabilities including age, intellectual impairment, extreme loneliness, depression, social isolation, or emotional neediness. Children who molest often use social and emotional threats to keep their victims quiet. "I won't play with you ever again, if you tell" is a powerful reason to keep quiet if the child-victim already feels lonely, isolated, or abandoned at home and at school.

Group IV children seldom express any empathy for their victims. Ten-year-old David, for example, repeatedly explained that he had to slap an eight-year-old girl and call her a bitch, because she would not stop screaming. "I told her to shut up," he said, "but she just wouldn't stop." The fact that the child was screaming because he was trying to penetrate her vagina with his finger did not seem to David to be particularly relevant or worth discussion. Even being discovered in the act of molesting another child does not necessarily break down the denial of responsibility. When his foster mother walked into the room where nine-year-old John was sodomizing his five-year-old foster brother, the older boy stated angrily, "I'm not doing anything."

As a group, these children have behavior problems at home and at school, few outside interests, and almost no friends. They lack problem-solving and coping skills and demonstrate little impulse control. Often, they are physically as well as sexually aggressive. In preliminary findings on children who molest no one—parents, teachers or peers—described any member of the group as "an average kid" (Johnson, 1988).

Even the bathroom games sometimes seen in group I children are markedly different from the disturbed toileting behaviors common in group IV. Some children who molest other children habitually urinate and defecate outside the toilet (on the floor, in their beds, outdoors, etc.). Although many group I children may mildly resist changing underwear, some children in group IV wear soiled underpants for more than a week or two and adamantly refuse to change. Some constantly sniff underwear. Many regularly use excessive amounts of toilet paper (some relate wiping and cleaning themselves to masturbation) and stuff the toilet until it overflows day after day. These children continue their disturbed toileting patterns even if their families have severely punished them for the behaviors.

Group IV children are often obsessively focused on toileting and sexual activities, the normal sexual curiosity and delight of young children in their bodies are absent. Instead, they express a great deal of anger, anxiety and confusion about sexuality.

Most sexually aggressive children who have been studied were victims of sexual abuse themselves, although the abuse had generally occurred years before they began molesting other children. All had been emotionally abused, and most had been severely and unpredictably punished by caretakers. All of these children lived in home environments marked by sexual stimulation and lack of boundaries, and virtually all witnessed extreme physical violence between their primary caretakers. Most parents of group IV children also have sexual abuse in their family history, as well as physical and substance abuse.

Although the sexual behaviors of group IV children generally cease or markedly decrease after focused therapy and support, the feelings that precipitated the behaviors are still very evident. Since sexual gratification is generally not the primary motivator of these children's behaviors, the sustained focus of therapy is underlying feelings, confused cognitions, sexual traumas and skill building. These children have paired intense feelings of loneliness, rage, and fear (each child has one or more such feelings) with sex, which itself has been paired with aggression. When they feel loneliness, they want to decrease the anxious and uncomfortable sensations, and think they can do so by acting-out sexually and/or aggressively. Although they experience momentary release, virtually all of these children feel worse after acting-out, and the intensity of the feelings remains.

Summary

The sexual behaviors of boys and girls ages twelve and under can be categorized into four groups, based on the level of sexual disturbance. Group I includes children engaged in natural childhood sexual exploration; group II is composed of sexually reactive children, group III includes children mutually engaged in the full range of adult sexual behaviors, and group IV includes children who molest other children.

Group I children are engaged in normal childhood exploration, and their sexual interest is balanced by curiosity about other parts of their universe. When they are discovered in normal sex play and instructed to stop, the sexual behaviors gradually diminish or cease, and may reemerge at a later developmental stage.

Many of the sexually reactive children in Group II have been sexually abused or overexposed to sexual stimulation, making it difficult for them to integrate their experiences in a meaningful way. They develop problematic sexual behaviors which manifest their confusion, anger, shame, or anxiety. These behaviors may represent an unconscious attempt to alert adults to their abuse.

Group III children have more pervasive and focused sexual behavior patterns and participate in the full spectrum of adult sexual behaviors. A distinguishing feature of Group III children is their matter-of-fact attitude toward sexual behaviors with other children—sex is often their way of relating to their peers. They are often victims of physical or sexual abuse.

Group IV children have pervasive, coercive sexual behaviors far beyond developmentally appropriate childhood exploration or sex play and their behaviors increase over time. The children in this group often link sexually aggressive behaviors with feelings of anger, loneliness, or fear. When Group IV children are not overtly abused, they live in home environments marked by sexual stimulation, lack of boundaries, and physical violence.

Depending on group membership, treatment needs differ. Some children require in-depth treatment to address not only the sexual behavior problems, but the myriad emotional problems that propel the behaviors.

References

Finkelhor, D. (1973). (Manuscript). *Childhood sexual experiences: A retrospective survey*. University of New Hampshire: Durham, NH.

Goldman, R., & Goldman, J. (1988). *Show me yours: Understanding children's sexuality*. New York, NY: Penguin.

Haugaard, J., & Tilly, C. (1988). Characteristics predicting children's responses to sexual encounters with other children. *Child Abuse and Neglect* 12:209-218.

Johnson, T. C. (1988). Child perpetrators: Children who molest other children: Preliminary findings. *Child Abuse and Neglect* 12:219-229.

Johnson, T. C. (1992). Child sexual behavior checklist revised. Unpublished.

Lewis, M., & Volkmar, F. R. (1990). *Clinical aspects of child and adolescent development*. Philadelphia, PA: Lea & Febiger.

Morgan, S. R. (1984). Counseling with teachers on the sexual acting-out of disturbed children. *Psychology in the Schools* 21(April): 234-243.

Terr, L. (1981). "Forbidden games:" Post -traumatic child's play. *Journal of the American Academy of Child Psychiatry* 20:741-760.

Yates, A. (1987). Psychological damage associated with extreme eroticism in young children. *Psychiatric Annals* 17: 257-261.

Yates, A. (1990). Eroticized children. In M. E. Perry (Ed.), *Handbook of sexology: Childhood and adolescent sexology*. New York, NY: Elsevier Science Publishers.

Yates, A. (1991). Differentiating hypererotic states in the evaluation of sexual abuse. *Journal of the American Academy of Psychiatry* 30(5): 791-795.

4

Etiologic Theories

Eliana Gil, Ph.D.

A great deal of research has been conducted regarding the incidence of sexual abuse in the histories of adult and adolescent sex offenders (Groth, 1979; Longo, 1986; Burgess et al., 1987). These data are often used to make predictions about the future offending behavior of children and adolescents who commit sexual offenses. Although there is evidence that adult sex offenders frequently report a history of childhood sexual abuse (estimates range from 10 to 80 percent), there is no evidence that all victims of sexual abuse in childhood develop offending behaviors as adults.

There is a significant gap in the longitudinal research of abused individuals. Recent research on "stress-resistant" children offers interesting insight into children's abilities to escape the effects of abuse relatively unscathed (Anthony and Cohler, 1987). Obviously, we need to continue formulating hypotheses about the psychological constructs that contribute to offending behaviors, and continue articulating what we learn from offenders themselves in addition to our own clinical observations. This chapter reviews the etiology of offending behaviors in young children. Although some of these theories draw from the offending behaviors of adolescents and may have limited applicability to younger sexually acting-out children, they are worth considering nonetheless.

Abuse Reactive and Sexually Reactive Children

The phrase "abuse-reactive children" was coined by staff at the Children's Institute International when they developed their 1985 program, SPARK (Support Program for Abuse-Reactive Kids). The phrase reflects a conceptual belief that children who molest other children are reacting to their early trauma in abusive, aggressive, and inappropriate sexual ways (Cunningham & MacFarlane, 1991). The underlying hypothesis was that most children who molest are themselves victims of sexual abuse. The literature has consistently documented persistent sexual behavior problems in sexually abused children, including sexually aggressive behavior (Friedrich, 1990a).   Two research studies were conducted with SPARK clients by then program director, Toni Cavanagh Johnson. Johnson found that in a sample of forty-seven boys ages four to thirteen, 49 percent had been sexually abused and 19 percent were physically abused, bringing the total percentage of known abused children to 68 percent (Johnson, 1988).   In another study of thirteen female children who molest, 100 percent of the youngsters had a history of sexual abuse (Johnson, 1989). We can hypothesize that some abused children tend to repeat or reenact the abuse that has been experienced.

The term "sexually reactive" has been used in different ways and has evoked some concern. Matsuda and Rasmussen (1990) defined sexually reactive children as "children, age 8 and under, who display sexually inappropriate behavior towards another which is harmful or unlawful . . . often in reaction to his/her own sexual victimization and/or exposure to explicit sexual stimuli" (p. 2). In a subsequent article, Rasmussen and co-workers (1992) expanded on that definition to include children "ages 9 to 12 who are acting out sexually and have a documented history of prior sexual victimization and/or exposure to explicit sexual stimuli" (p. 34). Friedrich (1990a) states: "By sexually reactive we mean sexualized behavior that appears to be in direct response to sexual abuse. This would include masturbation, increased sexual exploration, exhibitionism, and a temporary breakdown in the children's interpersonal boundaries" (p. 254). He differentiates sexually reactive behavior by stating that "[It] may or may not have an aggressive component to it but may simply be a heightened sexuality in sexually abused children, either transient or more prolonged in nature" (p. 246). In addition, he sates that it is often difficult to assess whether children are "sexually reactive vs. sexually aggressive or child perpetrators." It appears that sexually reactive behavior serves to explain not only one motive for sexually problematic behavior, but also includes a range and type of specific behaviors. Attempts to differentiate among types of sexually reactive behaviors are underway. Lane (1991) expresses concern that the term sexually reactive may sometimes be used in a way that "minimizes the nature of sexual behaviors that do involve some degree of coercion or an unequal power base"(p. 304). She says that the term may also be used to imply that being sexually victimized causes one to become sexually abusive, rather than viewing it as one factor that may contribute to abusive sexual behaviors. Lane advises that the term be used cautiously, and wonders if the popularity of the term doesn't relate to the greater acceptance of these children more as victims without negative intentions than as perpetrators who are choosing to exert their own power or control. Cunningham and MacFarlane clearly state that their term abuse reactive ". . . is not intended to imply a direct cause and effect relationship between victimization and perpetration or to de-emphasize accountability." They also state that their use of the term has never "served to lessen or minimize our awareness of the considerable harm done to their child victims."

It appears there is general consensus that the term sexually reactive does refer to a history of sexual abuse, and although no one professes a linear cause and effect, the history of abuse is seen as a relevant factor in children's development of unusual or problematic sexual behaviors. Since this theory has been validated by existing empirical data, it is safe to say that some sexually abused children will develop sexually abusive behaviors toward others. Therefore, service providers are well-advised to develop a concern for both victim and victimizer issues, since exclusive attention to one issue may be counterproductive. In consulting with service providers across the country, I have noted a disturbing tendency for professionals in child sexual abuse treatment programs to develop a rigid or polarized specialization, in which either victim or offender issues are addressed in an exclusionary fashion. This skewed treatment approach places children in positions of having to adjust to additional professionals and diffuse their treatment needs between providers with specific interests or expertise.

Several authors have made important contributions to the growing understanding of the impact of abuse and trauma on children's emotional, physiological, psychological, cognitive, and spiritual development. These theories or concepts are reviewed here with application to sexualized behaviors in young children.

Traumatic Sexualization

Finkelhor and Browne (1986) devised a conceptual framework for understanding the impact of abuse. They proposed the concept that child sexual abuse would result in "tramaugenic dynamics" and cited four separate domains in which a variety of psychological and behavioral concerns arose: traumatic sexualization, stigmatization, betrayal, and helplessness (pp. 186–187). For purposes of this discussion, the focus is on the first domain, traumatic sexualization.

Finkelhor and Browne state that sexually abused children are taught and therefore learn to behave in sexually inappropriate ways. Based strongly in learning theory, they propose that children learn through repeated conditioning with positive or negative reinforcement. Offenders exchange attention and affection for sex (positive reinforcement), or they withhold punishment in exchange for sex (negative reinforcement). In either case, the child learns to perform sexual acts for a variety of reasons. In my experience, the child learns that sexual behaviors can modulate anxiety and promote feelings of safety and well-being, despite subsequent feelings of shame, confusion, or isolation that frequently accompany sexual abuse.

Children learn that sexual behavior is necessary to meet their needs; sometimes the most basic of necessities are withheld until the child performs in a desired manner. One young child was not allowed to sleep or eat unless she first initiated and performed oral sex on her parent.

Inevitably, sexually abused children become confused about sexuality, and negative associations are formed between sexuality and caregetting and caregiving. In addition, children's normal development in the sexual sphere is thwarted by inappropriate and excessive focus on feelings and behaviors that would usually surface gradually during the child's development.

The emotional climate in which these "lessons" are taught may further create fear and anxiety in young children not yet capable of understanding the varied aspects of sexual arousal. Less obvious signs of sexual arousal in adults (the look in their eyes, the sounds they make) may frighten and disturb young children. The associations developed during overt sexual abuse tend to have long-lasting implications and often serve as a kind of imprinting in children's early learning about human sexuality.

Finkelhor and Browne state that overtly sexually abused children may therefore develop unusual or excessive preoccupations with sexual matters and may ultimately engage in inappropriate sexual acts with other children or adults.

As mentioned earlier, this conceptualization relies heavily on learning theory and focuses primarily on the resultant behaviors "learned" through conditioning. The basic tenet of the learning model is that children are taught to respond to specific stimuli in specific ways. Professionals who work in shelters where children are brought after an allegation of child abuse state that many children grab their genitals, make suggestive sexual remarks, and generally behave in sexually inappropriate ways that seem acceptable to the children. They are in fact drawing from a repertoire of learned behaviors.

At the same time, reliance on the learning theory alone may be insufficient. Garland and Dougher (1990) state, "The belief that sexual abuse causes sexual abuse, the so-called 'abused/abuser hypothesis' is simplistic and misleading." In their comprehensive critical review of the empirical data on the topic of victim-victimizer dynamics (i.e., whether adults who were sexually abused as children later abuse children) they conclude, "The fact that some relation, albeit a complex one, appears to exist between sexual contact with an adult during childhood and adolescence and sexual involvement with a child or adolescent during adulthood argues strongly for continued research on the issue" (p. 505).

Other theorists have complemented the behaviorists and the contribution of the learning model by discussing motivational and psychological forces behind observed behaviors.

Eroticized Children

Yates (1987) explains that sexually molested children become sexually experienced and "highly eroticized," regardless of their age. Since sexual responsiveness does not require cognitive skill, even very young children can become eroticized. Yates directs our attention to the family environments of molested children and asserts that separation anxiety, random physical abuse, or abrupt rejections intensify the importance of the sexual mode. "There are no alternatives; the sexual self becomes exclusive and central; the character is impoverished" (p. 259). Yates (1982) also notes that many preschoolers failed to differentiate affectionate relationships from sexual relationships and became aroused by routine physical or psychological closeness. In addition, erotic expression becomes so gratifying few comparable rewards exist for cessation. These children, she goes on to say, are often highly erotic, easily aroused, highly motivated, and readily orgasmic depending on the intensity or duration of the incest they have experienced. Based on this perspective, it appears that children develop a reliance on sexual exchanges to salvage a sense of integrity and self-esteem.

Post-Traumatic Play and Action

Terr (1990) recently wrote a ground-breaking book chronicling a longitudinal study with twenty-six elementary school children in Chowchilla, California. The "Chowchilla children," as they were later called, were kidnapped while riding home in their school bus and buried in the bus in a large tomblike hole underground. The children's resiliency and courage enabled them to make an amazing escape that eventually resulted in a successful rescue from what would have been an unthinkable death.

Terr studied the behaviors and responses of these children and other traumatized children for many years and found that such children have limited choices of how to process the horrific material: they reenact through either play or action. She notes that this type of play, called post-traumatic play, is very unique and has distinctive features, such as the tendency to be literal, repetitive, and morbid. Children compulsively and rigidly repeat the events before, during, or after the traumatic incident. As Terr cautions, the play can become dangerous if it fails to discharge affect or further focuses the child on feelings of helplessness and fear. Gil (1991) talks about the importance of creating opportunities for post-traumatic play when children don't spontaneously develop this play, but more importantly stresses the urgency of intervening in post-traumatic play when natural resolution does not occur, and when symptoms outside the therapy hour become exacerbated.

Behavioral reenactments (cited by Terr as another option to play reenactments) are more problematic in that children seek to repeat the elements of the traumatic event with other children—that is, they attempt to do to others what was done to them. Van der Kolk (1989) believes that children "seem more vulnerable than adults to compulsive behavioral repetition and loss of conscious memory of the trauma" (p. 390). This may be because other coping strategies are less available to children, and their cognitive capacity is more limited. Friedrich (1990a) says, "It's safe to say that children who are sexually abused who then become victimizers are making a powerful statement that their earlier victimization was not resolved" (p. 244).

The Trauma Model and Repetition Compulsion

The trauma model asserts that traumatic events need to be processed in order for an individual to return to healthy functioning. Yet according to the DSM III-R, trauma is highly linked to dissociation, a psychological defense in which there is "an alteration in the normally integrative function of identity, memory or consciousness" (American Psychiatric Association, 1987). Dissociation allows for the compartmentalization of fragments of an experience, which can further complicate the processing of a traumatic event. Janet (1889) believed that traumatic memories persist through (fragmented) memories of the trauma that can return as "physical sensations, horrific images or nightmares, behavioral re-enactments, or a combination of these." Van der Kolk (1989) agrees and specifies that trauma is "repeated on behavioral, emotional, physiologic, and neuroendocronological levels." He explains that "compulsive repetition of the trauma usually is an unconscious process that, although it may provide a temporary sense of mastery or even pleasure, ultimately perpetuates chronic feelings of helplessness and a subjective sense of being bad, and out of control" (p. 402). These feelings of being bad and out of control may be even stronger in children who are already susceptible to feeling bad, worthless, or unloved. Many young children with out-of-control sexualized behavior have confided, "I want to stop, but my brain thinks about it all the time and makes me do it."

A traumatized child keeps revisiting the traumatic event, focusing energy, and developing a kind of fixation. The traumatic event(s) have overwhelmed the child's psyche, and feelings of helplessness, terror, anxiety, and vulnerability persist. When the child "plays it out" or "acts it out," there may be an attempt at mastery or a more full integration of the trauma experience. The child goes from a passive to an active role (helpless victim to dominant perpetrator), and a temporary or permanent relief may ensue. Post-traumatic play or behavior may also be fueled by a desire to resolve the uncomfortable or problematic aspects of the trauma memory by achieving a gradual discharge of small and controlled affects. It is also clear that when the child reenacts through play or behavior, the child challenges his terror and pain by approaching the trauma memory while feeling safety and control (achieving partial or full mastery over time). In discussing adolescent sex offenders, Breer (1987) describes sexually aggressive behavior as an attempt to recreate past trauma in ways that lead to developing mastery and control over feelings.

Freud (1954) theorized that repetition gains mastery, but Van der Kolk insists that "Clinical experience has shown that this rarely happens, instead, repetition causes further suffering for the victim or for people in their surroundings" (p. 390). I agree that one motivation to abuse may be to master unresolved traumas, yet mastery can be elusive at best, and elicit more feelings of helplessness, coupled with guilt and shame.

Trauma Outcome Process

Rasmussen and co-workers (1992) believe that sexually victimized children have three possible responses to their trauma: (1) they can express and work through feelings associated with trauma to the point of acceptance (recovery), (2) they can develop self-destructive behaviors (self-victimization), and (3) they can identify with their aggressor and display assaultive behavior against others (assault). These potential responses to trauma overlap with the child's level of awareness. The crux of this theoretical framework is that once feelings reminiscent of a trauma arise, children make choices (conscious at some level and influenced by emotional factors) about how they respond. This trauma outcome process takes into consideration the children's "prior traumatization, lack of intimacy, impulsiveness, and lack of accountability," as precursors to their sexual offending. Rasmussen and co-workers also apply Finkelhor's four factor model to the development of sexually molesting behaviors in children (Finkelhor's four factor model discusses factors related to motivation to sexually abuse), and consider the applicability of this model when discussing sexually abusive young children.

Compensatory Exertion of Power and Control

Lane (1991) has found that adolescent offenders who begin their sexually abusive behaviors during preadolescence "exhibit coping styles that are characterized by power- or control-seeking dynamics that are already habituated and ingrained" (p. 316). Based on her experience with preadolescent children who molest, she has found that they exhibit a "compensatory response style" (for prior victimization) and "irresponsible use of power"(p. 301).

The "Adaptation" Perspective

Friedrich (1988) notes that sexual acting-out behavior in abused children can be viewed from an "adaptational perspective," stating that many "moderator variables" affect sexually abused children over time, including the children's developmental age, the children's coping strategies, family relationships, multiple assessments, as well as the social networks and other support systems that influence the family (p. 188).

Expanding on these ideas, Friedrich (1990b) discusses his "coping theory," which emphasizes the active nature of the child's and family's adaptation to this trauma. Clinicians are advised to assess the children's and family's functioning before the abuse; the nature of the trauma; and the initial response by child and family. He says that the degree to which long-term reactions occur is presumably dependent on all preceding events. Friedrich believes that instead of the coping theory diminishing the very real and negative sequelae of sexual abuse, it says something about the triumph of the human spirit and the healing potential of families.

In discussing sexually abusive and aggressive children, Friedrich (1990a) states that "The younger the child [engaging in sexual acting-out behaviors], the more likely the child has been sexually abused" (p. 249). He says that paired-associated learning is relevant to these children, in that a "behavior is more likely to be repeated if it is paired with an affective response that is pleasurable" (p. 251). Friedrich agrees that focusing on the abused child's victimization becomes an integral aspect of therapy.

Although many theories have been postulated, few have been systematically tested. At this point, it is best to have many theories to draw from and avoid using any one theory as exclusive.

In addition, most theories fail to discriminate between the motives that precipitate the behavior and the motives that sustain it. The actual experience elicits a range of internal and external responses that shape, modulate, and enhance the initial behavior.

Other Contributing Factors

In her study of thirteen "female perpetrators," Johnson (1989) considered the question of why her sample (who had all been sexually abused themselves) molested other children. This question was of particular interest because research indicates that young girls have a tendency to identify more with the role of victim, and young boys with the role of aggressor (Carmen et al., 1984; Jaffe et al., 1986). Johnson found that her sample had a "sexualization of personal and interpersonal experiences" as a result of their own abuse. The abuse they had endured was severe, chronic, and frequent; it involved individuals with whom they had a close relationship, and there was little support for them when they disclosed. In addition, family structures were unstable and the mothers had highly dependent personalities with histories of abuse. None of the children had a stable, nurturing mother or father, nor were they shielded from parental sexual activity. At the same time, parents lacked clarity about sexual issues or did not discuss the matter at all.

Johnson states that these childrens' sexual arousal differs from adult sexuality in that their arousal "was perceived by them as feelings of anxiety and confusion. Very few, if any, of the girls were looking for sexual satisfaction when they acted in a sexual way with another child. The girls were generally not looking for orgasm or sexual pleasure." Johnson says that "For the most part, the girls were looking for a decrease in the feelings of anger, confusion, and anxiety." Berliner and Rawlings (1991) offer diagnostic criteria with three levels of child sexual behavior disturbances: Level I is "coercive sexual behavior," level II is "developmentally precocious sexual behaviors," and level III is "inappropriate sexual behaviors." In their level II children, Berliner and Rawlings found the opposite from Johnson in terms of sexual arousal—a group of young children who "appear to be engaging in sexual behaviors because they find them intrinsically rewarding or gratifying or because they are reinforced." They speculate that these children may be "in the incipient process of developing a deviant sexual arousal pattern with children as preferred sexual targets," and they also find that these children (for whom sexual gratification is the primary motivation) would "not be expected to be involved in other antisocial activities and would more often have internalizing behavior problems" (p. 4). (In Johnson's sample of female children who molest, they were all diagnosed with oppositional or conduct disorder, similar to Berliner and Rawlings' children who have "coercive sexual behavior.")

The issue of whether children who molest develop a long-standing "arousal pattern" needs to be carefully approached. The reality is that we know very little about children's sexual arousal. We are not always privy to the sexual behaviors of children; thus we cannot say much about how transient the behavior might be. In addition, children do not always have the cognitive or linguistic abilities to report on their developing sexuality, or may have developed shame or guilt about discussing sexual feelings. Although it is evident that children's sexual apparatuses function and respond to stimuli, it is not certain whether children have less, the same, or more sexual pleasure than adults, and what kind of motivation emerges from the experiencing of premature sexual overstimulation.

Johnson found that in her sample, twelve of the thirteen girls who were victimized by family members chose victims in their own families or extended families. In each case, the child who molested described the sibling-victim as the "favored child in the family," which led Johnson to question whether the girls were showing their rivalrous feelings to their siblings in their molestations. In Garland and Dougher's review of the research (1990), they note that Stoller suggests that "Sexually compulsive behavior is the erotic form of hate." Stoller states that in some cases the sexual acts "represent the recapitulation of actual trauma directed at an individual's sex or gender . . . the means by which an individual symbolically attempts to gain revenge for and mastery over a childhood sexual trauma. As a result of identification with the aggressor, the individual, through such activities, is capable of temporarily turning a passively endured childhood trauma into an actively controlled triumph" (pp. 491–492).

In considering other factors that might contribute to childhood victims becoming adult victimizers, Garland and Dougher (1990) list characteristics of the child (e.g., age, socialization experiences, preexisting emotional disturbance or psychiatric disorder, interpersonal skills, sense of gender identity, prior knowledge about sex); family dynamics (e.g., family dysfunction); the sexual activity itself (nature and content, duration, and frequency); interactional features (number of perpetrators, age disparity, sex of the offender); as well as "social visibility of the sexual interaction, circumstances under which sex terminated, child's behavior following termination of sex, consequences for involved adult-offender, and reactions of others to disclosure" (pp. 496–509).

Schwartz (1991) says that traumatized children "internalize the perfectionistic, rigid, demanding, critical, and conditional love of their parents . . . the result is that they are self-abusive and often similarly demanding and cruel with others" (p. 45). All of these variables may contribute to the reenactments of abuse by child-victims who molest. Certainly, further research into these variables is relevant in prevention and treatment efforts.

Summary

In clinical literature, a great deal of speculation exists about the fact that abuse begets abuse—that is, that children who are sexual abuse victims will become victimizers. On closer examination, it becomes apparent that conclusions have been drawn either from retrospective data indicating that many adult sex offenders cite early sexual contact with adults or older children, or from a clinical sample of young sex offenders with a history of sexual abuse (Johnson, 1988, 1989). Garland and Dougher (1990) state that "A reasonable overall estimate of the percentage of adjudicated sex offenders of children and adolescents who report having experienced sexual contact with an adult during childhood or adolescence is approximately 30%" (p. 499). We do not know how many individuals who have this early sexual contact with adults or older children develop a pattern of repetitive behavior into adolescence or adulthood.

Learning theory postulates that children learn from observing significant adults in their lives, and that children can be taught through classical conditioning in which desired behaviors are reinforced and undesirable behaviors are punished or negatively reinforced. The fact that the ages of the children or adolescents with whom adult sex offenders become involved, and the types of sexual acts performed have been noted to correspond to their own previous childhood and adolescent sexual experiences with adults, advances the notion that learning occurs through observation and experience (Groth, 1979; Longo, 1986). It has also been noted by Garland and Dougher (1990) that "Male children and adolescents who have been sexually involved with an adult often recapitulate their sexual experiences, with the exception that they enact the role of the older individual." It appears that children can learn the victim-victimizer role simultaneously, as an interactive dyad, and may enact either role later. The role of the aggressor has inherent rewards, and many children prefer this role to the role of victim, with its resultant feelings of helplessness and fear.

Although the cognitive-behavioral theories of conditioning, reinforcement, and modeling have merit, intrapsychic issues may also contribute to our understanding of offending behavior in children who have experienced overt or covert sexual abuse. These psychological motivators include theories proposed by Finkelhor (traumatic sexualization); Yates (eroticized children); Friedrich (adaptational model); Terr and Gil (post-traumatic play); Janet, Van der Kolk, and others (the trauma model and repetition compulsion). In addition, the dynamics of families of children who molest suggest that issues such as family cohesion, parental nurturance, clarity of sexual matters, and appropriate sexual boundaries are necessary factors that contribute to the child's healthy sexual development.

It is tempting to generate a linear cause and effect for molesting behaviors in young children. It is clear, however, that to do so would be erroneous and premature since there is a paucity of empirical data about the nature of sexual offenses in this young population. At this point, we can submit a range of possible theoretical frameworks to aid in our understanding of the molesting behavior and to help us develop multilevel treatment responses.

References

Anthony, E. J., & Cohler, B. J. (1987). *The invulnerable child.* New York: Guilford.

American Psychiatric Association. (1987). *Diagnostic and statistical manual of mental disorders* (3rd ed. rev.). Washington, DC:Author.

Berliner, L., & Rawlings, L. (1991). A treatment manual: Children with sexual behavior problems. Unpublished. Seattle, WA: Harborview Sexual Assault Center.

Breer, W. (1987). *The adolescent molester.* Springfield, IL: Charles C. Thomas.

Burgess, A. W., Hartman, C. R., & McCormack, A. (1987). Abused to abuser: Antecedents of socially deviant behavior. *American Journal of Psychiatry* 144:1431–1436.

Carmen, E. H., Reiker, P. P., Mills, T. (1984). Victims of violence and psychiatric illness. *American Journal of Psychiatry* 141:378–379.

Cunningham, C., & MacFarlane, K. (1991). *When children molest children.* Orwell, VT: Safer Society.

Friedrich, W. N. (1988). Behavior problems in sexually abused children: An adaptational perspective. In G. E. Wyatt, & G. J. Powell (Eds.), *Lasting effects of child sexual abuse.* Beverly Hills, CA:Sage.

Friedrich, W. N. (1990a). Management of sexually reactive and aggressive behaviors. In W. N. Friedrich *Psychotherapy of sexually abused children and their families.* New York: W.W. Norton.

Friedrich, W. N. (1990b). Understanding the impact. In W. N. Friedrich, *Psychotherapy of sexually abused children and their families.* New York: W.W. Norton.

Friedrich, W. N. , & Luecke, W. J. (1988). Young school-age sexually aggressive children. *Professional Psychology: Research & Practice* 19:155–164.

Finkelhor, D., & Browne, A. (1986). Initial and long term effects: A conceptual framework. In D. Finkelhor and associates, *A sourcebook on child sexual abuse.* Newbury Park, CA: Sage.

Freud, S. (1954). Beyond the pleasure principle (1920). In J. Stracke (Trans. & Ed.), *Complete psychological works.* Standard ed., Vol. 3. London: Hogarth.

Garland, R. J., Dougher, M. J. (1990). The abused/abuser hypothesis of child sexual abuse: A critical review of theory and research. In J. Feierman (Ed.), *Pedophilia: Biosocial dimensions.* New York: Springer-Verlag.

Gil, E. (1991). *The healing power of play: Therapy with abused children.* New York: Guilford.

Groth, A. N. (1979). Sexual trauma in the life histories of rapists and child molesters. *Victimology* 4:10–16.

Jaffee, P., Wolfe, D., Wilson, S. K., et al. (1986). Family violence and child adjustment: A comparative analysis of girls' and boys' behavioral symptoms. *American Journal of Psychiatry* 143:74-77.

Janet, P. (1889). *L'Automatisme psychologique*. Paris: Alcan.

Johnson, T. (1988). Child perpetrators: Children who molest other children: Preliminary findings. *Child Abuse and Neglect* 12:219-229.

Johnson, T. (1989). Female child perpetrators: Children who molest other children. *Child Abuse and Neglect* 13:571-585.

Lane, S. (1991). Special offender populations. In G. D. Ryan & S. L. Lane (Eds.), *Juvenile sexual offending: Causes, consequences and correction*. Lexington, MA: Lexington.

Longo, R. F. (1986). Sexual learning and experience among adolescent sexual offenders. *International Journal of Offender Therapy and Comparative Criminology* 26:235-241.

Matsuda, B., & Rasmussen, L. A. (1990, November). Comprehensive plan for juvenile sex offenders: Preliminary report. Salt Lake City, UT: The Utah Governor's Council on Juvenile Sex Offenders.

Rasmussen, L. A., Burton, J. E., Christopherson, B. J. (1992). Precursors to offending and the trauma outcome process in sexually reactive children. *Journal of Child Sexual Abuse* 1(1): 33-48.

Schwartz, M. F. (1991). Victim to victimizer. *Professional Counselor* 43-46.

Terr, L. (1990). *Too scared to cry*. New York: Harper& Row.

Van der Kolk, B. (1989). The compulsion to repeat the trauma: Re-enactment, revictimization, and masochism. *Psychiatric Clinics of North America* 12(2): 389-411.

Yates, A. (1982). Children eroticized by incest. *American Journal of Psychiatry* 139:482-485.

Yates, A. (1987). Psychological damage associated with extreme eroticism in young children. *Psychiatric Annals* 17: 257-261.

5

Preliminary Findings

Toni Cavanagh Johnson, Ph.D.

Children who molest other children are variously referred to as children who molest, prepubescent offenders, abuse-reactive children, child perpetrators, sexually aggressive children, victim-perpetrators, sexually intrusive, and trauma reactive children. The variations in the names reflect conceptual differences in the understanding of these children, difficulty in categorization and diagnosis, as well as difficulty in consensus on how to refer to them.

Some do not like the term "perpetrator" used with such young children because it is stigmatizing. Others prefer focusing on the victimization the children have sustained, rather than focusing on their victimizing behavior. Some are reluctant to acknowledge the seriousness of the sexually offending behavior and therefore do not like to use terms describing that behavior. The confusion over labeling is further exacerbated by the fact that many professionals are still unclear about the exact group of children being referred to. Chapter three tries to clarify this problem by delineating four groups of children based on their sexual behavior. This chapter describes children who molest (group IV) by integrating information from three studies and my clinical experience with these children, their parents, and their families.

Data Sources

The first two articles describing children who molest other children were published almost simultaneously in separate journals in 1988. One article was entitled "Child Perpetrators—Children Who Molest Other Children: Preliminary Findings" (Johnson, 1988), and the other was entitled "Young School-Age Sexually Aggressive Children" (Friedrich & Luecke, 1988) (see Table 5-1). These first two articles were published by clinician-researchers who were unaware of the other's work, and yet they offer a startlingly similar picture. Separately, they defined a population of children whose sexual acting-out behavior was very serious and highly intertwined with aggressive behaviors. The authors found very similar sexual behaviors, histories, and parent and child characteristics. A third article was published in 1989, entitled "Female Child Perpetrators: Children Who Molest Other Children" (Johnson, 1989).

	Johnson Study 1	Friedrich Study 2	Johnson Study 3
Subjects	47 boys	14 boys 4 girls	13 girls
Ages	4–12	4–11	4–12
Race	44% Caucasian 28% Black 28% Hispanic		62% Caucasian 31% Black 7% Hispanic
Average age at intake	9.7 years old	7.3 years	7.5 years
IQ	Average to low average (no MR)	Range 70–139 Mean IQ 98	Average to low average (no MR)
Victimization history	50% sexually abused Pervasive harsh physical punishment	75% of boys 100% of girls were sexually abused	100% sexually abused Pervasive harsh physical punishment
Average age at first molestation	8.7 years old Range 4–12		6 years old Range 4–9
Average number of victims	2.1 Range 1–7	2 for boys 2 for girls	3.3 Range 1–15
Average age of victims	6.7 years old		5 years old
Average age difference between child who molests and victim	Boys and female siblings 4.5 years Boys and male siblings 3 years		Girls and siblings 4.2 years

Table 5-1   Description of Studies on Children Who Molest

The criteria used to include children in the Friedrich and Johnson studies were almost identical. Criteria included a pattern of sexually overt behavior in the child's history, an age differential of at least two years, and force or coercion used in order to obtain the participation of the other child in the sexual behavior. Although preliminary normative data on children's sexual behaviors has only recently been collected (Friedrich et al., 1992), both authors identified sexual behaviors that were more aggressive than the mutually exploratory sexual behaviors that are quite common between children. None of these studies use randomly selected subjects, and the children who are described represent referrals to mental health facilities in large cities in the western part of the United States. The studies do not claim to be representative of all children who molest. Interestingly, a description of sexually aggressive youth by the Department of Social and Health Services in Washington State shows those children to have very similar characteristics (English, 1992).

School Performance

The children had average to low average IQs. None of the children were mentally retarded, yet a large percentage had severe learning problems. Many were in special education classes at the time of evaluation. Although these classes were better able to meet the children's needs, extensive academic and behavioral problems were characteristic of their school performance. The children who were in regular classrooms were almost all experiencing extreme problems. Many children had attention deficit disorder, and many were hyperactive.

Peer Relations and Skills

Aggression, apart from the sexual problems, was also characteristic of most of these children. They had very poor peer relations, and very few, if any, had a best friend. Their relationship to other children was generally characterized by antagonism, fear, uncertainty, and continual disagreements. Social skills were few and these children had very limited ability to control their impulsiveness. Frustration tolerance was very poor. Problem-solving and positive coping skills were virtually nonexistent.

Evaluation using the Child Behavior Checklist (CBCL) (Achenbach, 1983), a paper and pencil inventory filled out by the child's caretaker, showed that their behaviors were more serious than the normative sample. T scores greater than 70 are considered clinically significant, and almost all of these children were above this cutoff on all scales. Scales on the Child Behavior Checklist for this age group include anxiety, depression, somatic complaints, hyperactivity, aggressiveness, and delinquency. Mean scores for children in study 2 were higher than the comparison group of sexually abused children on all scales. Sexually aggressive children as a group were above the cutoff for clinical significance on all scales except somatic complaints. On the sex problems index of the CBCL, which has a range of 1 to 12, Friedrich noted the girls had an average score of 6.8, the boys 5.9. His comparison group of sexually abused boys who had not molested had an average score of 1.3 (Friedrich & Luecke, 1988).

Sexual Preoccupation

Children in all three studies showed a high degree of sexual preoccupation. Friedrich (study 2) noted that on Draw-a-Person, Kinetic Family Drawings Test, the Rorschach, the Thematic Apperception Test, and the Robert's Apperception Test there was more reference to sexual themes or sexual content than is normally expected.

Children who molest more frequently draw genitalia on their human figure drawings than sexually abused children (study 2). The preoccupation of these children with sexuality is evidenced by their drawings, scribblings, and notes they wrote in school. Pictures of groups of people interconnected by their genitalia being inserted in different orifices of the others' bodies provide a graphic representation of sexual disturbance in these children.

On projective tests, these children see sexual content where others may not. For instance, Freidrich (study 2) noted that one child replied to card 4 on the Thematic Apperception Test, "They are going to kiss and go to bed and do sex." This card depicts a man and a woman standing together, with the man looking away as if to leave. On the Projective Storytelling Cards (Caruso, 1987), which pull strongly for sexual themes, the children see sexual and aggressive themes regularly.

The majority of these children did not report elaborate fantasies about sex, a few had frequent thoughts about consensual sexual behavior with same-aged peers or adults. Others fantasized about forced nonconsensual violent sex or physical aggression followed by sexual aggression. There were other children who had no conscious access to the sexual undercurrent of their thoughts, but were aware of the aggressive fantasies.

Diagnoses

Children in all three studies could be given a DSM III-R diagnosis. By far the most prevalent diagnoses were Conduct Disorder and Oppositional Disorder. Adjustment Disorder was less prevalent. In the Friedrich study, one girl was given a diagnosis of Dysthymia.

Although many of the children were depressed, few reached the level of Major Depression. Only one child had a thought disorder. Some children had suicidal thoughts, but this was not a persistent issue. Most of the aggressive feelings and destructive behaviors were directed outside the children.

Relationship to Adults

Most of these children had no satisfying relationships with persons of any age. In virtually all cases, a history of long-standing parent-child problems existed even before the child acted out.

The children's relationships to adults in the family and outside the family were generally stressed and fraught with conflict. Nurturance was clearly lacking in the relationship between the parents and children. Since most of the children lived in single-parent families headed by their mothers, this was the primary relationship from which to derive nurturance. Unfortunately, this was frequently not the case because the mother-child relationships were mainly characterized by highly ambivalent and strained feelings.

Friedrich (study 2) described only one of the mothers as having an emotionally supportive relationship to her child. Although some of the parents offered limited emotional support, this was generally not based on the needs of the child but on how the parent felt at the time. Generally no reliable method existed for the children to gain the approval of their parents.

These children were often the object of ridicule, scapegoating, or extreme blaming by their mothers. The majority of the mothers saw in their children characteristics of the children's fathers, who they hated, or other family members who they strongly disliked. These negative projections made it very difficult for the children to please their mothers or get positive support in any way. The mothers also projected their own negative feelings about themselves onto the children. In many cases, a history of maternal neglect was reported.

Victimization Experiences of the Children

The victimization experiences of the children included emotional, sexual, and physical abuse and neglect. In study 1, 50 percent of the boys were sexually abused, in study 2, 75 percent of the boys were sexually abused, and 100 percent of the girls had been sexually abused. In study 3, 100 percent of the girls were sexually abused.

Although there was little documentation of reported physical abuse, descriptions by children and their caretakers showed clear signs of severe and erratic physical punishment for the majority of the children.

Using a comparison sample of sexually abused children who had not molested, study 2 demonstrated that the sexual victimization of these children was more severe and protracted than the abuse in the comparison sample.

Most of the children, both boys and girls, were molested by family members, their fathers being the most prevalent offenders, yet few fathers were living in the homes when the children began their molesting behavior. Of the sixty children in studies 1 and 3, only one of the children was still living in the home with the offender when the sexually aggressive behavior was discovered and treatment began.

Eleven of the thirteen girls in study 3 were victimized by family members. When incest is defined as sexual relations between a parent and child, seven of the girls (54 percent) were victims of incest. In five of the cases, the perpetrator was the father; in one case, the perpetrators were both the mother and the father, in one case the perpetrator was the mother. Expanding the definition of incest to include the extended family, five other girls were molested by their uncle. Therefore, eleven of the girls (85 percent) were victims of incest. Twenty-three percent of these children were molested by females. The victimization of all of the girls, except one, occurred before they were five years old.

Sexual Behaviors

The sexual behaviors in which these children engaged included the full range of adult sexual behaviors. The sexually abusive behaviors noted in studies 1 and 3 were vaginal penetration with fingers, penis, and other objects; penetration of the anus with fingers, penis, and other objects; oral copulation; fondling; genital contact without penetration; exposing genitals; intercourse; and french kissing. The sexual behaviors of these children are comparable to those of adolescent and adult offenders. Significantly, Friedrich noted that the behaviors of the children he studied were more extreme than those seen in Fehrenbach and co-workers (1986) study of a large sample of adolescent sexual offenders. Twenty-three percent of the adolescents in Fehrenbach's study were involved in rape, whereas the majority of the behaviors of the young children in Friedrich's sample (study 2) could be classified as rape.

Data collected using the Child Sexual Behavior Checklist (see Appendix B) indicate that these children's lives are replete with sexual behaviors many of which are expected in all children but appear to be highly exaggerated in these children. (Although standardized norms for the Child Sexual Behavior Checklist are not currently available, it has been used with abused and nonabused populations. Children who molest show far higher numbers of sexual behaviors than nonabused children.) Examples are their pervasive interest in sexuality; the amount of physical contact they had with adults or children, for example, hugging or requesting hugs from adults and children or touching the breasts or genitals of adults or other children; frequency of masturbation; sexual or romantic talk; swearing; the imitation of adult sexuality using props such as stuffed animals, dolls, or toys; writing or drawing things related to sex and sexuality; and sexual contact with animals. Virtually all of the children had knowledge about sex and an interest in sex that the supervisory or parenting adults felt was beyond what was expected for children their age.

Many children who molest demonstrate a set of behaviors that at face value do not appear to be sexual in nature, but become sexualized due to the genital focus. The bathroom behaviors of these children were often highly charged. Some of the children refused, even after weeks, to change their underwear. They had frequent toileting accidents during the day or night, and some of the children urinated or defecated outside the toilet, with clear intent. Some of the children refused to clean themselves after toileting or used excessive amounts of paper with which they would trash the bathroom or make the toilet overflow. Voyeurism, sexual telephone calls, stealing of underwear, fetishism, and exhibitionism (outside the home) were less frequent than would be expected in an older sample.

Data on Molestation Behavior

Chart I shows that in studies 1 and 3, the average age at first perpetration by boys was 8.7 (range 4 to 12 years) and for the girls it was 6.7 (range 4 to 9 years). The average number of victims for the boys was 2 with a range of 1 to 7. For girls, the average number of victims was 3.3 (in study 2, the average number was 2), with a range of 1 to 15. The average age of the victims of the boys was 6.7, and for the girls it was 5. The girls had twice as many male victims as female victims. The average age difference between the girls who molested siblings and their sibling-victims was 4.2 years. The average age difference between the brother who molested and the sister-victim was 4.5 years. When the sexual behavior was between two brothers, the average age difference was 3 years.

Victim Selection

All of the children knew the children who they molested. The victims were all readily available to these children. In study 3, the first victim for ten of the thirteen girls was a relative. Of these ten victims, seven were siblings, three molested cousins. The three girls who did not initiate their molesting behavior in the family had no siblings and no contact with any relatives. Eight of these ten girls victimized only family members. All of the girls who were victims of incest chose victims in their own families, except the one girl who didn't have any siblings or cousins. This should alert officials that if girls molest extrafamilialy, there may be potential sibling-victims.

In the sample of forty-seven boys (study 1), 46 percent of the victims were siblings, 18 percent extended family members, 16 percent neighbors, 14 percent schoolmates, and 6 percent were other children in foster care. No clear relationship was shown between being an incest victim and molesting a sibling in this sample of boys.

Age of Sexual Aggression and Overt Victimization

An interesting aspect of the Johnson study of forty-seven boys was the relationship between sexual abuse of the children and sexually aggressive behavior. The children were divided into those who began to molest between four and six, those who began between the ages of seven and ten, and those who began between eleven and twelve. The data indicate that the children who began molesting at the younger ages were more likely to have been victims of sexual abuse. Seventy-two percent of the children who began molesting between four and six had documented histories of overt sexual abuse, whereas 42 percent of children seven to ten, and 35 percent of children eleven and twelve years old had documented histories of sexual abuse. The figures probably underestimate the number of children who had been overtly sexually abused because boys are reluctant to disclose sexual abuse. Also, some forms of sexual abuse by women are hard to pinpoint as abuse.

The molestation behavior by the children did not begin immediately after their victimization. In most of the children, a several year period occurred between the termination of the victimization and the onset of perpetration. As noted in Chapter three we need to distinguish between sexualized behavior and molestation behavior. Sexualized behaviors are more frequently noted in children currently being abused or soon after the abuse has ended. The intense anger, and its pairing with aggressiveness and anxiety, seen in children who molest, appears to take many years to develop and is generally not concurrent with the abuse.

Relative Age of Children who Molest and Victims

Although the criteria for inclusion in all three studies was that there be a two-year age difference between the child who molests and the victim, this was a poor premise. With older adolescent offenders, there is often a legal age difference criterion. In some locales, at least a 5 year age difference between two individuals must exist before it can be considered sexual abuse. The age difference criterion is not valid in and of itself for assessing children twelve years and younger (see Chapter two). Many children treated for molesting other children were the same age or significantly younger than their victims, some as many as four years younger.

Coercion

In studies 1 and 3, coercion was measured using four categories. Noncoercion was defined as instances in which the victims of the children who molested were so young that they did not know what was being done to them and therefore they did not need to influence the victim. Verbal coercion referred to children using bribes, threats, or otherwise verbally cajoling the victim. Physical coercion and excessive physical coercion referred to instances in which children used physical force to restrain the victim. An example of excessive physical force is the use of other children to restrain the victim. Relative to the sample size, girls used more force and physical coercion than boys in gaining compliance

Four girls who were cousins participated in the abuse of the brother of one of the girls. The male child was eighteen months old. They restrained him and orally copulated him. The abuse was so severe that he required medical attention. Each of the children had been previously forced to orally copulate their father or uncle.

Examples of the verbal coercion include seemingly mild or innocuous comments such as, "I won't play with you unless you let me suck your wiener." This type of statement is very meaningful to a young potential child victim who is friendless and has a history of parental abandonment and neglect. The following case example shows the quality and type of coercion used.

Jenny, age seven, was a highly sexualized and manipulative child whose thoughts and actions were pervaded by sexual themes. She masturbated frequently and openly, and often attempted to touch the genitals of adults and children around her. Her brother, Mark, with whom she had intercourse, was a passive, dependent, and frightened child who stated in the interview, "If I didn't do what she wanted, she would get mad at me. She would make faces at me, wouldn't talk to me, and would look so sad. I didn't want to do it [have intercourse] because I knew it was wrong and our parents would be mad. She would say, 'I won't be your friend.'" [Mark had been put up for adoption when he was three years old. His mother had openly stated that she did not want him. He was aware of this and also that his mother kept his brother. Upon entering group and family therapy, it was noted that Mark would not express any negative feelings about anything for fear he would not be liked or would be excluded by the adults or children.] Description of the acts between Jenny and Mark indicated that he had remained a passive partner while she stimulated and mounted him. Jenny said she had tried to stop because her brother didn't want to, but she couldn't. "I like his penis so much 'cause it's small and doesn't hurt like my dad's." She had been molested over a period of years by her biological father.

Unlike many adult pedophiles, the children did not slowly develop a caring, warm relationship with their victim and then take advantage of it. The vast majority of children who molest did not have conflict-free relationships with other children on which to build this type of relationship. Most children who molest take advantage of children who are more available, seem more vulnerable, and can be more easily forced, bribed or threatened into silence.

Differences Between Boys who Molest and Girls who Molest

Presently, it appears that a significant difference exists between the number of boys and girls who molest. Perhaps 15 to 20 percent of children who molest are girls.

One hundred percent of the girls were sexually victimized before molesting other children, whereas one-half to three-quarters of the boys had been sexually victimized. In the Johnson studies, sexual abuse sustained by girls was more intrusive, of longer duration, and on the average by a closer relative than that of the boys. The girls also had more abandonment experiences, deaths, and aggression in their homes. It appears that it may require a more severe history to push girls into the role of an abuser than boys.

During treatment, more girls seem to be ready to acknowledge their molesting behavior and their victimization than boys. Girls seemed to feel more guilt and shame and to experience greater psychic pain than boys, or at least it was more available for expression. Yet, for both boys and girls, empathy for the victim was mainly illusory, and fear of punishment was generally the most consistent reason for discontinuing the behavior.

The behavioral disturbances among girls were intense, but on the average, boys got in more trouble at school, where virtually all the boys experienced grave disciplinary problems. Although this was also true for most of the girls, a few did relatively well in school.

Girls expressed far less homophobic material than boys, yet all the children expressed strong negative feelings about homosexual encounters.

Same-sex sexual interactions were not uncommon among the children, yet neither boys nor girls appeared to relate their behavior to their homophobic discussions. When the children spoke of homophobia, it usually related to sexual behaviors between adults. As the boys got closer to eleven and twelve, there was heightened discussion of not engaging in sexual behavior with boys because it was "gross." Yet, particularly in the residential population, these discussions did not carry over into their daily activity as the boys engaged in sexual behaviors with boys subsequent to these discussions. It seemed they did not connect the behavior to homosexuality. When asked, they stated angrily, "I'm not gay." This appeared to be consistent with an impression that for some, the sexual behaviors had more to do with an expression of aggression than sexual expression. This was true for both genders.

A significant difference between boys and girls is the response of the criminal justice system. Not one girl was investigated by the police nor were there any police reports filed on the girls (Johnson, 1989). Although there were very few reports on the boys, police officers seem to view their sexual behavior as potentially dangerous and yet minimize the girl's sexual behavior. This was true, although one girl readily acknowledged to the police officer the aggressive sexual behavior, and a medical examination of her victim revealed positive medical findings (vaginal tears).

The difference in attitudes and perceptions regarding girls who molest also appears to affect child protective services. In sibling incest cases, it is rarely considered important to remove girls who molest. Boys are more often placed outside the home subsequent to abuse.

In several cases, girls appeared to be victims of younger, same-age, or teenage males, whereas after very careful evaluation, it became clear that the girl was encouraging the sexual contact. In several cases, this was part of the child's sexually aggressive dynamic. Because the interaction was between a girl and a boy, assumptions were immediately made about the boy being the instigator. It is more likely in our culture that when girls are engaged in sexual behaviors with males, suspicion falls on the males. This dynamic has not been evident with boys; however, it may also occur with them.

Characteristics of the Parents of Children who Molest

There was a preponderance of single-parent mothers in all three samples. Descriptions of the mothers indicate a propensity toward personality disorders and depression, with minimal evidence of psychotic processes. Many of the mothers suffered from Dependent Personality Disorder, Narcissistic Personality Disorder, or Borderline Personality Disorder. Many of the parents had a combination of these personality disorders, with varying intensity of each type. A substantial number of the parents were dysthymic at the time of the child's treatment. Some of the mothers had major depressive episodes. Virtually all of the mothers had some history of emotional and sexual abuse and had grown up in highly confused and disrupted environments.

The fathers of these children were mainly absent. Many of the fathers had been emotionally, sexually, and physically abused as children. Many had been involved in the criminal justice system. In some cases, the fathers were unknown because the mothers had multiple sexual contacts at the time of conception. Virtually no children had memories of a positive relationship to their father, and few children had any positive male role models.

A history of substance abuse was noted in the majority of the families. In twelve of the thirteen girls' families in study 3, one or more of the parents or grandparents of each child had been victims of physical abuse and/or sexual abuse.

Friedrich (study 2) obtained MMPIs from seven of the mothers of his sample. Anger was a predominant feature in each of the code types, as was family discord, impulsivity, impaired interpersonal relationships, and alienation.

Family and Home Environment

The vast majority of the children in all three studies lived with single-parent mothers. A very large number of divorces, relationships of convenience, and separations were noted in the parents of these children. Many of the mothers had a series of boyfriends who lived with them for a period of months or years. Sometimes these men drifted in and out of their lives and the lives of the children, were physically abusive to the mothers, and the children witnessed the abuse. Arguments over sex were likely to be the reason for the beatings, which were often accompanied by negative sexual comments. These beatings paired sex and aggression and were a part of the genesis of the sexually abusive behavior of these children.

Because of disruptions in the parents' lives, children were sometimes placed outside the home. In some cases, children lived with a relative for a while or were removed by protective services. Not infrequently, children who molested other children had multiple placements outside the home and subsequent replacements in the home. Sometimes when the child was replaced in the home, the parent was again unable to stay away from illegal substances, prostitution, or other illegal activities, and the child was again removed from the home. A subset of children who molest are in residential treatment facilities, group and foster homes, where they will remain until they are eighteen due to the parents' inability to care for them.

The families and homes of these children were generally very unstable. The emotional life of the family was chaotic. Relationships between family members were highly stressed and distrustful. Adults could not depend on the children to tell the truth, and the children could not depend on the parents to be consistently truthful. With some frequency, important things were kept secret from other members of the family. Some parents had other children of which the current children were not aware; in some cases, children were unaware of previous husbands of their mothers; incarcerations were kept secret, although the person had been living in the house at the time they were sentenced to jail. Parents made up stories about persons who disappeared, or children were told not to ask questions.

Child rearing was very rudimentary and generally based on an authoritarian model. Parents attempted to exert total control in an environment in which the parent was always correct and no questions were to be asked. Total obedience was expected. If there was not total obedience, parents had only physical punishment or negative statements about the child on which to rely. Virtually no parent of these children could draw more positive methods of child rearing from their own upbringing to change this pattern of relating to their children.

Some families had transient people living in their home. In some families, people coming to live in the home dislodged the children from their beds. During these periods, the children would have to fend for themselves, often ending up in the bed of siblings or on the floor.

Emotionally and Physically Intrusive Sexuality

Although the instances of reportable sexual abuse ranges between 50 and 75 percent in the two boy samples and 100 percent in the girls' study, there was also a pervasive quality in the families of very sexualized relationships. A covert sexualized atmosphere was found in virtually all the homes. The subtle and not so subtle sexualized relationship between adults and children was frequently the most salient force that sustained the children's sexualized and aggressive behavior. It was often difficult to determine whether the sexualized behavior in the home was reportable as sexual abuse. The lack of adequate sexual boundaries by many of the mothers would certainly have been considered abuse if done by males.

In many instances, it seemed that parents overstepped the boundaries of propriety because they were truly unclear about what was appropriate rather than being consciously abusive. Since the vast majority of the parents were themselves victims of sexual abuse and had experienced a similar lack of sexual boundaries in their own homes, it appeared they really did not know what was emotionally and physically intrusive. They were clear about the obvious forms of sexual abuse such as penetration, oral sex, and sodomy, yet they experienced more difficulty around more subtle issues.

Examples of this boundary issue around sexuality are varied. One mother slept unclothed with her three children. The children would say that her breasts would fall on them as she turned over. They described feeling uncomfortable in bed with her nude. Some parents entered the bathroom completely unannounced and lingered, under protest from the children, while children were bathing or toileting. Some parents entered the child's room without knocking or took the door off the child's room. Others were overly interested in the breast or penis development of their children and wanted to inspect the children's bodies. These types of behaviors would occur even after the parents had been in group therapy, where the rights of privacy had been discussed and examples given. Many of the parents continued to overstep the boundaries, and yet when confronted with their behavior, they responded as if they had just understood it for the first time. Protective services was kept apprised of the parent's participation in therapy and all risk factors.

Although highly questionable, it generally did not seem that parents were trying to be offensive to the children. Many parents had themselves been given no privacy as children and didn't understand. Parents used their children for confidantes, telling them intimate sexual details. One girl's mother regularly told her about her sexual interactions with her boyfriend including her frustration about his lovemaking style. It was not uncommon for the children to know about their mother's personal history of sex, conception, and contraception.

The information about the inappropriate behaviors by parents was readily revealed to therapists by the children. This appeared to be true because much of the sexually intrusive and inappropriate behaviors of the parents made the children very anxious, and they wanted it to stop. When working on the issue of privacy, both the parents' groups and children's groups were presented the same information. Interestingly, the children seemed to understand the information the first time they heard it. It often took three or four failures for the parents to understand (and then only intellectually) that these types of behavior were inappropriate. Curtailing this kind of emotionally and physically intrusive sexualized behavior was one of the most important aspects of the treatment process with the parents.

Sibling Incest

In study 1, 46 percent of the boys were involved in sibling incest. Analysis of the data reveals that in eleven of the cases the sexual behavior was between brother and sister; in twelve of the cases the sexual behavior was between two brothers. The average age difference between the brother who molests and the sister-victim was 4.5 years. When the sexual behavior was between two brothers, the average age difference was 3 years. (See Table 5-1)

Data from study 3 indicates that ten out of the eleven girls who were victims of incest, then committed incest themselves. The only girl who was a victim of incest and did not molest a sibling or cousin, had no siblings and she had never met any of her cousins. This should alert child welfare workers investigating incest cases to interview all family members to determine if the victim of adult-child incest may be sexually acting-out with a sibling. It is also possible that another sibling who was aware of the incest may be acting in a sexual manner with yet another sibling. The identified victim of adult-child incest is unlikely to come forward with this information. Because a great deal of disruption and unhappiness often occurs in the family when abuse is disclosed, sibling-victims are unlikely to disclose their victimization concurrently, particularly after seeing the results of the older child's disclosure of abuse. Since the disclosure by girls who molest of their own abuse was not received positively by the nonoffending parent, younger victims do not expect their disclosure to be any more favorably received.

In an unpublished analysis of thirteen cases (Johnson, 1990) of older brothers (twelve years and younger) who molested their younger siblings, the most common sexual behaviors were french kissing, fondling, vaginal intercourse, and oral sex. The mean age at the time of first molestation for the boys was nine years, seven months. The range of ages was seven to twelve. The average age difference between the brothers and their sibling-victims was five years. Seventy-nine percent of the victims were six and under. The average age of the victims was 4.5 years of age. None of the sibling victims had been previously victimized. In 39 percent of the cases, the abuse lasted for more than a year. Sixty-nine percent of the boys used verbal coercion, eight percent used physical force, 23 percent used no force or coercion as the victim was under two years. Generally, there was only a single victim for each of the boys. Sixty-nine percent of the children had only one sibling. Sixty-two percent of the boys molested sisters, 38 percent molested brothers; none molested both brothers and sisters. (Only two boys had both a brother and a sister.)

Three of the boys subsequently molested outside the family. During treatment, one boy was under the jurisdiction of the Dependency Court due to the molestation behavior. Two boys were on probation for the sexual behavior. Otherwise, there was no outside system support for the family.

Many commonalities were found in the families of these thirteen cases. All of the children had parents who were unsuccessful in their relationships to marital partners. The children's mothers had a series of adult male companions who were emotionally and physically abusive to them. Many had been sexually abusive as well. Substance abuse was frequent among the parents, and physically harsh management of the children was standard. The homes of these children had many people moving in and out. None of the children had ever been removed from their homes, and all had lived consistently with their mother from birth. The natural fathers had never been a significant part of any of the children's lives.

An outstanding characteristic of the mothers of sibling incest boys was their variable behavior and feelings toward their sons. Often the mothers were openly hostile to their sons when the attacks did not seem warranted. In many cases, it seemed that there was no way the boys could ever please them. The hostility toward their sons was in stark contrast to the mothers' appreciation of the sibling-victims. Whereas they would fawn over the younger siblings in front of the boys, the boys would get no encouragement or caring. The sons appeared to be the available objects of the mothers' intense hostility and fear of men. It sometimes appeared that the mothers would do to their sons what they could not do to the men who came in and out of their lives. Most of the mothers articulated their hatred of the boys' fathers, of whom their sons reminded them, and could acknowledge that their invective toward their sons was a displacement from their desire to retaliate against their fathers.

These mothers all had intense dependency needs. When they had no available adult male companions, they would frequently try to decrease their need for comfort, solace, and companionship by approaching their sons—a direct contrast to their general negative, hostile, distancing behaviors. This approach, although not overtly sexual, did emanate from the mothers' dependency needs, and given the confusion each of the mothers had around sexuality and boundaries, these occasions were highly confusing to their sons. The mothers might ask their sons to watch television with them or accompany them to the store or to the movies. The boys would console their mothers when they cried and felt lonely. They would become the men of the house and feel responsible for taking care of their mothers.

This relationship between the sons and their mothers would last until the mothers found adult male companionship again. The sons were then relegated to the outcast role and received the hostility; they lived in a never-ending struggle with intense jealousy, intense shame, intense need for love and understanding, helplessness and hopelessness, and intense confusion. Were they loved or hated? Were they the male companion-caretakers or the hated misfit superfluous boys? They never controlled their own fate. Whether they were needed or discarded depended on the men their mothers seemed to love more than them. And yet these men often beat their mothers, and the sons could not save them—they were always searching for a solution that was not within their reach. The terrible jealousy they felt toward the males with whom their mothers enjoyed themselves was compounded by the jealousy they felt toward their siblings, who were showered with love and praise by their mothers. If the men in the mothers' lives beat the boys, they could not rely on their mothers for consistent protection.

Each of the boys molested their siblings and had some awareness that it was their mother with whom they were angry. The anger was displaced onto the sibling because he or she was the favorite and had more consistent caring and attention from the mother. Because of the isolation of the family, the children were often playmates despite their ages. The sibling-victim frequently liked the sexually aggressive child and rarely wanted him removed from the home. This relationship was often very confusing for protective services. The boys all knew that by molesting their favored siblings, they could hurt (impact) their mothers. Whether the sons wanted to have sexual intercourse with their mothers, due to the highly confusing relationship they had to their mothers, and used the siblings as a substitute was unclear. The children generally had no conscious awareness of sexual desire for their mothers, but the relationships were fraught with extreme ambivalence and very strong emotions. The children were generally too young to pursue this line of inquiry with any diligence, but it remained a working hypothesis. Treatment of the mothers included intense work on the sexuality issues and their relationship to male companions, the sibling who molests and the sibling-victim.

A Very Preliminary Typology

Children who molest are a heterogeneous group. The following typology illustrates the diversity of boys who molest and the range in severity of their sexually-aggressive behavior. Although many of the etiological factors are similar, they show a wide variation in the way the problems are manifested. As researchers and clinicians continue to study children who molest, more will be discerned about them. At this time, a very preliminary grouping of these boys appears to have some clinical utility. This typology has not been empirically validated.

Although the categories described are not mutually exclusive, the groupings give the clinician some understanding of the dynamic issues that underlie the sexually aggressive behaviors of these children. Future study will modify and enhance these descriptions.

Incipient

These children have previously been in group II or group III (see Chapter three), but cross the boundary into coercive behaviors due to the internal conflicts and external stressors in their lives.

Subcategory 1

These children have previously been sexually reactive to their own sexual abuse or the sexually confused environment in which they lived (group II). A shift in the children's behavior occurs as they begin to seek sexual interactions with other children without consideration of the other child's rights or wishes. This shift may occur when the sexualized and/or aggressive aspects of the children's environment overwhelm their ability to cope and their needs for nurturance and stability cannot be met. Molestation behavior may be very infrequent as the fundamental drive toward sexual behavior relates more to anxiety and attachment needs rather than aggressive and destructive impulses.

Subcategory 2

These children who were involved in extensive mutually agreed upon sexual behaviors (group III) become more aggressive in their demands as they become more angry, resentful, and distrustful of the people in their environment and indifferent to punishment. A shift in their behavior occurs as they seek interactions with other children without consideration of the other child. They demand the other child's participation in specific sexual behaviors they want. These children may move between group III and group IV and therefore are hard to evaluate.

Conduct Disorder/Oppositional Disorder

These children molest other children that they know. They have witnessed a great deal of aggression between their caretakers. They have also lived in homes where there were very poor sexual boundaries. The parents of these children may be victims of child sexual and emotional abuse and are unclear about how to appropriately relate to their children. There are generally a succession of partners for the mothers of these children. Often physical aggression between the child's caretakers erupts without warning. The sexual and aggressive aspects of their lives have come together and been paired with one or more other strong feelings such as loneliness, fear, anger, loss, etc. Some of these children have been abandoned, and when the abandonment feelings arise they move to reduce the distressing feelings by acting in a sexual manner, often resulting in molestation. Although the sexual acting-out does not reduce the distressing feelings, it does interrupt the feeling. Most of these children say that any positive feelings are brief. Many feel worse, because they are aware they are not supposed to act in sexually aggressive ways. These children usually do not get along with adults, have severe problems at school, engage in lying, stealing, cheating, and property destruction. They are difficult to manage at home and do not get along with their peers. Many of these children have learning disabilities; all have learning problems. Virtually all of the children require special education services. Anger, anxiety, and confusion are pervasive feelings. They take little or no responsibility for their own actions.

Sibling Incest

These children often live in very chaotic home environments in which projections and distortions abound and scapegoating is endemic. Sexuality is a constant undercurrent in the home. The family has very diffuse boundaries regarding sexuality. Children who molest are often the recipient of highly charged negative projections from the mother. The mother's anger at the child's father, of whom the child generally reminds her, may be displaced onto the child. In sibling incest families, the victim-child is often the cherished child who can do no wrong. The mother may demand that the sexually aggressive child baby-sit or may blame the older child for things the younger child does. In some cases, there is blatant favoritism of the victim-child. The child's molestation of the younger child is often to retaliate against the mother for her lack of caring and love. Sexually aggressive children are aware, at least unconsciously, that they can impact the mother by hurting the child she favors. They generally feel totally incapable of impacting the mother directly. The relationship between mothers and the children who molest is highly enmeshed and ambivalent. Although the child is very angry at the mother, the child loves and needs the mother's love, attention, and caring. Due to the isolated nature of the children in these families, they often have a very positive bond to one another, as well as a very negative and jealous relationship. The sibling-victim often has very fond feelings for the sibling who molests, but wants the sexual aggressiveness to stop. This can happen in natural, step, and blended families. Sibling incest offenders may also molest outside the family.

Hopeless/Depressed/Angry

These children are generally in foster, group, or residential facilities or in the most emotionally vacant homes. Frequently, these children have been physically and/or emotionally abandoned, and emotionally, sexually, and physically abused. The children feel totally disconnected from family members. In fact, there may be no family members who care about them or visit them. They feel alone and isolated. Relationships to the children with whom the child lives are superficial. Relationships to the staff are equally as superficial. They have no attachment figures and feel this loss. These children may have been sexually abused in care or engaged in sexual activity with other children (group III) while in care, and now alternately befriend children and/or hurt them. They often have some status among their peers related to attractiveness, athletic ability, aggressiveness, or size. Other children are intimidated by these children; threats and physical coercion are used to keep the victims quiet. They may orchestrate other children to group together to hurt, molest, or intimidate another child.

Sexually Preoccupied Children

These children are preoccupied with sexual thoughts and fantasies. Although most children who molest do not have highly developed fantasies around sexual themes, these children do. Frequently, these children spontaneously begin to talk or act in sexual ways when the context does not warrant it. There is an erotic and sensual quality to the sexual behaviors of these children. They often describe receiving pleasure from the sexual interaction. Sexual arousal appears to be the reason for seeking the sexual behavior. If they were sexually abused by an adult or adolescent, they may not have perceived the sexual interactions as abusive; in fact, they may say they enjoyed it.

Sociopathic Children

These children have lived in very unstable environments from their earliest years. Their caretakers were unreliable, and frequent disruptions in the caretaking of the children occurred. Emotional abuse was chronic, with repeated episodes of either physical or sexual abuse or both. Some of these children appear to be socialized and may interact adequately with adults in authority and peers, but only in some settings, and at some times; their behavior can be so varied that adults in one setting can be puzzled how anyone would think the child is a problem. These children are highly manipulative and focused on their own needs. They have a very limited ability to see that others may have competing needs and almost no desire to help another, unless there is an immediate benefit to them. They have no empathy for their victims and little, if any, understanding of the concern of others about their molestation behaviors. They are very difficult to engage in the therapeutic process and have virtually no insight. Adults are usually seen as annoying and interfering unless they have something to offer the child. Right and wrong are defined entirely within the child's own framework.

Group-Related Sexual Molestation

These children are usually very aggressive and have very poor relationships with their parents. Most have been abused. They do not get along at home or at school and join together with other children to molest or physically intimidate or hurt other children. These children may act out alone as well as in groups. Some of these children seek membership in these groups to meet their intense affiliation needs because they generally have few social skills and no close friends. Group membership is not stable, and they may become a victim at another time. They do not trust adults and do not see adults as resources. Their parents have generally had multiple divorces, the family has lived many places, their father may be unknown or never lived with them. Some of the groups victimize much younger children, even infants. Physical coercion and force may be used. Threats are used to keep the victims quiet. Attacks occur on school grounds, in neighborhoods, and in the context of the family or extended family.

Violent Children Who Molest

These children have generally been severely physically abused and emotionally abandoned and battered from early childhood. They may also have been sexually abused. Generally, they have lived where there was explicit sex between adults, and perhaps children, to which they were privy and in which they may have been made to participate. Their early environment was filled with unpredictable and frightening aggression. The people who were supposed to protect them couldn't protect themselves, and these children were aware of this. These children are loathe to rely on anyone and feel highly vulnerable if they become emotionally needy or close to someone. These feelings quickly move to rage and a desire to strike out physically or sexually or both. The sexual behaviors these children engage in with other children are frequently violent and accompanied by verbal abuse or physical aggression. These children may physically hurt the other children while being sexual and may try to intimidate adults with whom they interact. Blame for the incident is placed on the victim for causing the aggressive child to act. They often have very violent fantasies that include dismemberment of people they know or are in contact with at the time. Verbalizations about sexuality are vulgar. They may say vulgar things about other childrens' mothers and fathers. Sex and aggression are firmly paired in the child's mind. These children have a deep intense rage that motivates many of their actions.

Adult Focused

These children seek out sexual interactions with women, often touching women's breasts, legs, and buttocks for pleasure. Because of their age, they can nestle their heads on the breasts of women without arousing attention and be hugged at will. Frequently, these children feel convinced that adult women are attracted to them as sexual partners. Fantasies about adult women pervade their consciousness both when awake and asleep. Some of these children also ruminate on same-age girls. Sexual arousal often accompanies the fantasy.

Summary

Data from three studies were used to described children who molest. These data are preliminary and may not accurately describe these children as a wider data base becomes available. Characteristics of the children included: age, race, school performance, peer relations and skills, sexual preoccupation, diagnoses, victimization, sexual behaviors, molestation behaviors, victim selection, coercion, and differences between boys and girls. Characteristics of the parents and the home environment, as well as sibling incest were discussed, in addition to a very preliminary typology of children who molest.

References

Achenbach, T. M. (1983). *Manual for the child behavior checklist.* Burlington: University of Vermont.

Caruso, K. (1987). *Projective storytelling cards.* Redding, CA: Northwest Psychological.

English, D. (1992). *Sexually aggressive youth study.* Department of Social and Health Services, Washington State.

Fehrenbach, P., Smith, W., Monastersky, C., & Deisher, R. (1986). Adolescent sex offenders. *American Journal of Orthopsychiatry* 56:225-233.

Friedrich, W., & Luecke, W. (1988). Young school-age sexually aggressive children. *Professional Psychology Research and Practice* 19(2): 155-164.

Friedrich, W. N., Grambsch, P., Damon, L., Koverola, C., Wolfe, V., Hewitt, S. K., Lang, R. A., & Broughton, D. (1992). Child sexual behavior inventory: Normative and clinical comparisons. *Psychological Assessment* 4(3): 303-311.

Johnson, T. C. (1988). Child perpetrators—children who molest other children: Preliminary findings. *Child Abuse and Neglect* 12:219-229.

Johnson, T. C.(1989). Female child perpetrators: Children who molest other children. *Child Abuse and Neglect* 13(4): 571-585.

Johnson, T. C. (1990). Commonalities in sibling incest cases when the perpetrators are boys younger than thirteen. Unpublished manuscript.

6

Sexualized Children

Eliana Gil, Ph.D.

From infancy, children are sexual beings capable of experiencing erotic pleasure through random autostimulation. As described in Chapters two and three, age-appropriate sexual development in children is progressive and influenced by a host of factors including the family's social and sexual functioning, overt or covert sexual abuse, cultural and religious values, as well as nonfamilial socialization experiences.

In the past, the terms "seductive," "precocious," and "inappropriate" have been used to describe explicit or unusual sexual behaviors in young children, particularly those who have been sexually traumatized. We have chosen to use the term "sexualized" to contradict the misleading notion that young children (whether sexually abused or not) develop "seductive" behavior. Seduction is defined in Webster's Dictionary as "tending to seduce, or lead astray." Children lack the intent implied in seduction; sexually abused children have been conditioned to exhibit sexual behaviors and display these behaviors in an effort to stay safe, decrease their anxiety, or negotiate their affection or attention needs.

The term "sexualized children" refers to young children who appear to be overly focused and compulsively drawn toward sexual matters when most of their peers do not seem to exhibit similar interest. These children may be sexually preoccupied, interpreting most situations as sexually charged. Their childhood drawings or stories may be replete with sexual content; conversations include an abundance of sexual references, and interactions are directed at sexual exchanges. They disregard other normal childhood activities, and parental or caretaker limits do not succeed in decreasing the children's sexualized behaviors, interpersonal exchanges, and activities. Children appear consumed with one pressing and exclusive interest: sexuality. Sexualized children may engage in excessive masturbation, causing pain or irritability; they may masturbate in public and may want to touch or be touched in their genitals by other children and adults. These sexual behaviors occur frequently and persistently despite parental limits, distract children from other age-appropriate activities, and may or may not be accompanied by other types of disruptive or aggressive behaviors.

Parents and/or caretakers become alarmed and may use appropriate or inappropriate discipline to curb children's behaviors. As the behavior continues, escalating in intensity, the parents' alarm increases and they may bring the children to the attention of mental health professionals, clergy, or medical personnel, looking for reassurance and directives. However, childhood sexuality is not well understood, and many professionals simply apply their own subjective criteria when assessing these situations: they may think about their own children, or their own experiences when they were children, to judge the appropriateness of childhood sexual behaviors. Needless to say, this subjective criteria is not sufficient and can create subjective evaluations of children's sexual behaviors.

Parents and caretakers have been exposed to a great deal of information regarding the sexual abuse of children. Included in this public information are "indicators" of child sexual abuse, or certain behaviors that should cause an adult caretaker to respond. Behaviors such as generalized fear and anxiety, depression and withdrawal, violent outbursts, or sexualized behaviors are frequently seen as red flags indicating potential child victims of sexual abuse. However, this information is often misinterpreted. Although specific behaviors *may* indicate a potential child victim of sexual abuse, the behavior must be assessed in a larger context. Other family problems (e.g., divorce or parental death) may also cause a temporary increase in overt sexualized behavior; child sexual behaviors may also be occurring naturally and may indicate little else than children enjoying their own body. Many parents have called me in a panic, afraid that their children's "excessive" masturbating may be a red flag for sexual abuse. The first step is to get a behavioral description of "excessive" masturbating, and often the parent reports age-appropriate masturbatory behavior. Excessive masturbation may be occurring when children do little else but masturbate, in private and public, avoiding a range of other childhood activities. Excessive masturbation may also cause physical problems such as blistering, bleeding, or secondary bacterial infections in the bladder or urethra. If children persist in inserting objects in their rectum or vagina, with apparent disregard to pain and self-injury, a comprehensive assessment is warranted.

Some typical sexual behaviors that precipitate referrals or consultations from concerned parents or caretakers follow:

Masturbatory Behaviors

Parents and others continue to feel uncomfortable with children's open masturbation. Depending on the parents' own experiences with masturbation, or if they have chosen to provide the child with responses opposite to their own, they have differing ability or willingness to observe, allow, or intervene in their children's masturbatory behavior.

As emphasized in both Chapters one and two, children explore their own bodies and go from random to more specific self-stimulation. Adult caretakers greatly influence children's perceptions of masturbation, conveying their approval or disapproval. Many young children have been threatened with catastrophic outcomes if they continue to masturbate (your penis will fall off); others have been severely castigated for open masturbation. I have seen many youngsters whose fingers were held to oven tops and burned by outraged parents who viewed masturbation as a sin. In my adolescent sex-offender groups, I noted a persistent tendency to deny masturbating and to view masturbation as a homosexual activity.

Some parents and caretakers are more neutral or positive in their reactions, simply distracting children from open masturbation or giving them the message that touching their own body is their right and it's better to do so in private.

Other parents seem to have an unusual interest in their children's masturbatory behaviors and may demonstrate masturbation to orgasm, masturbate their children to orgasm (to show how it's done), demonstrate adult sexual intercourse or ejaculation, encourage and observe their children's sexual coitus, or provide children with vibrators so that children can enjoy the pleasures of sexuality "to their fullest." In these cases, the parents are providing their children with information that exceeds the children's questions about sexuality. They are imposing their own sexual interests on the children who are being prematurely overstimulated. The children's normal sexual development is interrupted by these intrusive and inappropriate parental behaviors and may result in the emergence of problematic sexualized behaviors. Polarities in parents' or caretakers' responses will certainly have an impact on the progressive evolution of a child's sexuality.

Sgroi and co-workers (1988) define excessive masturbation in the following way: ". . . a child older than three years of age who continues to masturbate in public even when redirected, scolded or punished by a caretaker or authority figure" (p. 12). Sgroi and her colleagues believe that since the (masturbatory) behavior is purposeful, it may meet the children's need to feel in control and diminish anxiety, particularly if children have been sexually abused. In addition, excessive masturbation may serve to protect children from the stress of interacting with others since the masturbatory behavior tends to be isolating.

Ryan (1990) encourages parents or caretakers to label children's sexualized behavior in an empathic and nonjudgmental way, fostering empathic thought and consideration of others. For example, if the sexual behavior is touching another child's genitals, the caretaker would state the discomfort experienced by the other child. If similar or the same behavior occurs again, the caretaker confronts and prohibits the child from the behavior. If the behavior remains constant, a monitoring phase is undertaken. Ryan comments that caretakers and parents frequently have difficulty with the labeling response because there is a tendency to prohibit the behavior without discussion. This example clearly differentiates age-appropriate sexual exploration (which might be transient and responsive to limits) from sexualized behavior (which remains unresponsive to limits and may require further monitoring or assessment of underlying issues or concerns).

Two other responses to sexualized behaviors are worth noting. Hewitt (1990), assisting a young sexualized child with excessive masturbation, told the child: *"You are in charge of your penis and it's yours to touch. But you must touch it only at the right times and in the right places. You can touch it when you're alone but not in school, because that's not the right place and teachers won't like it. You may not touch it in public because that's not the right place. You may touch it when you are alone, maybe in your room or in the tub. It's your body and that's fine"* (p. 242).

Responding to a child with aggressive sexual behaviors, she used a similar approach: *"You have only one penis and it's the only one you'll get and it's a very important thing to have. You are in charge of keeping your penis out of danger. This means you have to be careful where it goes. . ."* (p. 242).

Hewitt acknowledges that this technique puts the boys "in charge," and by valuing the part of the anatomy that was devalued, it restores power in an area that had been rendered powerless.

Friedrich (1990) is convinced that how the family reacts to the child's sexual behaviors determines whether or not the behavior becomes of greater concern. His response includes five parts, and parental cooperation is required. The five part plan, using masturbation as a modal example, includes (1) assessing parental attitudes and behavior related to masturbation; (2) positive shaping of child's nonmasturbatory time; (3) creating a time and a place for children to masturbate; (4) normalizing the masturbation; and (5) dealing with the children's prior victimization if it exists. Age-appropriate masturbation in children does not in and of itself suggest a history of sexual abuse. Victimization experiences must be explored when children engage in excessive masturbation as previously defined.

Ordinarily, the response to excessive masturbation includes helping children establish control over their own body, rechanneling their energy into developmentally appropriate activities, and helping the family explore their own attitudes and develop appropriate parental responses (Reaney, 1987).

Inserting Objects into Genital Openings

Children are naturally curious and fascinated by their orifices. Youngsters are constantly sticking fingers in their ears, nostrils, bellybutton, anal opening, and vagina. When they inadvertently hurt themselves (e.g., children sticking a sharp object in their ear), the behavior usually decreases or stops. When the behavior is neutral (picking noses) or positive (touching genitals), it may continue.

Parents or caretakers may call a therapist, concerned that children are focused on intrusive behaviors of this type. If young children insert objects into the rectum or vagina (all the time or even a lot of the time), oblivious to any pain or injury the inserting behaviors may cause, do not respond to limits, and appear to have anger or anxiety associated with the behavior, an assessment is probably necessary. Because the human body is susceptible to bacterial infections, children may suffer from a variety of medical problems as a result of inserting foreign objects or unclean fingers.

Friedrich and co-workers (1992) found that when he compared the sexual behaviors of nonabused children to abused children, one of the distinguishing variables in sexually abused children was their tendency to exhibit inserting behaviors. Although the nonsexually abused children displayed a range of sexual behaviors, insertion did not appear with great consistency. This finding suggests that persistent inserting behaviors in young children may indicate underlying psychological concerns.

Sexual Language

Some children are referred to therapists or protective service workers because they use excessive sexual language with peers or adult caretakers. These children persist in using "dirty words," which they know are vulgar and unacceptable in most settings. Such language can be alarming because the children are very young and probably don't know the meaning of the words. One seven-year-old child was shocking teachers with his vast sexual vocabulary; it was later discovered that he had regularly watched pornographic videotapes with his baby-sitter. Another ten-year-old child had been hiding under his parents' bed while they made love. He could quite accurately mimic the sounds his parents made during lovemaking and repeated some of the phrases they uttered to his peers at school.

These children are not in need of therapy; rather, they need appropriate limit-setting. As mentioned in Chapter two, the response of parents can exacerbate or decrease children's use of sexualized language. It is important for consulting clinicians to inquire where children might have heard the language and what parental attempts have been made to stop the behavior.

Nudity

Children go through periods of inhibition and disinhibition regarding their bodies. Comfort or discomfort with nudity will probably change as children mature, although sometimes children's early preferences about nudity are taken into adulthood (i.e., children who are shy about showing their bodies may become adults who are uncomfortable with physical exposure). Since adults have varying degrees of comfort with nudity, children's nudity may trigger a host of responses. Teachers may frown on children disrobing in the classroom or at recess. Parents may be chagrined by their children's apparent exhibitionism during family parties or dinners. Parents or other caretakers may wonder if they should worry about their children's preference for nudity and may call clinicians to get advice about what to do.

Clinicians must assess when the nudity became apparent, whether other factors were involved (e.g., a divorce, a sexualized environment, overt or covert abuse, availability of sexually explicit materials, the death of a parent), and what parental attitudes and behaviors exist about nudity One six-year-old always wanted to be "naked like mommy" at school. Her mother was a practicing nudist and was generally disrobed around the house. The parent had to help the child understand that not everyone felt as comfortable with nudity as she did.

Nudity in and of itself does not represent a problem unless the nudity seems to be occurring in a vacuum (no one in the child's immediate family is modeling nudity), and the child or his or her family seems anxious, frightened, or concerned. Obviously, if the child's behavior is disruptive in the school or daycare setting, this may precipitate a phone call or visit to a mental health professional.

Peer Sexual Play

Play is a universal activity for all children. Using their ability to fantasize, and use symbolism, children naturally seek play either alone, with adult caretakers, siblings, or friends.

Some children initiate play, whereas others follow. Some children create games easily; others must be taught to play. Some children's play is self-absorbed and intense; others seek out the company of others and exhibit spontaneity and joy.

Children can play with toys, or they can play with each other. Often they experiment with each other sexually, imitating behavior they have observed in their parents, or what they have seen on television. They may enjoy playing "mom and dad," imitating parental fights or parental affection. They may want to look at each other's genitals and may display touching and poking behaviors. There are limits to the sexual behaviors that children try without first having observed such behaviors. Young children who do not know that a penis enters a vagina, anus, or mouth during lovemaking probably won't attempt those behaviors.

As described in Chapters two and three, children are sexual beings and experiment with sexual play during their sexual development. Parents need to view this curiosity as expected and not assume any abnormality in children engaged in sexual play.

When parents call with concerns, clinicians are advised to get a description of the play, the frequency and duration of the play, other childhood activities, and parental responses to children's sexual play. Sexual play can become coercive, aggressive, and scary to other children. If this is the case, a clinician can evaluate the situation and recommend a course of action.

Some evaluations result in a recommendation for therapy either for the parents or the child. It may be that the child's normal sexual play is unacceptable and alarming to parents with sexual problems of their own. It is possible that parents are overreacting to the sexual behaviors they see in their children and need some education about age-appropriate childhood sexuality.

Summary

Children naturally engage in sexual behaviors as they mature. These sexual behaviors can include masturbation, inserting fingers or objects in the genital openings, sexual language, nudity, and sexual play with peers. All of these behaviors are developmentally appropriate and require attention from parents and caretakers only if they become excessive, compulsive, unresponsive to appropriate limits, or escalate in frequency and intensity so they distract the child from other age-appropriate activities. In the latter situations, the sexualized behavior may manifest a host of psychological or emotional problems, including possible sexual abuse.

Clinicians must neither over- nor underreact to these situations and must assess the family dynamics, precipitating factors, and parental responses to children's sexualized behavior. Parents who respond in a harsh and punitive manner may create anxiety and fear for children who have felt pleasure with self-stimulation. Judgmental and frightened parents may elicit shame in children engaged in age-appropriate sexual activity.

Children who have been sexually abused have had experiences that associate anxiety, force, physiologic arousal, confusion, and emotional and physical pain with sexuality. When children are sexually abused by their parents, they may feel a range of physical sensations including pleasure, numbing, or physical pain and discomfort, in addition to loyalty conflicts and confusion. These child-victims of sexual abuse or exploitation may develop a range of sexual behaviors that reflect the internal conflict or confusion they feel. Children who molest and children with sexual preoccupations or problematic sexual behaviors were often abused themselves. Children's sexualized behavior therefore must be carefully evaluated to distinguish age-appropriate curiosity and experimentation from the sexual concerns of children who are exposed to overt or covert sexual abuse by family members or others.

In many cases that come to the attention of clinicians and authorities, parents and caretakers are reacting to normal sexual behaviors of their children with fear and grave concern. In these situations, parents and caretakers need education and guidance in developing appropriate responses to their children's developing sexual activity.

References

Friedrich, W. N. (1990). *Psychotherapy of sexually abused children and their families*. New York: W.W. Norton.

Friedrich, W. N., Grambsch, P., Damon, L., Koverola, C., Wolfe, V., Hewitt, S. K., Lang, R. A., & Broughton, D. (1992). Child sexual behavior inventory: Normative and clinical findings. *Psychological Assessment* 4(3): 303–311.

Hewitt, S. (1990). The treatment of sexually abused preschool boys. In M. Hunter (Ed.), *The sexually abused male*. Lexington, MA: Lexington.

Reaney, S. (1987). Traumatic sexualization of the school age child: Implications & guidelines for treatment. Unpublished Manuscript, University of Minnesota.

Ryan, G. (1990). Sexual behavior in childhood. In J. McNamara & B. H. McNamara (Eds.), *Adoption and the sexually abused child*. Human Services Development Institute, University of Southern Maine.

Sgroi, S. M., Bunk, B. S., & Wabrek, C. J. (1988). Children's sexual behaviors and their relationship to sexual abuse. In S. M. Sgroi (Ed.), *Vulnerable populations: Evaluation and treatment of sexually abused children and adult survivors*. Lexington, MA: Lexington.

7

Family Dynamics

Eliana Gil, Ph.D.

When we assess children whose sexualized or molesting behaviors have brought them to the attention of concerned professionals, we must immediately address the family environments in which these children live. Extreme and persistent sexualized and molesting behaviors do not emerge in a vacuum.

As stated previously, children's sexual interest and activity occur along a continuum, and most young children develop gradual and progressive attention to sexual matters. It is also apparent that children's interest or preoccupation with sexuality can be influenced or shaped by life experiences including exposure to explicit or inappropriate sexual material, sexual abuse or trauma, behavioral conditioning, and premature exposure to situations that they cannot process.

Exposure to explicit or inappropriate sexual material includes allowing or encouraging children to look at pornographic pictures or watch X-rated videotapes. Some adults may force children to watch them commit sexual acts, apparently using the children's observation as an aphrodisiac.

Sexual abuse includes any situations in which children are being used for someone else's sexual gratification, ranging from hands-on abuse, such as fondling, oral sex, or intercourse, to exposure to disturbing sexual material. Sexual abuse can be traumatic to children since it is an overwhelming, out of the ordinary experience, and elicits feelings of helplessness and instinctual arousal. Traumatic experiences cannot be "taken in" fully by children, and yet may be experienced during a physiologically aroused state; they may become repressed or stored in fragmented ways. For example, a frightened four-year-old who is forced to observe or be part of sexual intercourse between two adults cannot fully understand what is happening. The child may comply and "go through the motions," while emotionally he leaves his body or pretends to be invisible. The child's memory of the event may not be intact, yet he may suddenly repeat phrases he heard during the experience, have intrusive flashbacks of the adults' faces, or manipulate his penis as he "remembers" the adults doing. He also may suddenly become terrified in the presence of a male adult, or may refuse to go to bed, remembering on some level what previously occurred in that bed. These are ways in which children reexperience fragmented aspects of trauma through behavior, sleep disturbances, or post-traumatic stress symptoms, such as intrusive flashbacks.

Behavioral conditioning occurs when children are systematically taught to act in sexual ways by being given material things such as gifts or money, or emotional rewards, or are being allowed to meet basic needs such as eating or sleeping, in exchange for sexual activity.

Children's knowledge or interest in sexuality also can be swayed by exposure to explicit situations that are overstimulating or traumatic and cannot be understood or integrated by children, for example, parents who purposely have sexual intercourse in front of a young child, or adults who force a child to watch auto-erotic behavior.

All these situations can spark children's interest in sexuality as they provide explicit visuals complete with affective complements. Children asked to watch adults having sex may listen to grunts and moans, or observe a range of facial expressions. Young children may become frightened about the safety of adults having sex or may infer they are fighting with or hurting each other. Expressions of sexual arousal can be interpreted as expressions of physical pain and discomfort. These observations (which are stored into memory) may become associated with fear, anxiety, confusion, or anger.

Children's problematic behavior can be viewed as a call for help; our job is to listen to what is not spoken and decode their behavior. Once we find the clues, the puzzle may be solved. Once the puzzle is solved, the work of intervention begins.

Family Dynamics

In discussing the dynamics of families in which sexual abuse occurs, either between a parent and child or between children in the family, I propose there are two primary family types: overt or covert. Families in which overt abuse occurs engage in detectable (albeit secretive) behaviors; families in which covert abuse occurs create a sexualized climate where inappropriate attitudes are communicated verbally or nonverbally. Survivors of abuse have described these experiences and their impact, and several recent books have highlighted the occurrence of covert forms of sexual abuse (Adams, 1991; Love, 1990). This important covert dynamic can remain undetected for longer periods; there is little behavior to observe, and children are less likely to reveal its existence.

I have often heard clinicians who are assessing children with sexually problematic behaviors say, "Well I don't find any evidence of sexual abuse—the child clearly states no one has touched him [or her] in a sexually inappropriate way." Many children who develop symptomatic behaviors may be living in family environments replete with covert forms of abuse. It is critical to consider these dynamics, particularly when evaluating young children with problematic sexual behaviors since it is clear that these excessive or unusual behaviors do not emerge in isolation from interactions with family members, social contacts, and the family's cultural and religious values.

Overt Abuse

In cases of physical and sexual abuse, family dynamics have more similarities than differences. Individuals in families that physically and sexually abuse tend to have low self-esteem, impulsivity, low frustration tolerance, an inability to identify or meet needs, a lack of problem-solving skills, affective and expressive problems, communication deficits, feelings of helplessness and futility, frequent and unresolved losses, and isolation (both among family members as well as from the community) (Alexander, 1985). In addition, Friedrich (1990b) finds that incestuous families have high levels of personal, social, and economic stress, substance abuse, and exaggeration of patriarchal norms. These issues are frequently found in physically abusive families. Sexually and physically abusive families tend to develop and sustain unrewarding or problematic adult relationships that may include periods of estrangement. Intimacy is often compromised; there may be periods of physical, verbal, or emotional abuse. Parenting skills are characterized by high levels of frustration, punitive or harsh child-rearing styles, or triangulation. (Triangulation refers to the process of involving a child in an adult relationship to meet some goal, whether it is diffusing an argument or realigning the asking and meeting of needs.)

In speaking of incestuous families, Gelinas (1988) notes "pervasive relational imbalances" which are ". . . pre-existing, long-standing relational patterns of unfairness, progressively converging and focusing on the child who becomes the primary victim" (p. 25). I believe this dynamic also exists in families in which the person with the least amount of power (usually a woman or child) becomes the victim of physical violence. Gelinas describes that incestuous families engage in parentification—the child is "induced to assume, and does assume, premature and excessive caretaking responsibilities in her family" (p. 26). This "role reversal" has long been identified to exist in the interactions between physically abusive or neglectful parents and their children.

In these families there is much pain. Often, all family members share feelings of distress: No one cares about them, no one listens, they are alone, and they are helpless to change anything. They experience isolation, despair, and futility. When families cannot change these patterns, symptoms emerge as red flags, pointing to problems beneath the surface.

In cases of domestic violence between adults or physical abuse of children, the symptom is obviously violence. For whatever reasons, (often histories of this behavior in their own families of origin), these families resort to hitting, biting, kicking, and other physical expression of anger. As Lenore Walker has described, a "cycle of violence" develops that organizes the family's functioning. The momentum of the family's functioning is a pattern of hitting and forgiving; sequences of pain and comforting are metaphors for underlying issues.

Sometimes alcohol and other drugs can serve as a catalyst for violence. An observer can be persuaded that alcohol or other drugs cause the problem, when in fact they only take away one's inhibitions, allowing one to act on impulses that reside just beneath the surface and do not emerge during sobriety.

Family members who make emotional contact with each other through violent interactions learn behaviors designed to perpetuate the symptom. For example, an adolescent who lives in a violent environment may provoke and redirect violence toward himself in order to protect his parent from an inevitable beating. Or a mother may learn to anticipate a physical eruption, and may instigate the attack, in order to advance to the stage of comforting. A mother who provokes is not a sadist asking to be hit, nor is an adolescent who offers himself as a substitute "asking for it." These are family members who have learned strategies that meet their immediate needs, unfortunately doing little to change the system.

In families in which incest occurs, the symptoms of pain or helplessness may be manifested as deviant sexual behavior. Aside from prior history of specific forms of abuse, it is difficult to account for the selection of one versus another symptom. An incestual parent, not unlike a physically abusive counterpart, is typically isolated, in pain, passive yet dependent, helpless, and frustrated. The incestuous parent is also often rigid, secretive, dominant, with diffuse boundaries and role confusion (Green, 1988). Pittman (1987) describes incestuous fathers as sexually inadequate, unconcerned with the appropriateness of their behavior, and viewing themselves as playing "doctor" with a peer. Pittman finds the (nonabusive) mothers in these families emotionally uninvested in their children, with feelings of worthlessness and inadequacy. Both Green and Pittman note that incest fathers usually have a family history of victimization. Freeman-Longo (1982) asserts that deviant arousal patterns often develop as a result of learned behavior and social interactions such as sexual victimization or sexual trauma. Parents need to overcome their feelings of helplessness and may turn to a relationship in which helplessness immediately turns to feelings of superiority. The parent-child relationship provides the inequality in status and the necessary dependency the individual craves, and it is in this relationship that self-esteem momentarily returns, feelings of dominance prevail, some sexual gratification occurs, and pain finds a respite. However, most incest parents find themselves consumed with guilt and increased self-loathing immediately after committing incest. Unfortunately and paradoxically, these feelings may then be assuaged only by repeating the incestuous crimes.

The other partner or parent in an incestuous family also has his or her degree of pain and isolation. There is always the question of whether the "nonabusive parent" has had full knowledge of the incest crime and whether that parent is equally responsible for the victimization of children in the home. The nonabusive parent is an important figure in the incestuous family. That person is vital to the prevention of future crimes and restoration of some level of family functioning.

I can recall several incest cases in which the mother literally turned over her child to an abusive incestuous father as a replacement. In these cases, mothers refuse to participate sexually with their spouses and offer up their daughters to provide the service. These children have no safe refuge; they have two abusers and suffer the ultimate harm of parental abandonment. More commonly, the nonabusive parents are not fully aware of the child's victimization and may be shocked to discover that the incest crime has occurred under her very nose.

To explain this to myself, I have thought of a scenario in which a person is the surprise guest at a birthday party, and it is only after opening the door, seeing his or her friends gathered around a birthday cake, that the information that has been stored suddenly takes on meaning. The surprised guest suddenly realizes, "That's why you asked me to come to this restaurant . . . that's why Mary called this morning to ask what I was doing tonight . . . that's why there was wrapping ribbon in the trash." In this example, relatively meaningless pieces of information have been stored in memory and become available with new meaning to explain the situation (knowledge) the individual now faces. Likewise, a mother horrified to learn that her child has been sexually abused may say to herself, "That's why she hasn't been eating lately . . . that's why she's been wanting to spend weekend nights away . . . that's why she suddenly hasn't wanted to sit on her dad's lap." Does the mother have full knowledge of the incest in her home? I don't think so. Does this issue have to be discussed? Definitely. In fact, one critical treatment issue is the mother's ability to observe and respond to each and every occurrence in the home in a new way. Before the discovery, the mother used some aspects of denial present in most parents. No parent wants to consider the possibility that his or her child is being sexually used by the other parent. No parent wants to consider children kissed goodbye as they get on the bus will never return. There are so many useful forms of denial that we all employ every day to leave our houses, get on airplanes, jog along rivers, etc. When denial interferes with child protection, it must be challanged.

If we are working with an incestuous or violent family, and the children are being maintained in the home, we must take a rigorous position to assure that denial is broken and the family begins to meet the needs and heal the pain that exists beneath the surface of the "symptom" that brought them to the attention of the authorities.

Covert Abuse

Covert abuse is challenging to detect and respond to because the symptoms of the family's underlying problems never manifest themselves behaviorally. In these families, something interferes with the acting out of any aggressive or sexually inappropriate impulses. There is a level of restraint on the behavioral level, although on other levels, problems persist.

In families in which violence is the primary vehicle, there is a threatening environment replete with innuendo about the inevitability of violence. Whips, cattle prods, or other intimidating objects may be in plain view, and the parents may refer to the objects frequently, stand next to them, or clean them in front of the children. One client I worked with was petrified of her father, who almost daily threatened to "kill her in her sleep," and then had her sit and watch as he cleaned his guns for hours. She was never physically hurt by him, but the aura of threat existed nonetheless.

In cases of covert incest, a climate is created in which incest between adults and children or between peers can occur. Moreover, the climate by its very nature conveys an incestuous message. One adult survivor described the following nonbehavioral incest family:

"My father never laid a finger on me. He would just watch and watch and watch, with his ugly stare. I knew what he was thinking. I knew where he was looking. He just always looked and made a gargly sound with his saliva.

"My mother was always in bed sick or she was in the hospital. I don't ever remember her taking care of me or touching me really. He always took care of me, fed me, dressed me, bathed me. When he bathed me, he sat on the tub watching me, and he asked me to make sure I cleaned myself. I couldn't get out of the tub until I had cleaned my vagina and anus with a washcloth. He was watching me take a bath until I was twelve; after that I just refused and he never forced me. He took the lock off the door so I couldn't lock myself in to bathe, and he bought a transparent shower curtain to replace our linen one. Probably every other time I showered I would open the curtain to find his eyes staring through the door.

"Sometimes I would wake up at night and find him sitting on my bed watching me, or I would come into the house and find him in my dresser drawers touching my underwear.

"Luckily for me, he never touched me or said anything weird to me. In fact, he hardly ever said anything at all to me.

"When I was sixteen, I ran away and lived with my cousin and aunt. I saw him rarely after that, and even after my mother died I didn't have much contact with him. Even to this day, I can't stand my husband looking at me, and I'm still really anxious and frightened about anybody seeing my body."

In this case, the young girl was spared behavioral incest, and yet incest dynamics were still very prevalent. As a result, she later exhibited long-term consequences typical of incest survivors including bulimia, sleeping disorders, sexual aversion, and feelings of low self-esteem. Sometimes she would chastise herself for thinking about her father doing anything wrong and state, "Sometimes I feel guilty for thinking there was something wrong . . . after all, he was a good father and provider, and definitely seemed to take care of me. Maybe I'm reading something into it that wasn't there. Maybe I am bad for thinking about those things." She also stated, "If he had touched me or something then I could feel sure there was something sexual going on. Sometimes I feel like I'm making the whole thing up."

In my experience, victims of this kind of incest struggle greatly with the issue of whether it really happened. (In fact, even victims of incest who remember numerous physical contacts with their perpetrators often struggle with credibility issues.)

In most cases of nonbehavioral incest, one parent seems aloof or altogether absent while the other seems intrusive. The intrusion can be either emotional or verbal. One ten-year-old child experiencing emotionally intrusive nonbehavioral incest remarked, "Sometimes I feel like he's trying to get inside my head, like he wants to have all my feelings and be inside me."

Verbal intrusions include remarks that seem to focus on sexual issues. For example, one father constantly quizzed his twelve-year-old daughter, "Did he try to touch your nipple?" "Did he like your short skirt?" and was always buying sexy underwear for her that he would ask about. "Are you wearing the bra that separates and lifts up?" When the child leaned over he would always come over and try to peek at what she was wearing. The child complained vigorously to her mother, who seemed to trivialize the father's interest. "Oh honey," the mother would say, "he just can't stand to see his little girl growing up."

Patterns of Covert Dysfunction

Although overt sexual abuse has been described in detail in the literature, covert abuse has not been discussed as extensively. The following categorizations are not all-inclusive or self-limiting, yet they are covert abuse patterns I have found repeatedly among families with whom I've worked over the years, particularly families in which sexual abuse occurs between adults and children or between children.

The Transmission Pattern

Stierlin (1973) discovered that in some families of runaway youth, one or both adult parents shared the youngster's desire to escape although they had not acted on this feeling. The parent's hidden desire was somehow being transmitted to the child, and the child was acting it out "for" the parent.

Madanes (1981) revealed similar findings in her work with suicidal adolescents: when interviewing concerned parents of adolescents who had attempted suicide, it was not uncommon to find severe depression and suicidality in the parents. The suicidality was transmitted from parent to child, and while the parent did not attempt suicide, the child did.

This interesting phenomenon lacks a formal name, yet it could be described as a process of transmission whereby the parents, consciously or unconsciously, relay desires or frustrations to their offspring. The youngsters in turn do not seem content to allow the feelings to lay dormant, and instead act them out on behalf of their parents.

Family therapists would interpret this behavior as the child's attempt to "shake up the system" or obtain help for a silently troubled family system. The child can then bring the family to the attention of a mental health professional, who can provide help for the "real" troubled person in the group.

In families in which there is covert incest, a couple of important variables exist. The incest parent is frustrated, helpless, and in pain, and has chosen a child to meet his or her needs to feel superior, in control, and comforted. Although he does not act on these impulses, he may be conveying his desires to another (second) child, who he triangulates to act on his behalf. The parent does not cross the boundaries of the parent-child relationship by committing the incest crime, but the parent elicits the participation of another child in the family to act it out on his behalf.

One family with whom I worked was referred for treatment when the thirteen-year-old boy raped his eleven-year-old sister. In the initial family session, I asked who in the family was most and least upset by what had happened. Although the mother was distraught and suicidal over the incident, the father minimized it and called it "understandable" for an adolescent to be curious about sex.

It was later uncovered that the father had been "setting up" the adolescent boy for over a year by making statements such as, "Your sister is hot!" "Look at the way she moves those buns!" "Check out this chick. First guy to get into her pants is gonna be one lucky guy." The father constantly nudged the boy to attend as his sister walked by, and whenever the boy had a girlfriend the father would compare her to the boy's sister and discourage the relationship. Finally, the boy attacked his sister.

To treat this boy in isolation from the family would be a terrible mistake. The father had successfully broadcasted his incestuous desires toward his daughter, and although he could feel self-righteous for not committing the crime, he was nonetheless responsible for eliciting his son's interest and participation.

I once observed this same process in a physically abusive family in which the mother had singled out one of her children, a four-year-old, for physical abuse. She was a highly dysfunctional parent who alternately rejected and punished her children without apparent cause. All the children longed for her approval, and they waited on her hand and foot out of both fear and feelings of deprivation. Because she had beaten one child years before, and he was consequently removed from her care, she would not hit any of her children. She was, however, verbally and emotionally abusive.

The four-year-old child was particularly frail and sickly. The mother felt overwhelmed by his needs since she was used to a family system that catered to her. She began making statements such as, "Someone should shut that kid up" and "I wish someone would come and save me from that child." Eventually, her twelve-year-old son beat the four-year-old severely when the little one would not stop crying. When the child was quieted, the twelve-year-old was in his mother's graces for a time.

In this case, the mother did not act out her violent impulses, yet she elicited a violent response from her older child by transmitting the expectation that a valuable reward would follow if he took the necessary action. Luckily for the four-year-old, a public health nurse visiting the sickly child arrived shortly after one of the beatings and found the child bleeding and dehydrated. The youngster was placed in foster care and was eventually adopted. The other children were left in the home because they were not considered to be at risk, and the family was required to come to treatment.

These cases illustrate the necessity of assessing family dynamics fully. Questions must be posed to uncover these often inconspicuous configurations of family functioning. (See Chapter twelve.)

Sexualized Families

Sexualized children were described in Chapter six as those who develop an unusual or extreme interest in sexual matters. Excessive focus on sexuality does not evolve in a vacuum; it emerges because of exposure to inappropriately explicit sexual information, some type of direct sexual experience, poor parental guidance or lack thereof. Martinson (1991) states that "Erotic interactions that are seductive, exploitive, coercive, or manipulative and serve to use the child's sexual development behavior to meet the parent's needs have negative ramifications" (p. 78). Patton (1991) agrees that sexuality (gender and erotic components) is a fundamental dimension of family experience that can contribute positively or negatively to the development and well-being of the family.

Sexualized families are those family systems that seem to have an inordinate preoccupation with sex: They use sexual language, make sexual innuendos and double entendres, sexualize their intimate contact, respect few if any boundaries, stimulate each other with sexual information, "take in" a great deal of sexual information such as videos and pornographic magazines, and generally have a heightened sense of sexual arousal from the environment. Finkelhor (1978) categorizes families as sex positive or negative and high and low sexualized, which influence attitudes about sexuality, eroticization of family relationships, and the family's respect or disregard for boundaries. Herman (1981) found two family types, incestuous and seductive, differing primarily in the overtness of the sexual behavior by the incestuous parent (usually the father). Boat (1990) discusses the family dimension of eroticism, in which families are erotophobic or erotophilic. Parents on the phobic end may respond with anxiety or harshness to a child's sexual behavior. Erotophilic families may perpetuate sexual behavior in the child due to their own level of sexualization.

Mrazek and Mrazek (1981) emphasize that sexual behavior does not emerge in isolation—the child's family reciprocally influences the sexuality of the child. They discuss the need for a "psychosexual equilibrium," which occurs as a result of parental sexual adjustment, the child's developing sexuality, parental sexual adjustment vis à vis the child's development, and the exchanges that occur as the child's sexual development activates the parent's memories of and feelings about their own sexual development.

In families that are highly sexualized, nudity takes on dimensions of exhibitionism and voyeurism. Parents' nudity tends to be consciously or unconsciously purposeful: the intent is to arouse the viewer and make parents feel sexually attractive, even powerful. Sexualized parents make statements such as, "You can look, but you can't touch—Eat your heart out!" or "Someday you'll find someone with a body like mine, and then you can have your way with her." Imagine the impact of these statements on prepubescent children just beginning to feel sexual responses. Parents are conditioning children's arousal to their body, and are also satisfying a sexual need of their own.

Sexualized parents often insist on bathing with their children and encourage them to rub or scrub their genitals until they show signs of erotic pleasure. Parents may linger over their children's genitals, delighting in the youngsters' physical signs of arousal. When children become aroused, parents encourage further exploration, whether or not the children want to self-stimulate or touch or caress the parent. As children mature, they may seek periods of privacy and desire bathing alone. Parents at this point may either pull rank, humiliate and ridicule the child's request for privacy, or allow the child to separate, focusing instead on another child.

Once I treated a family that was referred because the preschooler was humping every child in the classroom, and the humping behavior was unresponsive to the teacher's direct admonitions. I quickly discovered that the child had ridden "piggy back" on his daddy's back while the father made love to the mother. The parents were surprised that I would question them about this behavior, and proceeded to explain (but not excuse) the fact that they had both been raised in a very repressed sexual environment and wanted their little boy to think of sex as nothing more than a natural function, such as eating and sleeping. After several months in therapy, the parents were ashamed to reveal that they had both enjoyed the child's presence in their lovemaking, and both felt more stimulated by having the child observe. Although these parents had not set out to use the child in a sexual manner, they were guilt-ridden uncovering the truth. The child stopped humping other children in school once the parents made clear to him that it was not acceptable behavior, and they stopped sharing their lovemaking with him.

I have seen many families in which children anywhere from four to ten years of age ask questions about sexuality. These questions range anywhere from "Why do boys have penises?" to "How are babies made?" to "Where did I come from?" Sexualized families often take these age-appropriate questions as invitations to demonstrate. One father whose nine-year-old son asked about erections demonstrated masturbation to obtain an erection and proceeded until ejaculation. He then had his girlfriend "sit" on his erection so his son could observe why the penis gets hard. Despite the lack of hands-on sexual abuse, the young boy in this example was nonetheless sexually abused. The child became obsessed with getting his penis hard enough so it could go inside a girl's vagina. He was referred for treatment when he tried to penetrate his preschool-aged sister by having her sit on his lap.

One mother was asked by her four-year-old, "Where does pee-pee come from?" The mother showed the girl her vagina, pointed out the clitoris, masturbated, and allowed her child to watch the pelvic thrusting of her orgasm. The little girl became fascinated with her vagina and was referred for treatment when she would not stop masturbating in her classroom and wanted to see other adults' vaginas.

Such families as these invite and encourage children to exhibit interest in sexual matters. Children watch pornographic videotapes and magazines, often as a family activity. One single father subscribed to three pornographic magazines for his eight-year-old son. When they arrived, the father would sit with his child (as if he were one of his peers) and review the latest array of sexually explicit material while drinking ale. Ultimately, the eight-year-old boy orally copulated a six-year-old girl, covering her mouth with tape so her screams could not be heard. Although he was never overtly sexually abused by his father, he was overstimulated by sexually explicit scenes that often merged sex and violence; he was subtly encouraged to behave in the ways depicted in the magazines and videotapes. At the same time, he was never provided with any guidelines or limits concerning his sexual responses, thoughts, fantasies, or behaviors. The boy was conditioned to obtain sexual arousal through the use of force, with the understanding and acceptance that men regularly behave in violent sexual ways toward women.

Unfortunately, sexualized families create an environment that is highly charged with sexual tension, and maintain this level of titillation and excitement through word or deed. They often seem indignant when there is outside intervention, believing they are liberated and sophisticated.

The boy was most certainly a victim of covert sexual abuse. Case and point, the father of this boy was outraged that he was being held in any way responsible for his son's "perverted" behavior, stating that he "never had to force any girl into giving it to him." The eight-year-old was subsequently placed in a foster home in which he seemed to thrive with appropriate, nurturing attention.

Sociopathic Families

A sociopathic family is one in which there is a perpetual level of ongoing criminal and illicit activity. Adults in the family engage in petty theft, selling or trading drugs, substance abuse, joy riding, amateur pornography, pimping and prostitution, selling stolen goods, etc. No sense of morality or family values exists; family members are unemployed, drifting, and without legitimate sources of income. Some individuals may collect welfare checks—the phenomenon of women having children to collect Aid to Families with Dependent Children (AFDC) checks is sadly not uncommon. Their houses or apartments are replete with transient friends or relatives. The environment is frequently grubby and in obvious disarray. New people appear almost daily. There is a lot of "partying" with heavy drinking or use of other substances. People are always looking for a quick buck and a quick fix.

In the midst of this chaos, children are raised without proper health care, nutrition, or structure. There are few guidelines for eating or sleeping; children may go to sleep whenever and wherever they wish. They frequently sleep where they can find room or where they are placed; they may be moved from one room to another to make room for someone who drops in. They eat whatever they can find. They may witness violence or disinhibited sexual activity. It is also possible they will become targets of sexual victimization by passers by who "crash" for a period. Parents or caretakers may disappear for weeks at a time, leaving children to fend for themselves. Other times, these children may watch their parents or other adults pass out drunk, and may be forced to act as caretakers for sick or inebriated adults. Strangers in the house may share drugs or alcohol with the children, or may ask the older children to pick up or deliver drugs for them.

In these families, sexual abuse, both overt and covert, "just happens" along with everything else. There is negligible supervision of children, and parents or caretakers have little contact with the larger community in which they reside. Children may or may not be sent to school. It is when they do go to school that they come to the attention of concerned teachers, principals, or counselors who may refer the child to protective services when they observe signs of neglect or abuse. The younger the child, the more likely it is that intervention will occur. Older children are more often seen as capable of caring for themselves as compared with young children who may be in need of protective services.

Sometimes contact from social services agencies causes families to move to another town. On occasion, social services may have enough evidence of neglect or abuse to file dependency petitions in the court, making the children wards of the state. These children will probably be sent to foster homes, group homes, or residential treatment programs.

Children from these sociopathic families are severely neglected, psychologically abused, physically abused, and may have exposure to, or direct experience with, sexual activity beyond their developmental level. They are undersocialized, malnourished, intellectually understimulated, and more often than not, developmentally delayed. Given the preponderance of deprivation they have experienced, these children can have a wide range of physical and emotional difficulties and require an array of educational, medical, and mental health services.

Repressed Families

In repressed families, sex is a taboo subject. Sex is sinful, shameful, and something to be hidden. Parents admonish their children against the evils of sex and use religious teachings to expound on the punishment that is forthcoming to those who think about, much less engage in, sex.

Children don't have freedom to ask about their bodies, and any sporadic self-touching is forbidden. One four-year-old child was referred to treatment because his father placed his hands on a hot burner when he caught the child masturbating. The child was removed from the home due to "cruel and inhuman punishment" and became extremely depressed in his foster home. During treatment, the child revealed his belief that he would burn in hell for touching his penis, and viewed the foster care placement as appropriate punishment for his sin. His comments revealed a pseudo maturity deplete of spontaneity and playfulness one would expect from a child his age. During family reunification, some headway was made with the parents and their views of sexuality, but certainly not enough. They conceded that the burning was an excessive measure, but held firm in their belief that the child's exploration of his body was sinful and would not be encouraged or allowed.

In families with repressed sexuality, both sexual thoughts and feelings are unacceptable. Clearly, a conflict will surface at some point when children raise questions about sex or if they appear curious, spontaneous, or light-hearted about sexual matters.

An interesting paradox can occur: When the subject of sexuality is forbidden and even thoughts are sinful, it takes on a greater appeal and mystery. Children who are raised in this manner may become agitated about the subject. They may feel compelled to seek out information or find peers who can provide answers. This quest may lead children to pornographic magazines or videotapes and to friends who are more knowledgeable or experienced. Out of frustration or intense fear of being caught, they may end up in situations in which they take sex forcefully, or in a hidden manner, without mutuality or reciprocity. These children have had minimal opportunity to develop a natural progression of sexual interest and/or activity, and they may feel acute curiosity coupled with a total absence of balanced moral guidelines about sexuality.

One eight-year-old youngster from a repressed family developed a great deal of shame because his parents were preoccupied with his "dirty thoughts and feelings." The parents had a habit of describing to the boy a litany of sexual activities they considered sinful in the eyes of the Lord. The child asked to see a counselor because he stated that the "dirty images" were on his mind constantly, day and night. When he told this to his parents, they could not get him to a counselor fast enough, distraught that the devil might be trying to gain possession of the child.

In treatment, the boy depicted every sexual act imaginable using the dolls in the playroom. Adults woke up having sex, stayed home from work to have sex, had sex before and after eating meals, and woke through the night to have sex. The boy's affect was anxious during the play, and the play always ended with all the bodies being burned in a bonfire.

After a thorough assessment with the child and the family, it became clear that the parents had in essence elicited this extreme sexual interest from the child by providing him with graphic descriptions of all the sins he should not commit. The parents were responsive to my instruction to stop these illustrative depictions and instead begin a new daily ritual of playing with the child in an age-appropriate way of their choice. The child enjoyed playing various games with his parents, and as time passed his sexual interest decreased sharply. In addition, I asked the parents to explain that children would not burn in hell for simply thinking about making love when they were married. (Mentioning this to the child was a major concession for the parents; luckily their concern for their child overrode any hesitation they had about discussing adult [married] sexuality with their child.)

The combination of withdrawing the sexual stimulus, removing the threat of burning in hell for sexual thoughts, and having the family spend time together (i.e., allowing the child to feel a part of the family, rather than an outcast because of his "dirty mind") helped the child develop a more balanced interest in sexual issues.

In some cases, repressed parents with few sexual outlets or an inability to feel satisfied by sexual contact may feel vicarious pleasure from observing their child's sexual acting-out. Children can perceive their parents' tacit approval of their behavior and continue to act out despite the parents' verbal admonitions.

Emotionally Barren Families

In some families, the environment is one of emotional deprivation; physical affection and nurturing behaviors are nonexistent. Children are neglected by their parents and left physically (and emotionally) unattended for extended periods. The parents in these families may be drug dependent, emotionally immature, infantilized, or borderline mentally retarded. They are in great emotional pain and often have a childhood history of severe deprivation. The parents are simply unable to give what has not been given to them. This is a tragic situation in that the parents are incapacitated and lack comprehension of the parenting task at hand.

Parents may be so needy that a role reversal occurs in which parents turn to their children to get their needs met. Children in these environments make great efforts to meet the needs of their parents and frequently show remarkable tenacity and perseverance, making great strides to "take charge." These children may then turn to siblings for comfort and physical nurturing so vital to their development. De Jong (1989) found that the physical or emotional absence of one or both parents is suggested to play a significant role in intensifying the mutual dependency or sexual curiosity of brothers and sisters. In addition, loose boundaries promote incest relationships.

A ten-year-old boy was referred for treatment when his six-year-old sister told her teacher that she always slept with her brother, and her mother wasn't always home at night. The mother was an alcoholic who had turned to prostitution to support her expensive daily habit. The children had witnessed their mother having sex with strangers in the night, but they always preferred having her home with strangers than simply not coming home. During the day, she was passed out on the couch and didn't seem to revive until the ten-year-old got home from school and made her a hot meal. The boy frequently ran a bath for his mother, undressed her, and helped her to the tub. The boy also made sure his sister got a proper dinner and took her bath before bedtime. For all intents and purposes, he was the "man of the house," as his mother was fond of telling him.

The boy was also extremely lonely and unhappy. He felt helpless in the face of his mother's alcoholism and despaired at being the primary caretaker for his sister, who was also frequently depressed.

At night he was usually alone with his sister and would rock her to sleep. The children gave each other the warmth and comfort they longed for. Still, they had been exposed to explicit sexuality, and they engaged in exploration of each other's bodies. The young boy had started to get an erection while cuddling with his sister and had mounted her and humped her while she slept. The sister shared some of what happened at home with the teacher, and a report of child neglect was made to the authorities. Both children became extremely distraught when they were placed in separate foster homes, and after each had been in therapy for six months, they were placed in a foster home together. In the foster home, sexual contact between the children ceased, and as they began to get their needs met by an appropriate and consistent caretaker, they blossomed. The mother was unable to change her life-style as required by the court, and although she continued to visit her children, a reunification never occurred.

In these emotionally barren families, children suffer great pain from acts of omission rather than commission. As a result, they may be vulnerable to seeking out sexual contact as a natural extension of trying to get their intimacy needs met. Sibling incest is under-identified and should be considered a very serious problem (O'Brien, 1991).

Summary

In all the families described in this chapter, there is severe parental dysfunction. Family boundaries are either enmeshed or disengaged. Parents are either reacting to children as if they are mates or as if they are small adults, capable of self-care. Elements of amorality or aggression are modeled or imposed. Children do not receive the appropriate care, affection, education, limits, and guidance they need to successfully complete their developmental tasks.

Children in these families may be exposed to graphic sexual materials, observe disinhibited sexual contact, or become victims of sexual victimization or pornography. Family environments are chaotic, disorganized, and inadequate. There may be a variety of substitute caretakers, and children may awaken to new residents daily.

Overt or covert sexual abuse may occur as well as overt and covert violence. Obviously, children in these families suffer from psychological abuse and neglect as well.

Often the children benefit greatly from a temporary transfer to a stable and caring environment, with caretakers able to provide structure, limits, guidance, nurturing, and supervision. Professionals must assess and treat the family to achieve reunification when and if possible and if in the best interests of the child.

Sexualized and molesting behaviors in children do not occur without cause and cannot be treated in isolation from the larger family system. As shown by the descriptions in this chapter, the sexualized and molesting behaviors of children are more often than not elicited by overt or covert abuse. In these cases, parents must alter their inappropriate behaviors if children are to be helped.

The following chapters discuss the salient therapeutic issues in individual, family, and group therapy. If family reunification is to occur, successful family treatment is vital.

References

Adams, K. M. (1991). *Silently seduced: When parents make their children partners.* Deerfield Beach, FL: Health Communications.

Alexander, P. C. (1985). A systems theory conceptualization of incest. *Family Process* 24:79–88.

Boat, B. (1990). Personal communication to Dr. William Friedrich, cited in Friedrich, W. N. *Psychotherapy of sexually abused children and their families.* New York: W. W. Norton.

De Jong, A. R. (1989). Sexual Interactions among siblings and cousins: Experimentation or exploitation? *Child Abuse and Neglect* 13:271–279.

Finkelhor, D. (1978). Psychological culture and family factors in incest and family sexual abuse. *Journal of Marriage and the Family* 4:41–49.

Freeman-Longo, R. E. (1982). Sexual learning and experience among adolescent sexual offenders. *International Journal of Offender Therapy and Comparative Criminology* 26(2): 235–241.

Friedrich, W. N. (1990a). Management of sexually reactive and aggressive behaviors. In W. N. Friedrich, *Psychotherapy of sexually abused children and their families.* New York: W. W. Norton.

Friedrich, W. N. (1990b). Understanding and treating the family. In W. N. Friedrich, *Psychotherapy of sexually abused children and their families.* New York: W. W. Norton.

Gelinas, D. (1988). Family therapy: Characteristic family constellation and basic therapeutic stance. In S. M. Sgroi (Ed.), *Vulnerable populations, Volume 2, Evaluation and treatment of sexually abused children and adult survivors.* Lexington, MA: Lexington.

Green, A. (1988). Overview of the literature on child sexual abuse. In D. H. Schetky & A. H. Green (Eds.), *Child sexual abuse: A handbook for health care and legal professionals.* New York: Brunner/Mazel.

Herman, J. L. (1981). *Father-daughter incest.* Cambridge, MA: Harvard University Press.

Love, P. (1990). *The emotional incest syndrome: What to do when a parent's love rules your life.* New York: Bantam.

Madanes, C. (1981). *Strategic family therapy.* San Francisco: Jossey-Bass.

Martinson, F. (1991). Normal sexual development in infancy and early childhood. In G. D. Ryan and S. L. Lane (Eds.), *Juvenile sexual offending: Causes, consequences and correction.* Lexington, MA: Lexington.

Mrazek, D. A., & Mrazek, P. B. (1981). Psychosexual development within the family. In P. B. Mrazek and C. H. Kempe (Eds.), *Sexually abused children and their families.* New York: Pergamon.

O'Brien, M. J. (1991). Taking sibling incest seriously. In M. Q. Patton (Ed.), *Family sexual abuse: Frontline research and evaluation*. Newbury Park, CA:Sage.

Patton, M. Q. (Ed.) (1991). *Family sexual abuse: Frontline research and evaluation*. Newbury Park, CA: Sage.

Pittman, F. S. (1987). *Turning points: Treating families in transition and crisis*. New York: W. W. Norton.

Stierlin, H. (1973). A family perspective on adolescent runaways. *Archives of General Psychiatry* 29:46-62.

8

Current and Proposed
Community Response

Eliana Gil, Ph.D. & Toni Cavanagh Johnson, Ph.D.

Current Response

Current responses to children who molest and sexualized children differ from state to state. A great deal of variation in identification, prevalence, and response to this problem exists, as illustrated in the following examples, taken from different states:

Mario

Mario, a nine-year-old boy, was referred to child protective services by a concerned neighbor and mother of five-year-old Wilma. The mother had entered the room to find Mario astride her daughter. Mario had little response to Wilma's mother entering the room and appeared oblivious that his behavior was in any way alarming or unusual. Wilma's mother called her pediatrician, who called child protective services to report an alleged child molestation situation. When child protective services called Mario's mother, she was surprised to learn that protective services had received a prior call about her son's sexual activity with another neighbor girl. This call had been investigated and found to be "normal sexual play between children." The child protective services worker told Mario's mother to keep him from playing alone with neighbor children since it sounded like Mario was "very sexually precocious." The mother provided supervision of her son and did not allow him to play with his friends. Wilma, on the other hand, did not understand or like her friends's sudden absence and kept asking for Mario, saying she wanted to "play house" with him again. When her mother asked what playing house meant, Wilma described that Mario got astride her, undressed her, and put his tongue in her vagina.

Wilma's mother was alarmed by this behavior and concerned for both her daughter and Mario. She called the protective services worker again to obtain advice and reassurance that there wasn't something else she should be doing for her daughter. The worker said that the mother should continue to prevent any unsupervised play between Wilma and Mario. Since the mother was willing and able to provide the supervision, the worker felt there was no current risk of abuse to Wilma. When the mother asked if there was something else she could do, the worker said the boy's behavior would "pass with time and appropriate supervision."

Wilma's mother continued to worry about her daughter and took her to therapy to assure herself that the sexual games had not been traumatic to her child. There was no intervention for Mario until the following year, when he attempted to sodomize a neighbor child whose mother interrupted when she heard her five-year-old screaming. Finally, the case was investigated and Mario's history of sexual acting-out was uncovered. Mario was referred for therapy.

Sammy

Sammy, an eight-year-old boy, had been trying to undress little girls in his church after services. Since his behavior was visible to many, someone made a report to the authorities after Sammy's mother denied that her child engaged in such behavior. Child protective services referred the call to the police since there was no identified victim and the child's actions occurred outside the home. The police handcuffed the child in his school yard and took him to the police station for interrogation. The child was released only after his mother reassured the authorities she would watch Sammy more closely. Police told Sammy that if he continued his "disruptive behavior" they might have to put him somewhere where he could not bother others. Sammy was taken to therapy six months later, when his mother found little girls' underwear in his room and he acknowledged that he liked to take off other childrens' underwear.

Gladys

Gladys, a ten-year-old girl, was sneaking looks at girls in adjacent bathroom stalls by bending down and putting her head under the separating walls. She asked numerous questions of her friends, including whether they stuck their fingers inside themselves, whether they let anyone "go down" on them, and whether they wanted to "touch teetees." This child rapidly became a nuisance to her friends, who talked to their teachers about the problem. The principal felt that Gladys's behavior could be indicative of a serious problem and called child protective services. The child protective services worker agreed that Gladys's behavior was unusual and made a referral to the police, who went to the school in street clothes and an unmarked car to interview Gladys. (In large jurisdictions it is customary for protective services to conduct investigations of familial abuse and police to investigate out-of-home abuse cases.) Gladys said she had learned the touching games from her mother's boyfriend, who was currently living in the home. Gladys described an array of sexual games she had learned from him. She was placed in an emergency foster home. An investigation revealed that her mother's boyfriend was a convicted sex offender.

The mother was initially annoyed with Gladys for bringing attention to herself and her family. Sensing her disapproval, Gladys recanted the allegations of sexual abuse by the boyfriend. The mother eventually agreed that her daughter's sexual games at school were "probably a little inappropriate," but immediately dismissed any possibility that her boyfriend had anything to do with Gladys's knowledge about sexual matters. In fact, Gladys's mother remarked that "Gladys just won't let up asking a whole lot of questions about sex—she's obsessed with it and watches soap operas as soon as she gets home from school. She probably learned all that stuff from the tube."

The police believed that Gladys had told them the truth initially and had recanted because of her mother's response. Although they could not charge the boyfriend with a crime, they felt that Gladys was at risk of abuse if she continued to live in the home. Gladys was placed in foster care and referred for treatment, along with her mother. The initial rift between them was mended when the mother's boyfriend was charged and convicted of molesting another child in the neighborhood.

Andy

Andy, an eight-year-old child, was nude, with erect penis, on top of his brother, Steve, six, who was also undressed, when their parents walked into the room. Andy became angry that the parents had entered the room, and Steve seemed frightened and had tears coming down his cheeks. When the parents asked Andy what was going on, he said "Nothing . . . we were just playing." When they asked Steve what was going on, Steve also said "just playing." The boys' father asked Steve if this had happened before, and Steve nodded yes. Steve would say nothing more, and Andy responded in a hostile and defensive manner.

When the parents discussed what they had seen, the father reminisced about his own sexual play with his brother but noted that they usually had fun when they played minor sex games. The father was concerned that Steve looked so scared and Andy so angry and defensive; the parents decided to call child protective services for consultation. After listening to the mother's description, the social worker determined that Andy and Steve were engaged in "mutual, consensual sexual exploration," which she deemed to be "perfectly normal" between siblings of approximate ages. The worker chose not to interview the children, and the parents were advised to provide them with separate rooms (which they already had) and have a talk with them to discourage them from sexual play since "they were the same sex."

The parents followed the worker's recommendation and told the children that they did not want them to be undressing together or rubbing their bodies together when they were nude. Both children agreed to stop doing so, and yet the parents were quite concerned with their younger child's overall compliance to his older brother.

They decided to bring the boys to therapy, concerned that there was a pattern developing in which Andy overpowered and controlled his younger brother. Because of the sexual issues that had surfaced, they sought out a therapist with experience working with children with problematic sexual behaviors. The therapist saw the children individually and during therapy sessions in the eighth or ninth month, Steve disclosed that Andy "stuck his pee-pee in my butt lots of times," and that he "didn't like it." Both Steve and Andy had initially denied that anything beyond undressing and rubbing their bodies together had ever occurred.

Andy had threatened to beat up his brother if he told anyone about the sexual abuse. Andy escalated his threats when they started therapy; as the months went by and Steve had not told his therapist about the sexual abuse, Andy stopped threatening him, confident that his brother was too afraid to tell.

The therapist reported the situation to child protective services, and a full investigation revealed that Andy had been sodomizing Steve for almost a year. A medical examination of Steve confirmed the suspicion. Andy was furious at his brother's disclosure and threatened to "kill him." Andy was referred to a residential treatment program, where he disclosed his own sexual abuse by a male adolescent cousin who baby-sat him when he was approximately six years of age.

As illustrated by these examples, the current system response is inconsistent at best and still in the developmental stages. The responses in these four cases point up the difficulties of responding to children with sexual behavior problems, particularly children who molest. There is still a tendency to label all children's sexual behaviors as sexual curiosity or sexual play. A typical response to these referrals is to increase parental supervision until the behavior subsides on its own. Many cases are never investigated because intake workers minimize the potential harm that a child may be able to exert. Often, intake workers and investigators are uncomfortable talking with children about sexuality and may allow linguistic problems to deter them from a detailed investigation. In Mario's case, Wilma was able to obtain a clear description of "playing house"; this opportunity to learn more could have been missed by someone who took the phrase "playing house" at face value.

The need for specialized treatment services for children with sexual behaviors is highlighted in Andy and Steve's case. A therapist inexperienced with sexual behaviors may not have seen the children alone, providing them with an opportunity to become familiar and trusting of the therapist; the therapist might have not focused on issues around sexuality that could have further delayed or prevented Steve's disclosure of this difficult material.

As mentioned previously, protective services usually investigate cases of intrafamilial child sexual abuse, and police investigate extrafamilial child sexual abuse allegations. At times, the police, accustomed to adolescents who molest, and the disparity in age between offender and victim and issues of consent required for molest charges, may assess young children with the same criteria. As discussed in Chapter two, children who molest may be the same age and yet be physically, developmentally, or emotionally unequal creating an opportunity for victimization. When police do not investigate, the child who molests does not receive needed services—these children often fall between the cracks.

In cases of sibling incest, protective service workers may be reluctant to label the children's sexual behaviors as "sexual abuse." Protective service workers may allow the parents to increase their supervision so that the children may remain safely in the home. However, sometimes the parents are not able or willing to make meaningful changes in their behavior so that the children remain safe. When there is a history of forced sibling incest, it is almost always safest to remove the child with sexually aggressive behaviors, possibly to a relative's home, until the treatment is under way.

Child protective services workers and police have been challenged by this type of referral, especially over the last few years, and recently they have been developing guidelines for assessment. Still, both agencies recognize the need for additional information and training in this area.

Current Community Responses

It is outside the scope of this book to verify and describe the individual responses of child protective services and police throughout the country. However, in preparation for this chapter, a number of child protective services workers and police officers were interviewed and asked to describe their responses and their perception of procedures when they receive referrals of children who molest or children with problematic sexualized behaviors.

Child Protective Services (CPS)

The protective services workers interviewed noted there has been a sharp increase in these cases in the last three to five years. The most typical cases involve sexually acting-out preschool children; sexually aggressive children in foster care; sibling incest; children who masturbate sometimes until they are raw; and children who have been molested or shown explicit pornographic material, who then act out what they've experienced or observed.

CPS workers reported that the average age for the referral of sexual behavior problems or children who molest is seven or eight, with ages ranging from three to twelve.

CPS workers stated that they try to go out on every case and interview the child-victim. They also interview children who molest since they also may have been victimized. They then consider the following:

1. The ongoing risk of continued abuse to the child-victim, and his or her emotional condition
2. The parent's ability/willingness to supervise the child
3. The type of sexual contact—is the sexual behavior a signal of previous or ongoing abuse or is the environment presenting the child with too much sexual stimulation?

If the investigation reveals a victimized child, the child usually is referred for (1) a medical examination, (2) psychotherapy, and (3) a petition for dependency (if the parent is unable or unwilling to protect the child).

Regarding the child who molests, CPS may (1) refer to the police; (2) in incest cases, require that the child is removed from the home if parents are unable or unwilling to protect the victim; and/or (3) refer for treatment. Children with problematic sexualized behaviors may also be referred for treatment.

Whether a case is "opened" or not, CPS workers encourage families to seek treatment of unusual behaviors in children. If the case is opened, the child-victim may be made a dependent of the court until the family is in a position to provide proper care and supervision of the child.

Police Response

The police officers interviewed said there has been a gradual and steady increase in the number of referrals involving children with problematic sexual behaviors and children who molest.

The most common type of referrals to police involves adolescents, although there appears to be an increase in younger children who are referred for alleged abuse as well. (This may be due to the fact that people are more likely to report adolescents who are abusive than they are to report younger sexually aggressive children.) Police officers said that the referrals include date rape, child molestation, and younger children initiating sexual behavior with other children.

Police reported that after referrals of adolescent offenders, the average age of children with sexual behavior problems was ten to twelve (higher than the average age seen by child protective services workers). When police determine an investigation is warranted, they do the following:

1. Talk to the child-victim and alleged child who molests

2. Refer the child for a physical exam when appropriate

3. Cross report to child protective services

4. Conduct a joint evaluation with child protective services whenever possible

5. Collect evidence for prosecution, when appropriate. There is infrequent prosecution of children under the age of twelve

When police investigate a case, they consider (1) the imminent risk to the child-victim and (2) the nature of the offense, including use of force, prior incidents, age discrepancy, and age-appropriateness of behavior. Most of the time, police make the following recommendations:

1. Psychotherapy

2. Probationary status (upon approval) for six months, with subsequent reevaluation

3. Out-of-home placement with extended family or friends

4. Residential treatment program for young sex offenders

5. Juvenile probation, juvenile citation, and reprimand

6. File charges (DA's office evaluate, and decide, whether to prosecute—unlikely with young children)

Summary of Investigation by CPS or Police

In an investigation, the primary goal is to gather sufficient information to evaluate a situation for evidence of a crime and need for child protection. The focus of the investigation is plain: child protective services is primarily concerned with whether a child needs protection; police are primarily concerned with whether a crime has been committed. The dilemma is that the crime may have been committed by a young child who is sexually aggressive as a result of prior emotional, sexual, or physical abuse or a host of family problems, not the least of which may be dysfunctional family patterns and child-rearing practices. Because of this complexity, child protective services and police officers attempt to provide services to the entire family, which can include abuse-specific psychotherapy for the child and family or referrals to specialized programs (alcohol and drug recovery programs).

The investigation in these cases is complicated since the alleged offender is a child. Investigators have long attested to the difficulty in communicating with alleged young child-victims and children who molest. For this reason, over the past five years training programs that take into account linguistic and developmental issues have been increasingly available to authorities.

Investigations naturally include interviews with parents or caretakers, school personnel, medical personnel or others involved in the care of both the child-victim and child who molests. Investigators find it particularly helpful to interview individuals who have ongoing contact with the child-victim or child who molests to establish any recent or unusual behavioral changes.

Child protective services personnel tend to receive referrals of in-home abuse with younger children. Police officers tend to receive referrals regarding older children who abuse children out of their own homes. Adolescents who commit sexual offenses are more likely to be referred for legal consequences such as probation, citations, or juvenile hall. In addition, when enough evidence exists (positive medical findings in the child-victim, and a child who is able to provide testimony in court), the district attorney may choose to prosecute the case.

Child protective services workers are primarily concerned with the child-victim and may or may not pursue the provision of services to children who molest. It is not unusual for the child-victims to receive services and children who molest to be neglected in terms of receiving referrals. Often, these children fall through the system cracks since they may not disclose. If there is no apparent victimization, the child's need for help may be over-looked.

Gender bias may exist in some authorities with regard to assessment of cases of sexually aggressive children. For example, both police and protective services workers may regard the sexually aggressive behavior of a boy as more serious than that of a girl. The bias may also extend to other professionals in positions of identifying and reporting suspected cases of abuse. There appears to be greater hesitation in reporting female offenders as compared with male offenders. In addition, most professionals tend to regard sexual acting-out of older children (thirteen and above) as more dangerous than the sexual acting-out of younger children. Some workers regard same-sex sexual acting-out as more perilous than opposite-sex sexual acting-out. All these biases can create problems in identifying, reporting, or providing services, and need to be acknowledged and carefully reviewed.

Referral Options

Child protective services and police have expressed frustration at the lack of resources for alleged children who molest. They complain that many mental health professionals prefer to take "victims," not "offenders," and clinicians often state they lack the expertise to treat children who have sexually molested another child.

To compound the problem, there remains a polarity among service providers: Victim specialists do not want referrals of children who molest; offender specialists frequently reroute victim referrals. Optimistically, there has been a recent trend toward viewing offender dynamics as related to prior victimization. This may increase the chances of clinical assessments of offenders exploring histories of victimization, as well as therapists addressing the potential to offend in their victim clients. This does not suggest a linear cause and effect; rather, it represents a clear understanding of the victim-victimizer dynamic and the need for resolution of traumatic childhood experiences.

Mental Health Referrals

Children who molest are referred for evaluation and treatment to mental health professionals in private or public agency settings. An increasing number of mental health providers have developed a specialization or interest in this population and have sought out additional education on the subject. Lane (1991) states that there are about thirty-five specialized treatment programs for sexually aggressive children across the country, and theoretical frameworks, treatment strategies, diagnostic tools, and unique props have been produced. (See Resources section.) Experience indicates that treatment providers need a firm grounding in victim and offender dynamics. Treatment for sexualized children who have been sexually abused can be addressed either in individual or group therapy. Special attention must be paid to the meaning of the sexualized behavior (e.g., reducing tension, coping with post-traumatic stress symptoms, feelings of helplessness, etc.). Treatment strategies are designed to both decrease the problematic sexual behavior and explore the underlying psychological concerns. The treatment offered to children who molest and their families must be focused on the sexually aggressive behaviors. (See Chapters ten, eleven, and twelve.)

Assessment

Mental health providers do routine diagnostic assessments to gain a comprehensive understanding of the child's symptomatic behaviors and underlying concerns. A rigorous family evaluation usually takes place, and a treatment recommendation is made after collecting data, conducting interviews, and observing the child's behavior during therapy sessions. (See Chapter nine.)

If the child's behavior seems high risk—that is, beyond the child's ability to control and the parent's ability to monitor or stop, a secured setting may be recommended. In some cases, family dynamics are so disturbed that professionals determine the child needs an outside temporary placement. In that case, out-of-home care alternatives are sought on a temporary basis. (See Chapter thirteen.)

School Involvement

School personnel frequently make referrals to authorities when they observe problematic behavior of children in the school setting. Because children attend school daily and engage in many interactions with peers, symptomatic behavior frequently surfaces in the school setting. Once school personnel report suspected abuse, they may receive only a modicum of information about the outcome of the investigation. However, in cases of children who molest or children who have developed problematic sexualized behaviors, it is critical for treatment specialists to be in touch with school personnel. Otherwise, the child may molest another child in the school setting, or expose children to explicit sexual behaviors or language. On occasion, a school policy may actually be counterproductive to the child's progress in therapy. For example, a young eight-year-old child had molested children in the privacy of the school bathroom and was now in a new school where her prior behavior was unknown. School policy dictated that children had to be accompanied to the bathroom by another child. In this particular case, allowing the child with molesting behaviors to go to the bathroom with another child was a high-risk situation. The child's therapist contacted the school with the parents' permission, and inquired about any problem behavior observed in the classroom. The teacher (who had noticed that the girl initiated aggressive wrestling) was advised to provide constant supervision and overlook the bathroom policy in this particular case. The teacher agreed that the child would be accompanied to the bathroom and called the therapist one week later to report that the child was no longer asking to be excused during class time. When the risk factor was controlled at school, the child began to make real progress in altering her impulsive sexual acting-out with other children.

Clinicians working with children who molest or act out are well advised to keep in contact with schools, where the problem behavior can be triggered. School personnel can also provide the best source of information about the child's progress, gauging academic performance, behavioral responses, and interactions with peers and adults.

Recommendations Regarding Community Response to Children Who Molest

The following recommendations are offered to establish a basic foundation for a coordinated community response:

Child Protective Services

1. Determine protective services policies for intake assessment of children who are referred with sexual behavior problems.
2. Develop a protocol for interviewing children who molest and children with sexual behavior problems.
3. Establish criteria for assessing cases of sexual activity between children under the age of twelve.
4. Define criteria for assessing risk factors in children who are molesting other children.
5. Determine protective services policies for providing services to children who molest in and out of their families.
6. Identify community resources providing services to child-victims.
7. Identify specialized community resources for children with sexual behavior problems, including children who molest.

8. Identify the settings providing diagnostic or treatment services to children who molest.

9. Use joint interviews with police whenever possible, avoiding multiple interviews.

10. Develop criteria for filing dependency petitions for children who molest, the criteria for removal, and a system for finding the most suitable out-of-home placement when necessary.

Legal Responses

1. Determine the laws that pertain to sexual offending behavior by children.

2. Develop and use an interview protocol for children who molest.

3. Establish a working relationship with probation departments regarding services to children who molest.

4. Establish joint interviews with child protective services workers whenever possible, avoiding multiple interviews.

5. Determine the circumstances under which prosecution or referral to probation or diversion program, and removal from home are appropriate or necessary for children who molest.

6. Identify the most effective way of using the authority of the legal system to mandate necessary treatment for children who molest and their families.

7. Identify community resources that specialize in the treatment of children who molest.

8. Identify the out-of-home care settings providing diagnostic or treatment services to children who molest.

School Personnel

1. Understand the duty to report suspected abuse by any person, including young children.

2. Establish criteria for differentiating between normal childhood sexual play and sexual behavior that can be considered abusive.

3. Cooperate with treatment specialists in providing a safe and appropriate school setting for children who molest. When necessary, school policies must be flexible to provide the additional monitoring these children may require for a period of time.

4. Identify and use community resources; maintain a list of therapeutic services available for children with sexual behavior problems.

A school-based treatment program called Teaching Acceptable Methods of Socialization (TEAMS) has been developed in Minneapolis. This privately funded program is administered through the Minneapolis Youth Division in collaboration with the Minneapolis public schools. The program trains elementary school teachers to handle sexual issues with children, identify sexual problems in young children that require mental health referrals, and decide which sexual problems need to be referred to protective services or the police. TEAMS employs a school psychologist who provides psychological assessments of referred children and school services as needed. TEAMS also provides group treatment of children with sexual behavior problems on the elementary school campuses. The program coordinates with protective services, probation, and police when indicated. This kind of creative program is exemplary and can serve as a model for a positive and preventive community response.

General Suggestions

The following suggestions may greatly enhance community response to this problem:

The availability of a person in every system (judges and court personnel, police, DA's office, probation, school, protective services) to be specially trained in sexual offenses by children and conduct multidisciplinary team assessments. These "in-house" specialists could provide ongoing consultation and training to their peers, review cases, and maintain a current community resource list. This multidisciplinary approach ensures that children do not fall between the cracks and receive the necessary response in a coordinated fashion.

The development of training programs, protocols, standards, and guidelines to be used with children twelve and under who molest other children. Included in these would be a definition of the problem, investigatory procedures, assessment tools to determine risk, evaluation and interagency coordination guidelines, treatment options, placement options, and guidelines for monitoring and supervising children. Although judiciary, law enforcement, social work and mental health professionals have different mandates, multidisciplinary training can promote enhanced working relationships and coordinated services using similar standards.

The clarification of the child abuse reporting law so professionals are cognizant of their mandate to report suspected abuse of a child by any person, regardless of the person's age. Physical and sexual abuse can occur by children against children. Like abuse between adults and children, peer abuses can occur within the family or outside of the family. School personnel and mental health professionals have noted some confusion about their reporting responsibilities when children are abusing. This matter needs to be clarified so children are protected when necessary, and so potential legal ramifications for failure to report are avoided.

After reports of children who have been victimized by other children are made to appropriate authorities, it is important to understand that problems emerge in the response system, since CPS is available to respond to the child-victim and not the child who molests. At the same time, children who molest may be manifesting their own victimization, and it is important that these children be assessed and offered services. Investigatory agencies must make sure that both the child-victim and the child who molests are referred for specialized treatment services. Coordinated responses by protective services and police are key to successful intervention.

The families of children who molest must be mandated into treatment. Professionals working with adolescent sex offenders have long recognized the need for the family's involvement in the treatment if the adolescent is to make the necessary progress. The family's involvement is even more relevant in cases of children who molest, since the family's cooperation is critical to eradicating the molesting behaviors in young children. Young children will not even be able to get themselves to therapy without a cooperative parent who brings them. But beyond that, the child's molesting behaviors did not occur in isolation from interactions and influences of the family. Families may have varying degrees of receptivity to attending therapy with their children, and their participation needs to be mandated by the courts.

Summary

Children with sexual behavior problems represent a new type of referral that seems to be increasing yearly. There is currently an inconsistent response regarding intake, investigation, and treatment.

The problems do not exist solely for those required to investigate; many professionals are uncertain about how to assess, when to report, and where to report these complex cases of children molesting other children.

Child protective services and police personnel make concerted efforts to respond to children who molest differentially. Most of the time, young children and their families are referred for counseling. Both child protective services and police consider risk of reoffending, children in need of protection, the severity of the sexual acting-out, and the family's willingness to acknowledge the problem and respond appropriately. After the investigation is complete, police and protective service workers may refer the children for treatment to individuals or agencies willing to treat a child's sexual acting-out or molesting behaviors; in some cases, the child's sexual behavior is age-appropriate and safe and requires no intervention other than parental education.

Police and child protective services workers frequently encounter mental health specialists who are available to provide services to child-victims but not to children who molest, even though they are often the same child.

The community response to children who molest or exhibit problematic sexual acting-out needs to be comprehensive, coordinated, nonjudgmental, and unbiased. Children's sexual behavior must not be viewed subjectively, but in the context of carefully thought-out criteria that established child sexuality along a continuum from developmentally appropriate to unsafe and abusive. If we are to learn more about the problem, a coordinated community response must exist so the cases are better identified and appropriate system responses can be implemented.

References

Lane, S. (1991). Special offender populations. In G. D. Ryan and S. L. Lane (Eds.), *Juvenile sexual offending: Causes, consequences, and corrections.* Lexington, MA: Lexington.

9

Clinical Evaluation

Toni Cavanagh Johnson, Ph.D.

When children are referred for treatment due to sexualized behavior, a thorough evaluation is essential to determine whether the children's sexual behaviors are within age-appropriate limits or whether they are symptomatic of problems that require intervention. The clinical evaluation also determines the treatment needs of the children and family (Friedrich, 1990).

The initial goal of the evaluation is for the clinician to determine whether children are engaged in sex play, are sexually reactive, are engaged in extensive mutual sexual behaviors, or are molesting other children (see Chapters two and three). Chapter one presents developmental lines along which to evaluate children's sexual development.

Children who have difficulties in the area of sexuality and sexual acting-out need to be evaluated by mental health professionals who specialize in child sexual abuse and have an understanding of child development and child sexuality. Although children may not have been sexually abused, sexual acting-out is frequently a symptom of sexual abuse and should be considered (Friedrich et al., 1988; Friedrich et al., 1992).

The procedures discussed in the following sections are suggestions that should be modified depending on the circumstances of the case, the ages of the children, the availability of the family members, the style of the clinicians, and the needs of the treatment program. These suggestions are specifically designed for the evaluation of problematic sexual behaviors and can be used in addition to a standard psychological and psychiatric evaluation.

Referral Sources

Referrals generally come from child protective services, police, teachers, daycare centers, neighbors, and concerned parents.

If children are at risk of abuse, initial attention is given to the need for reporting and engaging the services of child protective services and/or the police. Generally, a referral on young children engaging in sexually abusive behaviors is made to child protective services because the child is a potential victim of sexual abuse. In some locations, reports are made to the police because of the legal aspects of sexual molestation (see Chapter eight). If the community has a child abuse hotline, the hotline workers will be able to direct the call.

Professional Referrals

When a professional calls to discuss the sexual behaviors of a child, the intake person needs to determine the child's level of functioning, whether the child's situation needs to be reported, and whether the agency or the professional has the necessary expertise to provide services for the child and family.

If a child protective services worker calls, an assessment of the seriousness of the child's problem may lead the intake person to encourage the protective services worker to ensure an open case on the child. Some professionals refuse to engage in the treatment of children who molest without an open case in protective services or the criminal justice system.

Frequently, teachers are unclear when to become concerned about children's sexual behaviors. If a teacher becomes concerned about a child's sexual behaviors, all school personnel who come in contact with the child should observe the child and discuss their joint observations to assist the referral source.

Parent Referrals

Some parents' questions about children's sexual behaviors can be easily answered over the phone. However, if from early questioning of the parent, the child seems to be engaged in sexual behaviors that may require intervention, the clinician should determine whether the child has been seen at any other facility and/or is in therapy, and if they have been referred by social services or the police. If the clinician believes from the telephone intake conversation that the situation is very serious and there is reasonable suspicion that a child is molesting, he or she should encourage the parent to call protective services for assistance. If the parent is reluctant, the clinician can call protective services if sufficient data are available.

If the child's problematic sexual behaviors can be evaluated at the agency, and if it is not an emergency, it may be best to take information regarding the problem, the referral source, the family constellation, the child's demographic data, and other pertinent information for staff review. With this information, a more informed decision can be made about the suitability of the agency or professional's training and resources to do an evaluation and provide treatment.

Planning the Evaluation

Gathering Data from Outside Sources

When a referral is received for children with sexual problems, the evaluation must be planned. If protective services has interviewed the child, these records should be reviewed prior to evaluation. If the problematic sexual behaviors have been directed toward another child, and the police are involved, this information should be reviewed; data from previous therapists are also gathered.

If the child is in foster care or group care, the child's history, including information from all prior placements should be known before the evaluation. In addition, a history of the child's sexual behavior problems can be useful in determining the types of previous behaviors, their duration, and whether the behaviors are increasing or progressing in severity.

Who Will Attend the Evaluation

The greatest amount of pertinent information can be gathered if sexualized children are accompanied to the evaluation by their parents and any other primary caretaker who lives with them (e.g., grandparents or other people living in the home). It is also helpful to interview all children in the family.

If children are living in foster or group care, the primary caregivers should accompany them to the evaluation. If the children have regular visits with their family of origin or other relatives, decisions regarding when to interview the natural parents and other family members depends on the degree and quality of their involvement with the child. Because most children who are sexualized developed the behavior in the context of the family unit, it is important to get information from the family, as well as involve them in the treatment plan, if the child is to be reunified.

Length of Evaluations

The length of an initial evaluation with a family may take up to four, six, or eight or more hours. Because of the extensive data necessary to assess children with problematic sexual behaviors, and their families, it is sometimes useful to have several longer sessions than many hour-long sessions. Having more uninterrupted time can facilitate the process of gathering information and of developing a working relationship with the child and family.

Advice to Parents Before the Interview

Parents can be asked to bring toys, food, and whatever they need to be comfortable. In addition, parents can bring another adult to stay with the child while they are being interviewed. Clinicians can ask for the child's last several report cards if the child is in school, as well as some examples of the child's schoolwork, which will help them gain an initial idea about school functioning and developmental level.

Parents should provide their children with some information about the visit, for example: "We are going to see Dr. Toni. She works with children who are touching other children on their private parts. I called her to ask if she would talk to you. She has asked that all of our family go to her office to talk. She will talk with daddy and I, Johnny and Betty [siblings], and you. She has lots of toys to play with while you talk. She sounds nice on the phone. All we need to do is tell the truth and she will help us, if we need it."

The Order of Interviewing

Each clinician, or team of clinicians, must decide, based on the configuration of the family and the case information, the order in which the family is interviewed. For example, some clinicians interview the entire family first and then do separate interviews; others prefer to interview the child first and then the parents. Some interview only the identified child and the parents.

If there are two parents, the clinicians need to determine if one or the other adult will impede the ability of the other to be frank and open in discussing the necessary issues. The clinicians may want to begin the interviews with both parents and then separate them for further discussion. Many parents disclose for the first time in the interview for their sexualized child, a history of personal abuse. There is also the possibility that one or the other parent is emotionally, physically, or sexually abusing the child; therefore, separate interviews of the parents is more likely to allow this information to surface.

If sexual aggression has occurred between family members, and there is a fear of potential revictimization, the children should not be left together unattended in the waiting area at any time. The parents' attention to this factor is part of the assessment of their understanding of the problem and their ability to stay focused on the potential for problematic sexual behaviors between the children.

Observation of the Family in the Waiting Area

The sitting area and any playground area are the most natural settings clinicians often have in which to observe family interactions. Because the evaluation is regarding children with sexual behavior problems, the clinician's informal observations of the family focus on areas related to sexuality, aggression, boundaries, and parenting.

Diagnostic information can be gleaned by assessing what toys and/or food the parents bring to assist their children to cooperate during the initial interview. Parents' methods of reprimanding their children and setting limits can be observed in the waiting area. If there is more than one child in the family, are there differences in the manner in which the parents interact with them? How does the family interact? Do the parents have age-appropriate expectations of their children? Do they allow the children to run everywhere and get into everything? What are their interactional patterns regarding affection, aggression, and touching? What language is used in the family? Are there apparent role reversals? How much of the parenting is given over to other children? How does the identified child play, express sexual and aggressive behaviors, impulse control, frustration tolerance, and affect? What are the child's interactional skills? If there is more than one family in the waiting area, how does the family interact with them?

If someone accompanies the family to take care of the children while the parents are interviewed, the manner in which this person relates to the children also provides good information about the family's network of friends and support.

Confidentiality

Everyone who is interviewed must be aware of the limits of confidentiality as it relates to any newly disclosed abuse. The parents and children should be informed that if the clinician suspects that any abuse, either physical, sexual, or emotional is occurring, a report will be made to the designated authorities. A form can be developed that states the limits of confidentiality. This can be signed and dated by the parents, and children if it seems appropriate, and placed in the file.

Data Gathering Before the Interviews

Clinicians will generally want to gather information regarding the child's sexual behaviors at the outset of the evaluation. Open-ended questions or more structured formats can be used. If the evaluator decides to use a structured instrument, this can be given to parents or other primary caregivers before parental or child interviews. Helpful structured instruments include the Child Sexual Behavior Inventory (CSBI) developed by Friedrich (Friedrich et al., 1992) and the Child Sexual Behavior Checklist (CSBCL) developed by Johnson.

The CSBI (version one) is a thirty-six-item measure assessing a wide variety of sexual behaviors. It has been used successfully to discriminate between the sexual behaviors of children who have been sexually abused and children who have not been sexually abused (Friedrich et al., 1992). A copy of the CSBI, Version 1, is provided in Appendix C.

The CSBCL was specifically developed over a four-year period as an assessment tool for sexualized children, due to the extreme difficulty in collecting parental information about their children's sexual behavior problems. The CSBCL contains over 150 sexual behaviors of children ranging from natural and healthy childhood sexual exploration to behaviors of children experiencing severe difficulties in the area of sexuality. (See Appendix B.)

Additional paper and pencil assessment tools may be given later in the evaluation, depending on the level of severity of the problem and the treatment needs of the child and family (See Appendix D).

Interview with Parents

Parental Reactions, Feelings, and Levels of Concern

Parents often have difficulty discussing their child's problematic sexual behaviors and may be embarrassed, angry, or highly defensive. Clinicians should avoid placing blame on the parents, and decrease their feelings of shame regarding their child's sexual behaviors. Many parents of children who molest know almost nothing about the events that precipitated the need for the evaluation and have never openly or directly discussed the incident with the child. Some show a lack of concern about the sexual behaviors, general neglect of the child, shame, anger at the child, anger at the "system," guilt, and disinterest.

Due to the sensitive nature of the problem, parents often do not tell the interviewer about related incidents or concerns. In some cases, this may be purposeful or due to embarrassment. In other cases, this may result from a lack of understanding about related pertinent issues. Asking the parents for their reaction to their child's sexual behaviors and how they are currently managing the child may uncover behavior management techniques that may be detrimental to the child's self-esteem, including his or her own sexual self-esteem. This information may also help assess their parenting skills and level of concern.

No assumption should be made that the sexual behaviors, even including intercourse with a much younger child, or physical aggression against a defenseless child, is considered by the parent-caretaker to be very serious and, therefore, in need of intervention. Sometimes, what the child is doing may not be very different from what occurred in the parents' own history. Parents may believe that if they did it, or it was done to them, it can't be so bad, because they are alive. If the child is molesting other children, clinicians should ascertain the parents' level of concern and belief in the seriousness of the child's problems to help determine whether the parents can provide adequate supervision in order to protect other children.

During the interview, it is helpful to ascertain the parents' feelings about the child who is experiencing the problematic sexual behaviors. Negative feelings and projections can be brought into the open at this time. Parents are often relieved when a therapist speaks openly about the possibility of the parents' negative feelings toward the child. The therapist can empathize with the parents' difficulties and offer hope of a brighter future. In some families in which sibling incest occurs, the parents are less supportive of the victim than he or she needs. This may be due to a division of loyalties among family members. If this appears to be occurring, the clinician may want to talk about the difficult decisions of the parents, and encourage them to actively support the victim-child's disclosure in addition to supporting and encouraging the child with problematic sexual behaviors. Discovery of a problem can be the beginning of the healing and the end to the disruption, secrecy, and hurt in the family. This can be portrayed as a positive and mobilizing time.

Child's Early History

A developmental history of the child is important. Were there any difficulties with the pregnancy, birth, or early development of the child? How was the relationship between the child's parents during this period? How was the child's behavior during his or her early childhood? Who were the child's primary caregivers during this period? Where and with whom has the child lived? Were there any medical problems or other emotional or psychological problems? How does the child adapt to change? Have there been significant losses for the child? Have there been frightening occurrences for the child? Any serious accidents or deaths in the family? Does the child have friends? With whom does the child spend most of his/her time? Who is the child's confidante? How many friends does the child have?

How well does the child get along with other children? How does the child get along in the family? Who are the closest and least close family members? What is the role of the extended family in the lives of the family? When did parents first become aware of problematic sexual behaviors? All incidents of exposure to adult sexuality can be explored as well as questions related to all areas of physical, sexual, and emotional abuse.

Parents' History

Often a significant amount of turmoil exists in the background of parents of children who are sexualized. For this reason, in-depth interviews should be conducted about the parents' background and current functioning.

Questions regarding the parents' sexual history, including fulfilling relationships and negative experiences, provide valuable background information. The probability is very high that if a child is molesting another child that one or both of the child's parents is a victim of sexual abuse and other abuses (Friedrich & Luecke, 1988; Johnson, 1988; Johnson, 1989b). The parents' abuse history and coping style can assist the clinician's understanding of the parents' psychological needs and defenses, as they relate to the problems they are facing now with their own child. It may also aid in understanding the parents' level of available emotional and psychological resources.

Helping the parents explore the meaning of their own victimization may help build a bridge to the therapist and the therapeutic process. Some insight into the effects of their own abuse history often helps the parents appreciate the struggles of their children.

Physical Violence

The amount of abuse parents have sustained from partners, and the amount of physical violence children have witnessed, should be assessed. A significant factor in the background of children who molest is the high level of aggression they have witnessed and to which they have been subjected (Friedrich & Luecke, 1988; Johnson, 1988, 1989b). The pairing of the sexual and aggressive aspects of their childhood experiences is a very significant contributor to their sexually aggressive behavior. This variable is important to assess and modify early in the intervention process. Some parents use physical punishment to stop the problematic sexual behaviors. Use of physical punishment is contraindicated.

Genogram

It may help the clinician to draw a genogram to help understand the relationships in the family and the family history (McGoldrick and Gerson, 1985). The history of births, marriages, divorces, cohabitations, deaths, abuse, alcohol and drug problems, and incarcerations provide the context in which the child grows. Intergenerational patterns may emerge that aid in the evaluation and later in the treatment process.

Sibling Incest

In sibling incest, the parents' feelings about the sibling-victim and the child who molests are important to examine. Frequently, the relationship is more giving and caring with the sibling-victim and highly ambivalent and sometimes quite punitive with the child who molests. In group III children (see Chapter three), the parents may be distant from both of them. The relationship of the parents to the children, and vice versa, can often be best understood by observing the family's interactions in the waiting area and during a family interview.

Sibling incest presents parents with perhaps the most difficult situation possible. Because parents have strong feelings for both of their children, they often do not want anything to happen to either child. Parents should be supported in this dilemma. It is valuable for them to understand that there is help for them and for their children.

Many parents do not perceive therapists and/or child protective services as helpful, but as intrusive and unnecessary. Parents may try to impede the clinician's ability to gather pertinent information. Some parents tell the victim-sibling directly, and sometimes indirectly, to change what they have said to minimize the events already disclosed. Parents may also actively support any denial or minimization by the child who offended. When this happens, it is difficult to overcome parental influence.

In cases of forced sibling incest, the parents may be very angry at the child who has molested and feel protective of the victim, but be more angry at the interference of the clinicians and protective services.

In cases of sibling incest, the parents' major concern may be to protect themselves from any involvement by protective services. Parents should be encouraged to acknowledge the seriousness of extensive sexual behaviors between their children. Often, parents are aware of the family's need for help, but when it is given, they are so focused on the "intrusion" into their family, they cannot see its potential benefits.

When sibling incest occurs, almost all parents unrealistically believe that they do not need outside help to stop the behavior between the children.

Parents must be aware that the treatment process will involve all members of the family and not just the child. Parents should be gently informed that children who engage in forced or extensive mutual sexual behaviors are generally found to have a great deal of sexual confusion that emanates from aspects of the family environment, and that professional help is necessary to modify these aspects of the family life.

Boundaries

In some families of children with problematic sexual behaviors, parents have not provided a model of good boundary management for family members. Physical, sexual, and emotional boundaries are frequently blurred in these families, and information on boundaries can be important in initially assessing the treatment needs of the parents and the dynamics that may be supporting the sexual behaviors of the child. The issue of boundary-management is fundamental to the correction of problems in families of children who molest. Questions can be posed so that the focus is on the child's needs and requests. In this way, parents feel more comfortable to respond. For example: Does someone need to assist the child when he or she goes to the bathroom? Does the child need assistance when bathing? Does the child ask for assistance when dressing? The parents may be overly involved in the toileting and bathing of the child. Some children feel intruded upon by this behavior, but because they have not learned about adequate personal space, they cannot articulate their discomfort.

Not infrequently, parents bathe several children together to save water, time, and energy. Children who have been sexualized often find this over-stimulating. If the child bathes with siblings, this should be discontinued until the sexualized child feels more in control of the behaviors.

Does the child want to sleep with the parents? If a sexualized child is sleeping with the parents or with other children in the family, this should be discontinued. Not infrequently, the child feels sexualized by the body contact with the parents. It has been found that some of these parents' actions and sleeping attire are very confusing and inappropriate. If the child with problematic sexual behaviors is sleeping in the bed with other children, this can also be highly stimulating and confusing. In some cases, parents have several children sleeping with them. This is too stimulating and confusing for the child with problematic sexual behaviors.

The need for separate sleeping arrangements is sometimes difficult for the parents to comprehend and follow through on, because it may also meet some of their own dependency needs. When there is a lack of space because of financial constraints, or the children are afraid to sleep alone, parents should be encouraged to use sleeping bags on the floor near their bed or make a bed with blankets and pillows. Parents should be told to curtail their sexual activity while the child is in the room, even if the parents are sure the child is asleep. Although historically, millions of children have slept with their parents and not been adversely affected, children with problematic sexual behaviors can be adversely effected due to their confusion about sex and sexuality.

Religion

An assessment can be made of the religious background of the parents and the role of religion in the family. In some cases, religion plays an important role in exacerbating sexualized behaviors. The attitude about sexuality may be very charged: Sex is not to be mentioned, sex is only for adults, children who engage in any sexual activity are sick and dirty, and in some cases, it is believed that children are damned to hell for sexual behaviors. Clinicians should determine whether masturbation is considered to be sinful or if it is allowed. In some families, such strong negative feelings exist about masturbation that touching one's own genitals produces enormous guilt.

Some parents, rebounding from sexual excessiveness, may be so full of religious fervor that they have renounced sex, just as they have renounced the devil. In this atmosphere, the tension level may be so highly charged that the young child acts out the repressed sexuality of the parent. In some highly repressed homes, parents consciously or unconsciously appear to set up circumstances for the children to act out sexually. The highly repressed parent seems to get vicarious pleasure from the sexual behaviors of the children. For example, when asked why two highly sexualized children are allowed to bathe together, when it is clear they feel great tension when undressed in the same room, the parent may be unable to explain his or her actions. Positive aspects of the family's religious beliefs are also explored and integrated into the treatment approach.

Culture

A clinician must be cognizant that a person's ethnic heritage brings with it important cultural values. In addition, the family's friends and relatives, as well as their church, and the neighborhood in which individuals live, contain value systems that influence the family and their behavior. This culture in which a child lives determines normative behavior, and evaluators must understand and respect this variable in order to conduct thorough and effective evaluations.

Interview of Other Adults Who Live with the Family

Often people in the same households have different perspectives of life in the home. Clinicians can profit by as many perspectives as available to understand what may be prompting or sustaining a child's sexual behaviors.

Since all adults who are in caretaking roles to a child with problematic sexual behaviors will be part of the change process for the child, an initial interview to gather information about them, their lives, and struggles is important. Sometimes other adults who live in the family may themselves be struggling with issues in their own lives that may be influencing the child's behavior.

If the CSBCL or other behavior checklists are used, significant differences in frequencies of sexual behaviors that are observed by nonparental adults versus the parents should be carefully evaluated.

In addition, nonparental adults who are living in the home need to be interviewed because it is possible that they may be engaging in inappropriate sexual interactions with the child.

Interview with the Siblings

When a child is referred for problematic sexual behaviors, it is helpful to interview all the other children who live in the same home. In this way, data can be gathered from other children about the sexual behaviors of the child and it can be determined if there are current or past victimizing behaviors by adults or children in the family.

If the child with problematic sexual behaviors lives in a foster home, the foster siblings can be assessed during this interview. If the child lives in a group home, the other children in the group home can be interviewed. Very valuable information that is often unknown to the foster parents or group care workers may come out of these interviews. Permission to do interviews is obtained from children's protective services workers.

The overall goal in the interviews is to determine if problems in the home are causing distress to the siblings. Interviews with the siblings help alert the children that the family will be working on its problems, and that their concerns and perspectives are of importance to the clinicians. Siblings often feel very encouraged that there will be no more secrets, and that it is time for the family to be open about its problems.

It is not infrequent to find that the siblings of children who molest have a significant number of emotional and behavioral problems. For this reason, many programs include these children in the treatment, which can be individual, group, or family therapy.

The overall informational objectives of the interview are to determine the following:

Distress children feel in the home. Do siblings feel comfortable with the level and type of sexual expression and expression of anger in the home, and does anything in the home make them uneasy. For example, the clinician can ask: "Do things happen in your house that you worry about? Sometimes kids get scared when their parents get angry, does that happen in your house? Some children tell me that they feel kind of funny when people do sex stuff in front of them at home? Do you?"

Issues related to the behavior of the child with problematic sexual behaviors. Has the sexualized child touched other siblings in a way that was beyond age-appropriate sex play? Has the sexualized child made the siblings feel uncomfortable or unsafe in any way (e.g., coercion, bribery, manipulation, hitting, threats; this need not be restricted to sexual behavior)? Do siblings feel safe living with the sexualized child? Are siblings aware of sexual behaviors of the sexualized child? How long have they been happening?

Issues related to abuse. Has any sibling been sexually, physically, or emotionally abused or aware of abuse to anyone else in their family? This can be asked informally: "Has anyone ever touched you on your private parts in a way that you didn't think was okay? Do you know if anyone in your family has ever been touched on their private parts in a way that made them uncomfortable? Does anyone have any secrets about touching private parts in your family?"

Since interviews are confidential, clinicians should not disclose any information to the siblings that they did not know. In the final interview with the family, problematic sexual behaviors are disclosed to the extent necessary, and a plan is made about how to respond to them.

Interview with the Alleged Sibling-Victim

If a sibling has been victimized, the sibling should be interviewed before the child who molested him or her. In this way, the clinician will have more information and, therefore, be more helpful to the child who molested. When the child who molested knows that the interviewer is aware of at least some of the information, he or she is less tempted to try to fabricate or deny the behaviors. (This interview should not be confused with the investigatory interview conducted by child protective services or police to determine if sexual abuse occurred.)

Interviewing the sibling-victim first also alerts the child that the clinician is very interested in him or her and that his or her needs are important. If the sibling disclosed the abuse, this can be discussed as a very positive move toward getting help. The clinician can confirm that the sibling-victim's safety is important to everyone, and that every effort will be made to provide for it. The victim can be encouraged that the family will be a safer and happier place for everyone when there are no more secrets.

The overall informational objectives of the interview are to determine the following:

Issues related to the abuse by the sibling. The clinician should find out what sexual behaviors occurred, how frequently, and where; the extent and type of the threats, force, coercion, manipulation, or bribery, if any. Were the sexual behaviors mutually engaged in at one time and then progressed to the use of coercion or force by the other child? Was the child physically hurt? Were there games or feelings the child found pleasurable? Were there any other children involved? Where were the parents when the behaviors occurred? Were the parents ever aware of any of the sexual behaviors?

Emotional relationship to the abusive sibling. Siblings who are involved in incest generally have some aspects of their relationship that are positive. The interviewer can find out about all aspects of the relationship. This can help clarify situations in which protective services intends to remove a child for molesting a sibling, and the sibling says he or she does not want the abusive child to leave (see Chapter five).

The child's comfort in the home. Is the child fearful for his or her safety at home? Is the child comfortable with the expression of sexuality and anger in the home? Does the child think his or her parents believe what happened and will be protective?

If a child has molested a sibling, the child who molested should, under virtually all circumstances, be removed from the home for a period of time. It is perceived as a punishment if the child-victim is removed and the child who molests remains. Although it is more difficult to find a suitable placement for the sexually aggressive child than the victim, the wrong message is given if the victim is removed. The parents also need to be clear about the responsibility for the sexual activity and that the child who molests is to be admonished, not the victim.

Interview with the Alleged Nonsibling-Victim

If the information on referral indicates that the child who has been referred for sexual behavior problems has likely molested another child, and the victim is not in the home, every effort should be made to gather information from the victim or someone who interviewed the victim, before the interview. If protective services or the police will be interviewing the child, it is prudent to wait for the results of their investigation before interviewing the child who molests.

Interview with the Child with Sexual Behavior Problems

Style and Manner of the Interviewer and the Interview

The manner and style of the interviewer are important. The approach that facilitates disclosure is open and direct. Interviewers should speak matter-of-factly about sexual behaviors with children and encourage them to talk about their problematic sexual behaviors—children sense immediately any interviewer reluctance to talk about sexual material. Some children like to know that the interviewer has heard these things before and will not be shocked.

Sitting on the interviewer's lap or touching or hugging the interviewer should be actively discouraged, because children who have been sexualized can easily misperceive the adult's intentions. The clinician might say for example, "We do not know each other well. Hugging and sitting on laps is for people you and your parents know well."

Children should know that if they get uncomfortable while talking about sexual behaviors that there is time for a break or the door can be opened (if confidentiality can be maintained). Some sexualized children experience sexual, aggressive, sad, or other feelings while talking about their sexual behaviors, which can make them very uncomfortable. Children may confuse the interviewer's intentions for talking about the sexual behaviors, because many of them have parents who are psychologically and sexually intrusive, and many have been sexually and emotionally abused.

Rapport building is important. These interviews are difficult for children because they often feel they are in trouble and are reluctant to talk. Children can be told briefly what the therapist knows about them and the sexual behaviors, and then given a chance to talk about school, favorite toys or games, and sports activities. However, children should know at the outset that it is important for the interviewer to know as much as possible about the sexual behaviors before the interview is finished. Some children like to talk about the sexual behaviors right away, others like to wait until they are more comfortable. Either is fine. The clinician should pace the interview to the child's needs and circumvent power struggles by the use of empathy, choices, and firm and active containment of the child's behavior.

If the evaluator feels that the child's young age, developmental level, vocabulary, or reticence to speak about matters related to the genitals would be aided by a discussion of all the body parts, this can be done in the early part of the interview. Some people like to use a doll and have children identify the body parts on it; others use a drawing on which children can point out body parts (Groth, 1989). If the evaluator does not feel that all the body parts need to be used as a method of introducing the subject matter of the genitals, it is useful to ensure a mutual language for the genitals, rectum, breasts, and buttocks.

A common vocabulary also needs to be found for when one child touches another child. One strategy is to talk about "the touching." (It should be clarified that "touching" refers to the touching of private parts or of other behaviors related to sexual activity.) If it is determined that the touching is a concern, and the child will be entering treatment to work on it, the term "touching problem" can be used. The purpose of the term is so the child and evaluator know they are talking about the same thing and do not have to spend time redefining each time they discuss problematic sexual behaviors.

Sexualized Behaviors During the Initial Assessment

Some children become stimulated or get erections while discussing the sexual behaviors and want to leave the room to go to the bathroom. Some children get very angry and leave the room, slamming the door. It is generally more helpful for children to take a break from the interview and allow the feelings to dissipate rather than trying to talk it through when agitated. After the child has had time to discharge the immediate feelings, it is helpful to discuss what happened and put it in perspective for the child. In some instances, the arousal experienced by the child may mimick previous abusive situations. This will need clarification so that the child does not become apprehensive in the treatment situation.

Some children begin to masturbate while talking about victimizing others or having been victimized. If the behavior is obvious and the child is aware of it, the clinician may suggest that he or she stop talking about the sexual behaviors for a bit to see if the child's desire to touch his or her genitals decreases. (The therapist does not want to give children the impression it is not all right to touch their genitals, but that this is best done in private.) With some children this provides an excellent opportunity to talk about the feelings attached to the sexual behaviors: "How were you feeling when you wanted to touch your privates [or whatever term for genitals is most comfortable for the child]? Did any thoughts go through your head that made you want to touch your privates? Were there thoughts or pictures in your head when you wanted to touch yourself?" This can be an opportunity to teach the child that sometimes children touch themselves or other people when they are sad, or mad or glad, or for other reasons.

This situation can also provide clinicians with an opportunity to ask if they said or did anything to make the child feel like touching his or her genitals. If children mention sexual abuse or make other affirmative statements, clinicians need to reassure children that they will not be touched and they are safe. If children feel that clinicians are being intrusive, it may be best to stop the interview and continue in the presence of the children's parents, or any other person with whom the child feels comfortable. Clinicians can also choose to complete this part of the interview in a group therapy setting.

If the child starts to masturbate or rub his or her genitals, but it is not obvious and the child is most likely not aware of it, the clinician may choose to overlook the behavior during initial interview situations. Bringing it up may cause children to feel intruded upon, since they may not believe it was occurring. Children may feel the clinician is making it up, which may be reminiscent of sexual discussions with the persons who molested them or with others who have inadequate sexual boundaries.

Plethysmograph Use with Prepubescent Children

The plethysmograph is an instrument that measures the client's sexual arousal patterns. A ringlike band device is put around the shaft of the penis. Visual images or auditory stimuli with explicit sexual content are presented to the client and sexual arousal is measured by the degree of tumescence of the penis.

There are serious objections to the use of this device on prepubescent children—the basic assumptions for the use of the plethysmograph are not met with prepubescent children. One basic assumption for the use of plethysmographs is that offenders are sexually aroused to the victim. With prepubescent children, there are no available data that substantiate that they molest because they are sexually aroused to their victim (although this may or may not be true, or may be a factor with some children and not others). Another basic assumption in the use of plethysmographs is that clients have an established sexual arousal pattern—a pattern of sexual arousal to specific people or things. No available data confirm consistent sexual arousal patterns in prepubescent children.

In addition, another basic assumption in the use of plethysmographs is that demonstrated sexual arousal on one test predicts future sexual arousal to the same stimuli. No available data exists to substantiate this factor. Data on the use of plethysmographs with adolescents who have been sexually or physically abused show increased sexual arousal with no specific patterns to the arousal (Becker, 1992). Since this occurs in adolescents, the same arousal levels in prepubescent children could be equally non-discriminating, especially since prepubescent children may be responding to a novel (visual and auditory) stimulus.

An ethical consideration in the use of plethysmographs with prepubescent children is the use of visual or auditory sexual depictions. In my opinion, children who molest have already been prematurely overexposed to sexual information that they were unable to understand or control. Because the basic assumptions for the use of plethysmographs are not met with prepubescent children, there appears to be no justification for further exposing children to sexual material—this exposure to explicit sexual material could be experienced as another victimization.

In a recent Arizona case, a hospital program for sex offenders used the plethysmograph on an eleven-year-old boy. Slides shown to the boy included pictures of nude children, adolescents, and adults, and bondage. Parental permission was not obtained before using the plethysmograph. The use of plethysmographs with prepubescent children can not be justified unless all the basic assumptions in the use of plethysmographs can be met. Clinicians who are treating and assessing prepubescent children with sexual behavior problems must remain aware of the children's sexual development. Although the plethysmograph is very useful in the assessment and treatment of adults offenders and some adolescent sex offenders, it remains totally unproven with prepubescent children.

Goals of the Interview with the Sexualized Child

The goals of the interview with the sexualized child are not presented in any particular order. Some of the topics suggested may be more pertinent than others, depending on the group membership of the child. Evaluators will find different question areas more or less consistent with their own approach and choose those that suit them best. Evaluators will be further guided by the referral issues, the age and developmental level of the child, the immediacy of the problems, the background information and the number and type of previous interviews.

All of the suggested topic areas may not be covered in one interview. Evaluators may want a second session. In some cases, if it is determined the child will enter group treatment, some of the questions may wait until the child is being prepared to enter the group.

Specific Goals

The overall goal of the interview is to determine the child's group membership (see Chapter three) and the needs of the child and family for protective service, police involvement, and treatment interventions. This overall goal can be reached by assessing the following areas:

The nature of children's problematic sexual behaviors. When interviewing the child, the clinician is likely to already have knowledge from the parents or others about the child's sexual behaviors. The behaviors the child discloses may be quite different from what the adults know. Communication between the child and the parents may not be very open, particularly around areas of sexuality.

The clinician can help the child talk about the problematic sexual behaviors by saying, "I understand that your parents are a little bit worried about the touching you are doing. They told me that sometimes you like to touch [Suzy, yourself, etc.] and that maybe you are doing that too much. They asked me to talk to you about the touching so we could all decide if maybe you need some help. One of the things I do a lot is talk to children about touching. Do you think you have a problem with touching?" This approach is suitable when children are most likely group I or II (see Chapter three). With children in group III or IV in which the level of disturbance is greater and there is a higher likelihood of denial, minimization, or misrepresentation of the truth, the following type of statement may be more suitable: "I have spoken with your parents and [social worker, police, teacher, etc.] and I know some things about you. We have spoken a little about your school, your friends, and how you get along in the family. I have also asked about the touching you have been doing. Even though I know some things about you and the touching, I would like you to tell me in your own words. Only you really know what has been going on, so you are really the very best person to hear from. It is important that you tell the truth. If you feel like you want to say something that is not true, I would rather you tell me you don't want to answer right now. If we are both telling the truth, we can trust each other. If for some reason you are having a hard time telling me the truth, you can tell me why it is hard to tell. Maybe you are afraid someone will be mad, or you will get in trouble, or someone won't like you. The reason we are here is to see if you and your family need help, not to get mad at anyone."

If children have possibly engaged in some abusive behavior, there are issues that need to be assessed. What were the behaviors? How long did they go on? How many children were involved? Was there coercion involved? Were there any threats? Was there any physical harm to the other child? Was any force used? Were there any adults involved? Whose idea was it to do the sexual behaviors?

If the child acknowledges sexual behaviors with other children but says it was by agreement, the evaluator may ask where the behaviors occurred, why was it in those locations, where parents and other adults were, and whether the child wanted the other child to keep it quiet and why.

Additional questions include: "Who decided what the touching stuff would be? Who decided when it would start? Who decided when it would stop? Who decided who else could know? Did the other child get to make any decisions about what and where the touching stuff would happen? How do you like the other child? Do you generally play together? Are you good friends? Do you ever feel mom is nicer to the other child? Do you ever feel kinda jealous of the other child? When you get mad at the other child, what do you usually do? When you did the touching stuff, what were you trying to do to the other child? How long did you plan it before you did it? What did the other child say when you were doing the touching stuff? What did you say to the other child?"

The evaluator needs to understand that, in general, only the tip of the iceberg is known before the evaluation. It is also common that only a slightly larger part of the tip is discovered during the evaluation. More of the information will come out during the treatment process. Some of the information may never be disclosed.

Children's motivation for the problematic sexual behaviors. Very few children can answer a question about motivation whether it concerns sexual behavior, stealing, lying, or anything else. Children do not generally think about why they do things—they just do them. Nevertheless, the question can be asked and some children do answer it. Some children who are engaged in sex play answer the question, "Because I was curious." One ten-year-old girl who had molested her sister for two years said, "Because my father taught me to put things in her vagina while he watched. After he went to jail, when

I would feel mad at him for putting things in my vagina, I would do it to her. Yes, I know it hurt her, but she deserves it. She is a pain in the neck."

Clinicians can encourage children's responses by asking: "All children have different reasons for doing things. Any ideas why you touch Robbie on his penis?" Children may say they don't know. The clinician can then say "kids have told me that they touch other kids 'cause they want to, 'cause they feel mad or bad or sad, 'cause they like to, 'cause the other kid likes them to do the touching, 'cause it feels good, and for other reasons. Any idea about why you touch Robbie on the penis?" (The younger the child, the fewer choices given.)

If the questioning does not lead to an answer, the issue has been raised that there are reasons for touching and that children can figure them out. This gives children hope that they will understand the motivation for their touching behavior and bring it under control.

Children's feelings about sexuality. One of the discriminating features between children in the four groups (see Chapter three) is their affect regarding sexuality. Group I children often are giggly or silly about sexuality. Group II children experience more shame and guilt and anxiety about sex. Group III children may experience anxiety or guilt, but they frequently also have a cavalier or ho-hum attitude and do not understand the concern of the adults about their sexual behaviors. Group IV children's affect around sexuality is frequently volatile, and generally has very aggressive and anxious features. In some children, feelings of rage are associated with sexuality. Other group IV children's associations are fear, grave sadness, jealousy, extreme loneliness, or other uncomfortable feelings.

Who else knows about the problematic sexual behaviors? This question can help the evaluator determine how widespread the sexual behavior is and whether there are other children or adults involved. In some cases, the sexual behaviors between the children are being orchestrated by an adult for the adult's sexual pleasure. In other cases, the adult is no longer using the children in this abusive manner, but the children continue to engage in the behaviors.

When the question is asked, it is sometimes discovered that other mental health providers or community agencies have been involved and that the parents have neglected to disclose this or the evaluator neglected to cover this thoroughly with the parents. This question may also elicit information about the parents' knowledge of the sexual behaviors. In some cases, the parents have been aware of the behaviors and not taken steps to change them until people outside the family became aware of them.

Children's desire to change their problematic sexual behaviors. Many children report a high desire to change their sexual behaviors. Although this is good prognostically, the reason the child wants to change should be assessed. Some children's desire is based on not wanting to hurt other children, whereas others have a desire not to get in so much trouble. Some children say they want to stop so that they will not get so many spankings. This information will be helpful in guiding the parents about how to react to the children's problematic sexual behaviors. The clinician can ask, "Do you think you need help to stop the touching?" "Do you think you can stop the behavior?" "Who wants you to change the most?"

Denial, misrepresentation, or minimization of problematic sexual behaviors. Because children do not like to get in trouble, they sometimes do not tell the truth about what they have done. Because it is likely that children will deny they did something others perceive as wrong, it is important for the evaluator to have all available information on the child's problematic sexual behaviors. Even though evaluators tell children at the beginning of the interview the outline of what they already know, children may still say the behaviors didn't happen. The evaluator must assess why there is such a powerful reason for the child not to tell the truth. The evaluator can ask: "What would it mean to you [about you] if you did the things people say you did? What would happen to you if you said you did the touching? Why would someone say you did the touching, if you didn't?"

If the evaluator determines that the reason for silence is the child's fear of punishment, this needs clarification before the evaluation is completed.

If evaluators have obtained mistaken or incomplete information, they need to ask for additional information. The child will benefit from seeing that the evaluator is honest and pursues the truth. The child will learn that the evaluation setting is a new and different place in which he or she can build or loose credibility, independent of previous history.

If the child absolutely denies the behaviors, and there is no way to gather the substantiating data at that time, the child can be told in a positive manner that the evaluator will contact the people who may have more information and meet with the child again. If there are reports from protective services or the police they can be read (judiciously) in the child's presence.

Should it appear that a child has molested another child and the child is reluctant to acknowledge having a touching problem to the clinician, the child can be encouraged to disclose some part of the behaviors, because that is necessary for the child to enter a treatment group. Since most children who molest look forward, with some relief, to being in a group in which all the children are openly working on the touching problem, they will often disclose some part of the behaviors.

Do children understand others' concerns about their problematic sexual behaviors? Depending on the environment in which children were raised, and other cultural and social factors, they may or may not understand others' concerns about the problematic sexual behaviors in which they are engaging. If children feel the behaviors are normative, and yet the larger culture does not, changing the behaviors will be more difficult.

Children may be mirroring sexual behaviors that occur in the home or neighborhood. Although the parents are unlikely to voluntarily disclose this information, children may tell the evaluator and be relieved that someone else is now aware of the situation. The evaluator needs to handle this information carefully. Further questions to the child may prompt concern for the appropriateness of the home environment and may or may not necessitate reporting to child protective services.

Children's willingness to accept responsibility for their problematic sexual behaviors. Many children want to blame others for their behavior. This phenomenon is not unique to sexual abuse or to children, yet in the area of sexual abuse, the seriousness of the denial of responsibility is especially grave. Phrases reminiscent of those used by adults and adolescents can be heard from children as young as five: "She wanted me to do it. She asked for it. It wasn't my fault."

The degree of responsibility individuals take for their actions is often learned from the environment in which they live. Generally a high correlation exists between parents and their children in this regard. Parents need help to see the relationship between the child's acceptance of his or her behavior, and their own willingness to acknowledge the child's problem and take responsibility for any changes they may need to make.

Children's feelings about the child with whom problematic sexual behaviors occurred. Determining the relationship and feelings between the sexualized child and the child with whom the sexual behaviors occurred often helps the evaluator decide the group membership of the child (see Chapter three). If two children are engaged in sex play together, they will have an ongoing mutually satisfying play relationship. If the play relationship is mainly aggressive and antagonistic, the sexual behaviors may well have the same dynamic. If the children do not have a play relationship at all, it is unlikely that they would choose each other to engage in sex play because this generally occurs between children who are friends.

Children who molest do not generally engage in sexual behaviors with friends, because many have no friends. They often seek someone they feel jealous of or about whom they have underlying negative or highly ambivalent feelings. Many choose vulnerable children who are lonely, sad, and seek companionship. Clinicians can ask, "Why did you pick that child?"

In sibling incest, the two children may have some positive feelings toward one another. This may be particularly true of the younger or emotionally weaker child for the stronger or older child, yet there is generally an underlying anger or jealousy that gets played out in sibling incest. Frequently, the emotionally stronger or older child is displacing anger at the parent onto the weaker child, because the weaker child has a favored relationship with the parent. The sibling sexual behaviors may also be mutually agreed upon.

After children are aware that it might be hurtful to another child to engage in sexual behaviors, do they feel sorry that they might have hurt the other child? Do they feel any concern for the other child? Does it seem that they have the capacity for feeling empathy?

Do children have fantasies or daydreams that may propel them to act out sexually and/or aggressively? Children who molest frequently have very intense fantasies about aggression; some have full-blown fantasies about sex, others have fantasies that combine sex and aggression. Many children report no sexual fantasies. Children who are living outside their homes frequently daydream about their parents, what their parents did and did not do and their feelings of loss, frustration, and anger. Some of these fantasies cause children such anxiety that they act out sexually to decrease the feelings generated by the fantasies.

Although this information may be hard for children to disclose in an initial interview, the content of their fantasies provides useful information for assessing their probability of reoffense and degree of dangerousness. It is hypothesized that the more sex or aggression in the fantasies, the higher probability of acting-out. These types of fantasies generally do not serve to sublimate feelings in young children. Although this may be so in some children, it may not be true in others. An evaluator can inquire about fantasies by saying: "Some kids tell me they day dream alot. I think what they mean is they sort of space out and think about things, like when you are at school and you are bored. Some kids say it is kind of like having a movie running in their head. Sometimes they are in the movie and sometimes not. Do you ever day dream? Some kids say they think about touching stuff in their day dreams. How about you? What things do you day dream about?"

Clinicians should determine if children engage in masturbation during the fantasies, and if so, how often this happens, exactly what the fantasies are and whether the children have ever played out the fantasies.

Children who share fantasies can be asked if they have ever seen their fantasy played out (e.g., in real life, on television, in videos or pornographic magazines). The clinician can ask, "Have you ever heard others describe this kind of fantasy? Have you ever experienced something similar?" These kinds of questions may lead the interviewer to discover abuse of the child by someone else. It is also a useful way to discover if there is access to sexual material in the home.

How children feel before and after engaging in the problematic sexual behaviors. This is a question that is pursued in great detail if children enter therapy. At the initial interview, children who are aware of the feelings preceding sexual behaviors generally have a better prognosis than children who have no idea or even get angry at the question. If the feelings that precede the sexual behaviors are deep anger or rage, the overall prognosis is more guarded. This level of aggressive feelings, which may also be associated with such feelings as despair, frustration, and distrust in children, is hard to diminish. Although many children stop the sexually aggressive behaviors, they may continue to act in socially aggressive and destructive ways.

Have children witnessed sexual behaviors in vivo, on videos or television, or in printed matter? Children who behave in a sexualized manner may be imitating behavior they have observed. Clinicians can ask: "Where did you learn about sex and touching?" Some children who have lived in communes or more liberal environments that include more nudity engage in more sexual behaviors than other children (Friedrich et al., 1992). Some children who have lived in highly sexualized environments that have caused them to become overstimulated show more sexual behaviors (Johnson, 1990b). Whether children have witnessed sexual behavior is frequently a baseline question by police and protective services. If the question is answered in the affirmative, some persons feel they then have an adequate explanation for the sexual behaviors, and concern for the children can be dismissed with no further explanation. Although this may be true in some situations, this is not always the case. Many children witness sexual behavior and it does not cause them to behave in a manner that brings them to the attention of mental health professionals, the police, or protective services. In cases in which the children's behavior has alerted outside authorities, and there is an initial evaluation, this generally indicates sexual behaviors that are out of the norm. This may signify more than too much or uncontrolled observation by children. A thorough evaluation of the children and their family is important.

Have children been sexually, physically, or emotionally abused? What is their response to the abuse? The most intuitive belief is that if a child is acting in a sexualized manner, the child is a victim of sexual abuse. In children who molest, the number of boys molested ranges from 50 to 75 percent in different samples (Friedrich & Luecke, 1988; Johnson, 1988). One hundred percent of the girls studied by Johnson and Friedrich had been molested (Friedrich & Luecke, 1988; Johnson, 1989b). Approximately 60 percent of victimized children show sexual behaviors beyond what is considered a normative level (Friedrich et al., 1992).

Excellent materials have been developed regarding interviewing children about abuse (see for example, Jones & McQuiston, 1988; Garbarino & Stott, 1989; Hoorwitz, 1992). Clinicians should ask open-ended questions when asking children about being touched in a way they think may not have been okay. Evaluators should be open to any and all information. Children may have been abused several times and have only disclosed one instance or part of one instance. Sometimes there have been multiple perpetrators and only one is known. There may be current abuse that remains undisclosed.

If children do not report abuse when first asked, this does not necessarily mean that they have not been abused. Clinicians need to respect the children's report and give them the time and space they deserve. If professionals create an environment in which children feel comfortable, they will disclose uncomfortable, confusing, or unjust behaviors to them. Children must not be made to feel that the only justifiable reason for sexualized behavior or sexually aggressive behavior is having been abused. Evaluators need to be aware that not all sexualized children or children who molest have experienced events that reach the threshold for reporting, or designation as abuse, by protective services or the police. Clinicians have found that highly sexualized environments can produce feelings and actions in children that are consistent with those found in some children who have been sexually abused (Johnson, 1991b). Although sexualized environments are generally not considered abusive for purposes of reporting, they can feel very confusing to children and cause sequelae consistent with sexual abuse.

Sexual abuse or highly sexualized environments are not the only antecedent to problematic sexual behaviors. Psychological and emotional abuse, physically harsh punishment, and erratic caretaking may all be precursors to sexually aggressive behaviors. Physical abuse is an important precursor to the sexually aggressive behavior of children who molest (Friedrich & Luecke, 1988; Johnson, 1988). Many of the children have not only been physically beaten but cruelly treated. This is an important etiological factor in the rage that many of these children feel.

If a child is molesting another child, it is most profitable to separate the questions about victimization from questions about the child's own sexually aggressive behavior. Although the two may be intimately connected, linking them may not be beneficial to the child. If the child sees one as the precursor of the other, it may feel inevitable to the child that he or she will molest.

The victim-to-victimizer cycle has gained currency in the American culture and carries with it a meaning that can have unfortunate consequences for some parents and children. This cycle was described to aid our understanding of the precursors to problematic sexual behaviors; however, the child's parents may believe that perpetration is an inevitable result of victimization. If parents believe the victim-to-victimizer cycle, they can develop negative feelings toward their child and believe the child to be damaged and unredeemable. They may feel their child will inevitably grow up to be a perpetrator or will have intense sexual problems. This may have the effect of making them pull away from the child. Out of fear and misunderstanding, some parents do not touch their child in the same way they did before they discovered the child was abused. Some parents even blame the child for being abused. The child may have overheard this assumption on the part of the parents, or may also have this misconception. This takes away the child's hope and makes him or her a further victim of the victimization that already occurred.

Rational discussion about this "cycle" may help the child and parents. Reassurance can be provided with the knowledge that if every abused child were to become a perpetrator, the number of perpetrators would be impossibly enormous. Recent data indicate that far from all perpetrators were victims of sexual abuse (Wolf, 1985; Burgess et al., 1987; Becker et al., 1987). This information on the sexual abuse histories of known offenders is important for parents to understand if they are struggling with the victim-to-victimizer cycle. The way in which victimization is an antecedent to perpetration, when it is, is not well understood. Important research in the field of physical abuse has begun to examine the often-held belief that victims of physical abuse become perpetrators of physical abuse. Recent research indicates that this is far from inevitable, and that many circumstances can mitigate this from occurring (Egeland, 1988). Research on sexual abuse victims indicates that an important factor in mitigating the effects of abuse, is a confidante (Gilgun 1991; Prentky et al. 1989).

If parents want to mitigate the serious aftereffects of sexual abuse, they need to consider the following important factors:

1. When child-victims feel loved, understood, and believed after the disclosure of abuse, the abuse is much less likely to result in sexual acting-out

or any other long-lasting negative sequelae. However, if children's disclosures are met with doubt or disbelief, and no help is sought when needed, children can feel entirely undermined.

2. When the perpetrator is not firmly given the message that his or her behavior is wrong, children who are victimized may feel that their rights have been seriously eroded.

3. When child-victims are subtly encouraged to retract their statements about abuse, so the offender will not be prosecuted or a sibling will not be removed from the home, this is very likely to cause serious aftereffects. The aftereffects may not be perpetration but anger, guilt, shame, fear, isolation, vulnerability to further abuse, self-destructive behaviors, and depression.

Do children feel that people in their home environment are overly sexual? Most children are not aware of living in a sexualized environment, unless it is very blatant. Boundary issues regarding personal space are generally too subtle for children to understand, particularly if poor boundaries are all they know and they have no other point of reference. Evaluators can ask: "With whom do you sleep? Does anyone help you clean yourself in the bath or after you go to the bathroom? Can people enter the bathroom when others use it? Do people have privacy to change their clothes?"

Because of the importance of sexual boundaries and sexual confusion among sexualized children, it is important to ask both the children and the parents similar questions. Discrepancies should be clarified. Depending on the level of intrusiveness of the behavior, changes can be made during the early part of the treatment. If the child is sleeping with other children or with the parent, or if no one is allowed privacy for bathroom or changing, suggestions for immediate change are important.

As the treatment progresses, these areas will need to be reviewed many times. Often it's not the children but the parents who forget the rules. The children may disclose the information to get help from the therapists.

Where and with whom do children feel most safe and least safe? Many children who are demonstrating uncommon behaviors are doing so because of distress in their lives. The behaviors are a signal that the children cannot contain within them all the feelings they are experiencing. The feelings may deal with neglect or emotional, sexual, or physical abuse. Sometimes the feelings deal with what the children see, hear, smell, or taste each day.

During the evaluation, a preliminary assessment of the child's safety can be made with the help of such questions as: "Where do you feel most safe? Do you ever feel like something bad might happen? Have you ever worried that you might get hurt? Have you ever seen anyone hurt? How do you feel when people start to yell? In your house, when you do something wrong, what happens? Where do you feel safest? Is your neighborhood safe? Who do you like to stay with most? Who don't you like to stay with? When you do something wrong, what's your worst punishment? Do you feel lonely when no one is home? What do you do when you are left alone?" Answers to some of these questions will begin to form a picture of the environment in which the child lives and who the protective and nonprotective adults are for the child. This type of assessment may lead the evaluator to caution the parents about the child's safety or may lead to a report to protective services.

Assessing for children's developmental and intellectual level. Screening developmental and intellectual functioning is important for purposes of school placement. Part of the treatment plan may be a screening for referral to the school system for evaluation for special services. Many children who have experienced traumatic childhoods, and have behavioral problems, experience developmental disruptions that require special education services. Children with learning disabilities and cognitive deficiencies can be more susceptible to emotional stressors. In all communities, children who qualify are entitled to special education services. If the school has not identified the child's needs, a referral from the therapist can be the first step in qualifying.

If the child's emotional and cognitive developmental levels are significantly below the child's age, this may cause a problem for group therapy. Generally, a fairly narrow age grouping functions best for group therapy. If a child is twelve, but developmentally delayed, being placed in a group with eight-year-olds generally does not work. Intellectually and emotionally it may be suitable, but because of the child's physical development, the child's interest in sexual matters may already be more adolescent. It is inadvisable to introduce adolescent and preadolescent thinking into a group of eight-year-old children. It is better to search for another child with similar problems. A group can be formed from two members.

Assessing children's strengths and weaknesses. Assessing children's strengths is very important. Frequently, evaluators focus on negative aspects of children who may already feel guilty and ashamed. Addressing children's strengths and weaknesses can be done during the early part of the evaluation by asking a balanced mix of questions such as: "What are some of the things you do the best? What are some of the things you do that make you happy about yourself? Are there some things about you which you think are not so great? Are there any things you would like to change about you? What is the best thing you ever did? What is the worst thing you ever did? What makes you feel the proudest? What was your biggest disappointment?"

Assessing other areas of emotional and behavioral difficulty described by children. The interviewer should try to include time and space for issues children may want to raise, for example, "If someone were to come here and say you could make three wishes and get what you wanted, what would you wish for? What makes you happiest? What makes you saddest? Are there any things you have a really hard time with? Are there some people you just don't like? How about friends? Do you have some friends you really like to play with? What would you like me to know about you? Your family?"

Determining children's perception of their school performance and peer relations. The evaluator can say: "Some kids like school, some kids hate school and some kids are kind of in between. What about you? Do you like school? What is your favorite thing to learn? What is your worst thing to learn? Do you have friends at school? Does the teacher ever ask you to leave class?"

These questions are fairly objective. If the child's answers are different from the answers of the parents, it may give an indication of the child's need to be perceived in a positive light, the child's lack of insight, poor self-appraisal skills, or other characteristics. When children give information that is opposed to reality, other information generated in the evaluation needs to be assessed in the same light.

Assessing children's willingness and ability to connect with the therapist and their suitability for group therapy. Some children have various problems that make it very difficult for them to profit from group therapy. Children who have been very severely abused or have been raised by parents with severe psychiatric and personality disorders may have great difficulty sharing the therapist with other children. It may be best for them to start in individual therapy and gradually move to simultaneous individual and group therapy.

Some children appear so damaged that they find it very difficult to relate positively to adults. These children can be given an opportunity in individual therapy and in group. Sometimes the intimacy of the individual session is too great for them. In group, they often are too disruptive and they may try to organize the children against the therapists. A highly structured group is best. If the therapist feels the child may have little conscience, no empathy, and very disturbed object relations, and/or has engaged in seriously coercive sexual behaviors, the group may not profit from the child's participation. If children are very easily distracted, a group situation is difficult for them. Often the child's teacher can be of assistance to let the therapists know whether the child can learn in the group situation.

If the child is taking medication, the medication may wear off by the time the group starts. This should be discussed with the parents and possibly the physician. Children with Attention Deficit Disorder and/or hyperactivity find it very difficult to maintain and profit from group, if they are not taking their medication.

Assessing for psychiatric disturbances. Although all evaluators need not diagnose a client using psychiatric nomenclature from the Diagnostic and Statistical Manual of Mental Disorders (DSM III-R), it is incumbent on the evaluator to assess for levels of disturbance other than problematic sexual behaviors.

The evaluator needs to be aware of depression, anxiety, thought disorders, or confusion in reality testing. Some children may be experiencing Post-Traumatic Stress Disorder or dissociative phenomena. Somatic concerns or sleep disorders may be present. Some of the basic information is gathered through the use of the Achenbach Child Behavior Checklist (CBCL), which the clinician can use as a guideline for further questioning.

An awareness of any possible self-injurious behaviors is important. Some children may be thinking about suicide and a brief assessment is warranted (Madison, 1978; Orbach, 1988). Questions like "When you feel sad, what do you think will make you feel better?" may be helpful. If the evaluator gets any inkling that children may have thought of terminating their lives, questions such as the following can be asked: "Have you ever thought you would like to be dead? Sometimes children tell me they feel so badly they just don't want to be here anymore. One child had even thought of killing himself [herself] to make the pain go away. Have you ever thought of anything like that?"

Depending on the evaluation results, an assessment for hospitalization or medication or a more intense therapeutic intervention may be important. Although the assessment is for problematic sexual behaviors, other problems must be assessed and addressed.

Drugs and alcohol. Because children are becoming involved in substance abuse at ever-decreasing ages, and because of the more pervasive use by adults, the evaluator can ask the child any of the following questions: "What drugs do kids at your school try? Do kids at your school sell drugs? Has anyone ever tempted (asked) you to try marijuana? How about cocaine? Do any kids at your school drink alcohol? Did you ever try it? Have you ever seen people drink too much? Do you think it might be fun? Do your friends want to try it? Do people in your neighborhood ever take drugs? Do you know what a drug looks like? Have you ever seen cocaine? Have you ever been scared when you saw people use drugs or alcohol?"

Organizing Assessment Information: Making a Plan

After the assessment with the child, the evaluators need to integrate the information from the interviews with each of the family members. It is helpful to do this before a final interview. In the final interview, the recommended plan for the child and family can be discussed. As the evaluators organize the material from the interviews, the following questions, along with looking at the Risk Index (see following section) are important:

1. Does the child, based on the sexual behaviors and related issues, belong in groups I, II, III, or IV? (see Chapter three)

2. Which specific lines within the child's sexual development are distressed? (see Chapter one)

3. Has any abuse happened to this child or other family members?

4. Has the child abused any other children?

5. Is there a need for reporting to child protective services or the police?

6. If the child has molested, how high is the risk that it will happen again?

7. Is the child safe where presently housed?

8. Are other children safe?

9. What are the treatment needs of the child, and other family members, if any, and how can these needs be best met?

10. What are the strengths and weaknesses of the parents in relation to the child's problems?

11. What do the family members need to know about the child's behaviors?

12. If the child can remain at home, how can the child's behavior be best managed?

Risk Index

Various factors related to the abusive sexual behavior, the child, the family, and the home environment can be evaluated to estimate the seriousness of the child's problematic sexual behaviors. The greater the number of factors present, the more serious the behavior and the higher risk of a further offense.   This index is based on clinical experience and has not been empirically verified. Future research will result in a weighting of the factors.

Risk Factors Related to the Child

- Displays oppositional behaviors
- Has poor peer relations/coping skills/self-concept/academic record/few, if any, friends
- Disregards rules and regulations at school, at home, in the community
- Is aggressive at school, home, or neighborhood toward adults and/or children
- Destroys own property and/or the property of others
- Threatens others with harm
- Behavior is beyond parental control
- Has no (apparent) positive affective connections with adults or children
- Extremes of affect, poor modulation of affective responses
- Is cruel to animals; sets fires
- Displays volatile temper, or rage reactions; manipulative behavior
- Has witnessed physical aggression directed at his or her primary caretaker
- Is a victim of physical, sexual, or emotional abuse, abandonment or neglect
- Has low cognitive ability (in conjunction with aggressive physical and sexual behaviors)

Risk Factors Related to Problematic Sexual Behaviors

- Denies the sexual behavior, although there is good evidence that it occurred
- Dislikes or has a highly ambivalent relationship to the other child
- Has no relationship to the child with whom he or she engaged in the sexual behavior
- Planned the sexual behavior without the knowledge of the other child

- Doesn't seem to care that the other child might be hurt physically or emotionally
- Other child is highly vulnerable
- Blames other people or circumstances, takes no responsibility for the sexual behavior
- Has a history of sexual behaviors apart from this incident
- Caught multiple times for coercive sexual behaviors
- Hurt the other child while engaging in the sexual behavior
- Has very intrusive sexual behavior
- Recruited other children to engage in the sexual behavior with him or her
- Doesn't think it was serious to engage in coercive sexual behavior
- Used physical strength to gain compliance of other child
- Bribed, teased, coerced, or threatened other child
- Used threats or other leverage to reinforce secrecy

Risk Factors Related to the Family

- Parents-caretakers with very confused sexual boundaries and confused notions about sexuality; poor physical and emotional boundaries in the family
- Parent-caretaker uses child to meet his or her own dependency and sexual needs
- Spousal battering
- Mother with a personality disorder with dependent, narcissistic, and borderline characteristics, and depressive features
- Psychiatric diagnoses in parents
- History of prostitution; history of living in motels, the street, or cars
- History of violence and impulsivity in the family to which the child has been privy
- History of emotional, physical, or sexual abuse to parents themselves; history of emotional, physical, or sexual abuse to other family members
- History of child protective services or police involvement with the family

- History of perpetration in the family
- History of family disruptions including divorce, out-of-home placements
- History of drug and/or alcohol abuse; history of inadequate parenting to the child (i.e., inconsistently meeting the child's needs)
- Parents know little about the offense or deny the child committed the offense or do not see the offense as a real problem
- Parents dislike the child and project negative attributes onto the child
- Victim was a favorite child in the family
- Father is incarcerated or otherwise involved with the law
- Absent father who was authoritarian and distant from family members and emotionally/physically abusive to mother
- Multigenerational sexually abusive family
- Role reversals in which the child feels the intense need to care for the parent who cannot care for himself or herself without the child's assistance
- Single parent with other children in the home

Risk Factors Related to the Environment

- Child who molests lives with the victim
- Child who molests has access to vulnerable children
- Economic stressors
- Poor supervision
- No sense of orderliness or predictability in the child's life

Reporting Child Abuse

If it is determined that a child abuse report is to be made, the evaluators need to decide how they wish to do this. Some clinicians call before the family leaves the agency or clinic, particularly if a child has disclosed abuse by someone with whom he or she lives. Some clinicians inform the family first, if the abuse is extrafamilial, and then call.

If the child has victimized another child, a report to protective services needs to be made. Informing the child and the parents prior to calling is advisable. In this way, the call can be made before the child and family leave and the evaluator can try to determine with protective services or the police what course of action will be taken subsequent to the referral.

If the child poses a danger to a sibling or other child, decisions regarding the placement of the child need to be made.

Elements of the Treatment Plan

Finding the most suitable placement. When there are vulnerable children in the home, it is safer for the child with a significant touching problem to live elsewhere for a period of time. Sometimes there is a relative who does not have vulnerable children with whom the child can live while treatment progresses.

Some children cannot be maintained safely at home, a foster home, a group home, or a residential facility due to the lack of specialized services and supervision. Some children may need intensive hospitalization for a brief period while a secure environment is sought with access to specialized treatment.

Treatment for children with touching problems. All treatment for these children must be focused and specialized. Group therapy is generally the most beneficial for working with molesting behaviors. Individual therapy is very helpful for intrapsychic conflicts and other issues. Family therapy will be essential as the treatment progresses. Therapists who have a solid background in child development and the treatment of sexual abuse are preferable.

Working with the child's caretakers to assist them in providing the necessary guidance to reduce and finally eliminate the problematic sexual behaviors. Caretakers need a great deal of assistance from the treatment staff to teach them how to help to reduce the child's problematic sexual behaviors. This may be in group, couple, or individual contact with a therapist who is working with the sexualized child. Some programs provide parents-caretakers with education on child development, child sexuality, and parenting in intensive sessions at the beginning or throughout the treatment process. If the child remains with the natural parents, a minimum of weekly contact is necessary; more contact provides more support. Group therapy for the natural parents coinciding with the treatment of their children is very helpful (see Chapters eleven and twelve). Family therapy will be necessary as the treatment progresses. Many parents profit from individual therapy, because many have had intense difficulties in their lives.

Medical evaluations. Depending on the history of sexual behaviors, medical evaluations may be required. Physical examinations should be conducted by a medical professional with experience in assessing child sexual abuse.

Some children can profit from an evaluation for medication from a child psychiatrist. Some medications have been found to decrease problematic sexual behaviors of young children.

Intervention with school, daycare, or after-school care personnel. Depending on the level of seriousness, people in these agencies may need to be contacted regarding the touching problem and an intervention plan coordinated between the agencies, parents, and therapists. Children at school or in the community should not be exposed to a high risk of molesting behaviors by a child. This should be explained to parents to gain their approval and assistance. All releases should be signed and placed in children's files. Evaluation of school performance to determine suitability of classroom placement and whether there is a need for additional services through the school system is necessary.

Treatment for sibling-victims. Initially, sibling-victims are best served by individual or group treatment that is specifically focused on victimization. Later, family therapy will be essential.

Supportive interventions with other siblings. In some treatment programs for children with touching problems, siblings participate in special, separate groups with the objective of ongoing observation and evaluation for problems and prevention lessons.

Final Interview with the Child and Family

Based on the information to be shared, the evaluator determines who should be at the final meeting. Should the whole family meet for the entire session, or does some information need to be shared with just the parents, or just the parents and the child with the touching problem first, and then bring the family together? Since boundaries are generally an issue in families in which sexual issues arise, this should be carefully considered.

In the family session, the problems of the child and the family are discussed, and the suggested treatment plan is elaborated. It may be important for the child with problematic sexual behaviors to tell the parents directly about his or her sexual behaviors, if they are not aware of the extent of the sexualized behavior. This depends on the group status of the child, the relevance for meeting therapeutic goals, such as taking responsibility and acknowledging problems, and the need of the family members to know for prevention and treatment purposes.

Neither the sexualized child, nor anyone else, should be made to feel badly in this discussion. The sexual behavior problem should be stated matter-of-factly. The evaluators should assure that there is clarity and openness between family members regarding the child's problematic sexual behaviors, understanding of the level of seriousness of the problem, and that all family members can help the child stop the behaviors. Stress can be placed on the necessity for there not to be any secrets in the home. Everyone is encouraged to be open and forthright about all family problems.

If the problematic sexual behaviors are coercive, an initial plan can be made in this final evaluation session regarding the following issues:

1. Targeting specific abusive sexual behaviors.

2. Determining the consequences for further occurrences.

3. Agreeing on rewards for no inappropriate sexual behaviors.

4. Agreeing on any restrictions for the child, such as being alone with other children, bathing, changing, or sleeping with others.

5. Developing a list of substitute behaviors. Substitute behaviors are used if children feel as though they may want to engage in probematic sexual behaviors. When children have the feeling, they can engage in a substitute behavior to divert attention (see Chapter eleven).

6. Supervising children. If a child with abusive sexual behaviors is to remain in the home with other siblings, all elements of supervision of the children in the home are discussed in detail.

If there are vulnerable children in the neighborhood, and the child who molests is to remain in the home, very detailed plans are made in this session for managing the behaviors, supervision, and the safety of all vulnerable children. The child who molests must not be isolated as "bad"; instead the emphasis is more that the child is manifesting some of the problems in the family (Johnson, 1991a).

7. Reporting sexual behaviors. A plan can be made regarding family members reporting any sexual behaviors of the child and to whom the behaviors should be reported.

All plans should be clear and explicit. Parents and children can brainstorm together to develop them. It often helps for the entire plan to be written down. This is as much to help the children as the parents. This plan will be updated, and any necessary modifications made throughout the course of the treatment.

Areas that will be the initial goals of treatment are elaborated. All family members are encouraged to ask questions at this time. After discussion, the parents and treatment providers should agree on a plan for the child and family. Commitments should be sought for adherence to the plan.

Report Writing

Evaluations may be requested by Protective Services or the Courts. Reports should include information regarding children's history and current functioning; sexual behaviors, including seriousness and risk of further occurences; family dynamics, and the child's relationship with family members (Haverbush, 1992). Reports also should include the following information:

Background and current functioning of the child and family. The evaluator provides information on past or current alcohol and drug use; incarcerations; physical, sexual, and emotional abuse; neglect or abandonment; and describes the home environment. In addition, information is given on children's past and current functioning in the home, school, and community, including aggressive, oppositional, or conduct disorders. Children's medical history, special needs or disabilities, and/or DSM III-R diagnosis are provided.

Incident that brought the child to the attention of the system. The evaluator provides a description of the current incident in the context of the child's previous sexual behaviors, describing the use of force, coercion, bribery, or trickery. In addition, the evaluator lists the number of children victimized by the child who molests and their relationship to each other; in sibling incest cases, information is included on the children's relationship to each other, and to their parents.

Parental responses. The evaluator discusses the parents' cooperation and whether or not they understand the seriousness of their child's molesting behavior. In addition, in sibling abuse cases, the parents' ability and willingness to protect the child-victim, and cooperate with the treatment plan for their children is noted.

Areas of strength and concern for children and their family. The evaluator documents areas of strength in the children and other family members, as well as concerns which may foster or sustain children's maladaptive behaviors.

Summary and recommendations. This section contains a brief summary of findings, and the evaluator offers specific recommendations based on the clinical evaluation.

Summary

Evaluating children with problematic sexual behaviors requires careful attention to preliminary information gathering, deciding who is interviewed and when, the interviews themselves, and developing a treatment plan.

Clinicians should gather all available information regarding children's general and problematic behaviors before the evaluation. This data comes from protective services, police, foster or group home providers, mental health professionals, and children's caretakers if they are currently living outside their homes. Children's natural parents should be interviewed and provided treatment services if reunification is planned. Other adults who live in the home provide valuable information on the functioning of the child. The clinician must pay special attention to existing family characteristics or environmental factors that may foster or sustain problematic sexual behaviors in children.

Clinicians are encouraged to interview all children in the family before interviewing children with problematic sexual behaviors. When interviewing the child with problematic sexual behaviors, the interview is detailed and specific to sexuality as well as other areas of the child's life.

After interviewing everyone, the clinician determines the group membership of the child, distressed areas of the child's development, and risk factors, in order to formulate a treatment plan for the child and his or her family. A treatment plan includes generating placement alternatives if children with problematic sexual behaviors cannot remain in the home, and suitable medical, educational, and therapy interventions for children and their family.

References

Abel, G. G., Becker, J., Cunningham-Rather, J., Rouleau, J., Kaplan, M., & Reich, J. (1984). *Treatment of child molesters: A manual.* New York State Psychiatric Institute. Unpublished manuscript.

Achenbach, T. M. (1983). *Manual for the child behavior checklist.* Burlington: University of Vermont.

Becker, J. (1992). Profile. *Violence Update* May:3–7.

Becker, J. V., Cunningham-Rathner, J., & Kaplan, M. (1987). Adolescent sexual offenders: Demographics, criminal and sexual histories, and recommendations for reducing future offenses. *Journal of Interpersonal Violence* 4:431–445.

Burgess, A., Haxelwood, R., & Rokous, F. (1987). *Serial rapists and their victims: Reenactment and repetition.* In New York Academy of Sciences Conference on Human Sexual Aggression: Current Perspectives. New York.

Egeland, B. (1988). Breaking the cycle of abuse: Implications for prediction and intervention. In K. D. Browne, C. Davies, & P. Stratton (Eds.), *Early prediction and prevention of child abuse.* New York: J. Wiley and Sons.

Friedrich, W. (1990). Evaluating the child and planning for treatment. In W. Friedrich *Psychotherapy of sexually abused children and their families.* New York: W. W. Norton.

Friedrich, W. (1991). Sexual behavior in sexually abused children. In J. Briere (Ed.), *Treating victims of child sexual Abuse* . New York: Jossey-Bass.

Friedrich, W., Beilke, R., & Urquiza, A. (1988). Behavior problems in young sexually abused boys. *Journal of Interpersonal Violence* 3(1): 21–27.

Friedrich, W., Grambsch, P., Damon, L., Koverola, C., Hewitt, S., Lang, R., & Wolfe, V. (1992). The Child Sexual Behavior Inventory: Normative and clinical comparisons. *Psychological Assessment* 4(3): 303–311.

Friedrich, W., & Luecke, W. (1988). Young school-age sexually aggressive children. *Professional Psychology Research and Practice* 19(2): 155–164.

Garbarino, J., & Stott, F. M. (1989). *What children can tell us.* San Francisco: Jossey-Bass.

Gilgun, J. (1991). Resilience and the intergenerational transmission of child abuse. In M. Patton (Eds.), *Family sexual abuse: Frontline research and evaluation.* Newbury Park, CA: Sage.

Groth, N. A. (1989). *Anatomical drawings.* Dunedin, FL: Forensic Mental Health Associates.

Haverbush, D. (1992). *Sexual offender assessment report guidelines.* Toledo, OH: Lucas County Juvenile Court.

Hoorwitz, A. N. (1992). *The clinical detective: Techniques in the evaluation of sexual abuse.* New York: W. W. Norton.

Johnson, T. C. (1988). Child perpetrators—children who molest other children: Preliminary findings. *Child Abuse and Neglect* 12:219-229.

Johnson, T. (1989a). *Curriculum in human sexuality for parents and children in troubled families.* Los Angeles: Children's Institute International.

Johnson, T. C. (1989b). Female child perpetrators: children who molest other children. *Child Abuse and Neglect* 13(4): 571-585.

Johnson, T. C. (1990). (Manuscript). Commonalities in sibling incest cases when the perptrators are boys younger than thirteen.

Johnson, T. C. (1991a). Children who molest: Identification and treatment approaches for children who molest other children. *The Advisor* 4(4): 9-11.

Johnson, T. C. (1991b). Understanding the sexual behaviors of young children. *SIECUS Report* (August/September).

Johnson, T. C. (1992). Child sexual behavior checklist revised. Unpublished.

Jones, D. P. H., & McQuiston, M. (1988). *Interviewing the sexually abused child.* London: Gaskell Psychiatry Series.

Longo, R. E. (1982). Sexual learning and experience among adolescent sex offenders. *International Journal of Offender Therapy and Comparative Criminology* 26(3): 235-241.

Madison, A. (1978). *Suicide and young people.* New York: Houghton Mifflin.

McGoldrick, M., & Gerson, R. (1985). *Genograms in family assessment.* New York: W. W. Norton.

Orbach, I. (1988). *Children who don't want to live.* San Francisco: Jossey-Bass.

Prentky, R., Knight, R., Sims-Knight, J., Straus, H., Rokous, F., & Cerce, D. (1989). Developmental antecedants of sexual aggression. *Development and Psychopathology* 1:153-169.

Wolf, S. C. (1985). A multi-factor model of deviant sexuality. *Victimology* 10:359-374.

10

Individual Therapy

Eliana Gil, Ph.D.

Rationale for Individual Treatment

Children with problematic sexualized behaviors or children who molest exhibit compulsive, disinhibited, and persistent sexual behaviors that elicit concern from adults in caretaking positions. Some children with sexualized behaviors "grow out" of problematic behaviors, respond to limit-setting from their parents, develop more appropriate ways of exploring their sexuality, and learn to use their own internal controls to curtail their disruptive behaviors. When clinical assessments indicate that children's sexualized behaviors are out of the range of age-appropriate sexual interest or behavior, remain unresponsive to specific limits to decrease the behaviors, or gradually progress to molesting behaviors, professional interventions become necessary.

It appears that the most effective treatment plan for children with sexual acting-out may be consistent with the treatment provided to older children, adolescents, and adults who commit sexual offenses—that is, a combination of individual, group, and family treatment, with group therapy the pivotal component of effective treatment. In working with adolescent sex offenders and younger children who molest, family therapy is a close second in value and importance. Family assessment and treatment have been found to be critical components of working with adolescent sex offenders (Ryan, 1991; Thomas, 1991), and may even have greater importance for the younger child in treatment for problematic sexual behaviors.

Another treatment model with implications for the treatment of children who molest is the approach used with children with conduct disorders. Kernberg and Chazan (1991) assert that "No one perspective is sufficient to account for the diversity of constitutional, family, intrapsychic, interpersonal and cultural factors that produce and perpetuate this disorder." They recommend a combination of individual supportive-expressive play therapy, parent training, and play group therapy. This is the core of the treatment model proposed in this chapter. (It is interesting to note that most children who molest are diagnosed as conduct-disordered children.)

The younger the children who molest, the more dependent they are on the family for supervision, limit-setting, and guidance. The younger child's family yields more influence on the child; peers play a greater role as children enter a child-care (preschool) program or a school setting. Young children's sexual acting-out behavior is likely to be more closely related to family dynamics, at times a literal reflection of the behavior of family members. Specific family dynamics (e.g., overt or covert abuse) may elicit or exacerbate the child's sexual acting-out. The clinician's access to the family of children who molest is critical to the success of treatment, since the children's behaviors do not occur in a vacuum.

Individual therapy serves specific purposes within the overall treatment plan. Children with sexualized behaviors that do not involve other children are best treated in individual or family therapy. As discussed in Chapter six, many of the behaviors of sexualized children may decrease by providing the parents with education about age-appropriate sexuality for their children and teaching them the skills to set appropriate limits when necessary. Some sexualized behaviors may have been learned by children through exposure to overstimulating and explicit sexual information such as witnessing sexual intercourse, pornographic videos or pictures, and so on. In addition, some children develop sexualized behaviors as a result of their own victimization (overt sexual abuse) in or out of their families, or through covert abuse in the home. Clinicians design services based on these factors and may need to take specific action (e.g., file reports of suspected child abuse, treat the family to stop covert abuse, recommend the child's removal from the home when the family is unresponsive and children's needs are not met) or children continue to be exposed to inappropriate and overstimulating sexual stimuli. Children's sexualized behavior can decrease gradually if parents follow clinical directives, remove inappropriate stimuli and receive treatment as warranted. Children with sexualized behaviors that reflect prior victimization respond well to individual therapy or group therapy for victimized children. (Placing sexualized children in groups with children who molest is contraindicated.)

Children who molest seem to benefit greatly from group therapy. Clinicians have a unique opportunity to make interventions with inappropriate behaviors as they occur. Often children who molest are stimulated to act out sexually in the presence of other children and the group setting provides an opportunity for needed clinical interventions.

Individual therapy is also beneficial in a number of ways. The individual therapist prepares the child for group, addresses specific concerns that arise in group therapy, and provides a safe therapeutic environment for children who cannot be treated within a group context. In addition, because the children's molesting behaviors often serve as red flags for possible prior victimization or underlying psychological concerns, an individual therapist may provide more in-depth or long-term work on other issues that may surface as the acting-out subsides.

Criteria for Providing Individual Therapy

Friedrich (1990) finds that individual therapy for abused children is most likely to be effective when: "(1) ongoing support of the child is provided by a primary parent figure; (2) a sense of safety has been or is being established for the child to protect against future victimization; (3) the therapy with the child is occurring concurrently with therapy that is creating systems change and the nonabusing parent is having regular contact with the therapist; (4) the therapist is skillful, goal-oriented, conceptually clear, and willing to be directive in a supportive manner, and (5) the child is able to communicate regarding the abuse and can tolerate the intensity of the therapy process" (p. 132). When individual therapy is provided to sexualized children or children who molest, these criteria apply. In addition, parents or caretakers must provide a sense of safety for children who molest by carefully monitoring their problematic sexual behaviors, ensuring that other children are not victimized. Parents must exhibit a willingness and an ability to recognize the problematic aspects of their children's sexual behaviors, as well as follow the therapists' clear directives. If children who molest are living out of the home, therapists must provide caretakers with suggestions about addressing their problematic behaviors in that setting. Clinicians should make every effort to develop or refer children who molest to group therapy. Often, therapists can start smaller groups with two or three of their own clients, if larger groups are not available.

General Treatment Issues in Working with Abused Children

Clinicians who provide services to children who molest, and sexualized children, need to have a foundation in general treatment principles with abused children. In recent years, abused and neglected children have been the focus of many research studies. As a result, the impact of abuse on children's emotional and psychological well-being is better understood.

Many studies have been scrutinized for methodological problems, and critics encourage researchers to both refine their methods and better define their samples by ethnicity, age, type of abuse, the use of control groups, and so on. At the same time, much of the available data seems reliably consistent and presents an overview of the types of emotional difficulties experienced to one degree or another by most child-victims of abuse. Hibbard and Hartman (1992) note that sexually abused children are generally more symptomatic than nonabused comparison subjects and appear depressed and unhappy, moody, aggressive, demand attention, exhibit strange behaviors, do poorly in school, have trouble sleeping, worry, and are secretive. In addition, Hibbard and Hartman note that several behavioral problems can serve as indicators of sexual abuse including eating disturbances, fears and phobias, antisocial behavior, sexual behavior problems, anxiety, somatic complaints, and low self-esteem. Several studies have established that sexually abused children have more sexual behaviors than neglected, physically abused, or psychiatrically disturbed children (MacVicar, 1979; Friedrich et al., 1988; White et al., 1988). Walker and co-workers (1988) specify that children with significant traumatic sexualization are likely to have distorted views of sexual norms, sexual identity confusion, sexual aggression, heightened sensitivity to sexual issues, and associate highly negative feelings with any sexual activity or arousal. Finkelhor and Browne (1986) and Marvasti (1989) describe the merging of affection and sex resulting in confusion between caregetting and caregiving and sexuality. Physically abused children frequently exhibit low self-esteem, withdrawal, oppositional and aggressive behavior, hypervigilance, compulsivity, impaired socialization skills, defensive responses, learned helplessness, and pseudomature behavior (Martin, 1976; Kent, 1980; Reidy, 1980). Neglected and psychologically abused children often have feelings of deprivation, affect inhibition, emotional disturbances, anxious attachments, self-destructive behaviors, fear and distrust, behavioral problems, and impaired ability to empathize (Polansky et al., 1981; Garbarino et al., 1986). As a result, abused and neglected children often have developmental delays and learning difficulties.

In recent years, several authors have contributed their clinical expertise and experience by outlining critical treatment issues for traumatized or abused children (James, 1989; Donovan & McIntyre, 1990; Friedrich, 1990, 1991; Terr, 1990; Gil, 1991). Although these books are different in scope and perspective, they have striking similarities in their view of hurt and injured children. The authors agree that children must undergo a reparative process that strengthens their sense of self, mastery, feelings of increased control, trust, ability to attach, and hopefulness for the future. In addition, because traumatized children develop psychological defenses that often serve to compartmentalize the injuries and their associated thoughts, feelings, and perceptions, clinicians must be able to assess and treat dissociated states, including multiplicity. It appears that although young injured children require, deserve, and benefit from a therapeutic experience, some of the work must be "abuse-specific" or directed at the resolution of the trauma. Since unresolved traumas can contribute to symptomatic and acting-out behavior reminiscent of the trauma, these issues become particularly relevant in the overall treatment of children who molest, or children with problematic sexual behaviors.

Lane (1991) states: "Ultimately however, defining causation is secondary to the needs of the perpetrating child." I believe that in most cases, causation is primary to establishing a treatment plan that has long-lasting effects. Although therapy for children who molest must initially focus on their unacceptable behavior, attempting to change behavior without a clear idea of the cause of children's behavior (i.e., the meaning and purpose it may serve) may result in (1) temporary changes that are susceptible to acute or chronic stress, (2) lowering of defenses and the emergence of repressed memories that cause persistent relapses, (3) revictimization, or (4) other situations or sensory-motor stimuli that elicit the emergence of fragmented memories causing an increased sense of helplessness. In other words, the special behaviors of children who molest must be *decoded* so the treatment is comprehensive and addresses not only behavior but underlying causes, as well as children's initial and maintained (internal and external) motivators.

Special Therapy Issues in Working with Abused Children and Children Who Molest

Dissociation

The therapist who is unfamiliar with both normative and pathological dissociation is at significant disadvantage in work with all patients, but especially with children. Dissociative phenomena are so pervasive in childhood as to be normative. As such, they are part and parcel of a world the therapist must understand and be able to manipulate.

Denis M. Donovan and Deborah McIntyre

Dissociation is a defense mechanism that allows the individual to protect against harm by splitting the emotional self from the physical self.

The DSM III-R (American Psychiatric Association, 1987) defines dissociation as "a disturbance or alteration in the normally integrative functions of identity, memory and consciousness." Dissociative states occur along a continuum: normal dissociation occurs during periods of boredom, fatigue, or while performing routine tasks (e.g., automatism or "highway hypnosis"). An individual can also have dissociative episodes in situations of extreme stress, or during trauma with its induced feelings of helplessness and instinctual arousal. More severe forms of dissociation include fugue states (physical flight without memory), depersonalization (losing the feeling of reality), or psychogenic amnesia (losing memory for specific periods or events). The most extreme form of dissociation is multiplicity, in which at least two discrete personality states exist, with one personality state taking executive control of the person's behavior.

Abused children often report feelings of depersonalization and psychogenic amnesia for prior events. They may be observed to "space out," staring into space for periods of time. Children who dissociate may not remember what has occurred; this is particularly relevant because entire therapy sessions may be forgotten, and children may be unable to remember their own victimization or victimizing others (during dissociated states). Gil (1991) discusses the need to address dissociation with children who are clients by developing a language for it, talking about when it is and is not helpful, identifying times when children would rather not dissociate, helping them to learn about their own unique way of dissociating, understanding patterns and early cues for dissociation, and then learning what to do instead. Children often view this as a game, particularly when the clinician asks them to "pretend" to dissociate, and children learn how to continue or interrupt their ability to dissociate. The goal with child and adult clients who dissociate is to help them feel more control over where and when they dissociate. In this way, a clinician can help children maximize their experience in therapy.

Dissociation is relevant in the treatment of children because it's important to recognize when children are dissociating in individual and group treatment, since they will be unable to hear, understand, and process what is being discussed. Children who dissociate typically have difficulties remembering previous therapy discussions. In addition, children who dissociate can develop pervasive feelings of depersonalization and although they may not necessarily report discomfort, they may develop problematic symptoms in order to cope with the condition. For example, one eight-year-old abused and abusing child, cut his arms to see his blood. Once he saw the blood he felt human again since his depersonalized state led him to expect that he had wires like robots do, inside his body. Self-injury became the symptom that alerted me to his concern with depersonalization.

Multiplicity

The most extreme form of dissociation is multiplicity (or Multiple Personality Disorder). Multiplicity is usually diagnosed in adults, but it originates during childhood, usually under the age of six. A group of clinicians (including Richard Kluft, Frank Putnam, Gary Peterson, Pamela Reagor, J. Fagan, and P. McMahon) have highlighted the need for enhanced skills in the assessment and treatment of childhood multiplicity. Since the correlation between severe child sexual abuse and multiplicity is indisputable (Putnam, 1989), it behooves any clinician working with children with histories of severe and chronic abuse (including children who molest) to have a clear understanding of this phenomenon. Clinicians wishing to become better informed on dissociative disorders and multiplicity, can subscribe to a cutting-edge publication entitled *Dissociation*.[1] Two recent articles (Reagor et al., 1992; Kluft, 1992) as well as prior articles (Peterson, 1990, 1991) discuss this important issue.

Post-Traumatic Stress Symptoms

The symptoms of post-traumatic stress vary by individual and can include intrusive flashbacks, emotionality, explosive outbursts often followed by numbing, nightmares, and physical sensations. The classic feature of post-traumatic stress is that the individual can feel disoriented and remain unaware of the precipitating original traumatic event. Individuals with post-traumatic stress often feel the intensity of the original trauma, at times without having any clear memory. For example, one of my child clients hyperventilated when she smelled alcohol, without realizing that the man who had raped her was very drunk when he committed his crime.

I often explain Post-Traumatic Stress Disorder in the following way: For children (and for many adults as well) traumatic experiences are too

---

1. *Dissociation* is the official Journal of the International Society for the Study of Multiple Personality Disorder, c/o Ridgeview Institute, 3995 So. Cobb Dr., Smyrna, GA   30080-6397

overwhelming to be integrated in any cohesive manner. This is particularly true for children who are limited in their cognitive, emotional, and physical strength and abilities. Traumatized children therefore absorb the trauma in a fragmented way. As a metaphor, imagine a mirror that has shattered into many small fragments, yet the fragments remain glued to the backing. Each small piece, or fragment, is one separate yet connected piece of the mirror. Children who integrate an experience in shattered pieces may find that the separate pieces, or fragments, contain one element of the experience. One fragment may contain perceptions, the other smells, the other physical sensations, the other sounds, and so on. These separate yet connected fragments can remain repressed in this fashion for years: it's as if they are frozen in time and place. And yet the little fragments can dislodge and surface into consciousness, causing great concern for the individual. For example, if one of the fragments contains the physical sensation of pain, an individual can suddenly feel stinging and pain across the face, as if he or she has just been slapped. At the same time, the person may feel startled, unaware of any current events that could account for the sudden painful feelings. The detailed treatment of Post-Traumatic Stress Disorder (PTSD) is beyond the scope of this book and is discussed in greater depth in other writings (see, e.g., Van der Kolk, 1984; Eth and Pynoos, 1985; Figley, 1985, 1986). When working with children who may be more perplexed and frightened by their symptoms, it is important to educate them that the symptoms are the body's way of remembering and offering information. The puzzle-piece metaphor may be helpful. Clinicians can instruct clients to write down the various things they feel or think or see and bring them to therapy for discussion.

Assessing and responding to symptoms of post-traumatic stress is important in working with children who molest, because PTSD surface randomly and acutely, keeping children in the emotional climate of their past trauma and often producing increased feelings of helplessness and vulnerability. These feelings may in turn propel children to act in aggressive and inappropriate ways. Acting-out behavior is therefore the manifestation of unresolved traumatic experiences (unconscious reenactments) and begs for attention, not only to the problematic behavior that must stop, but also to the chronic underlying distress of an unassimilated trauma that must be processed. To direct most or all therapeutic services to changing the child's behavior while ignoring or minimizing nightmares, flashbacks, emotionality, or other symptoms of trauma-related stress is a great disservice to the child and counterproductive to instituting long-lasting changes. A nine-year-old girl who was abused by her father and adolescent brother, molested her two younger brothers. She was an intelligent child who understood why it was important for her to stop molesting her siblings. She would often verbalize her strong urge to molest whenever she had intrusive flashbacks of her own abuse. "I hate what they did to me. I hate what they did to me," she yelled, "And I don't care if it hurts them when I do it, I don't care if it hurts them!" In this particular case, the treatment focused equally on her molesting behaviors and her post-traumatic symptoms, which reinforced her feelings of helplessness and elicited angry responses toward her two younger brothers. In addition, the parent's cooperation was pivotal to making sure this child could remain safely in her home without victimizing others or being revictimized.

Unconscious Reenactments

This has been discussed in the previous section and yet can be illustrated through the following examples. A teenage girl was brought to therapy by her mother because she was being beaten up by her boyfriend on a regular basis. This teenage girl had been physically abused during early childhood by an alcoholic father who was now deceased. This child had learned the lessons of violence too well. In our initial meeting, she quietly asserted, "My mom is exaggerating. Doug just gets mad sometimes. He doesn't mean anything by it; he really does love me, and he's always sorry when he gets carried away. My mom is making a big deal out of nothing." When I asked her a few more questions about Doug, she offered, "He's not weird or anything, he's just a guy, you know, they get mad sometimes."

This teenager had learned firsthand that love and violence go hand in glove. She expected and tolerated violence as being "part of the territory," in an intimate relationship. She was not seeking out violence, but unfortunately, she unconsciously selected a mate who shared her beliefs and behaved in a manner consistent with what she knew. She experienced a certain comfort in the familiarity of a violent man, and she unconsciously contributed to reenacting a pattern from her past. In addition, this teenager had already solidified certain beliefs about her self-worth that negated any external messages that she "deserved" better.

The early lessons of abuse that become so well integrated and help shape the abused individual's self-perception and expectations contribute to the development of behavioral scenarios that replicate that individual's past experience. That is why it has become so commonplace to find that adult survivors of abuse frequently interact with others in the position of victim, perpetrator, or rescuer. These three roles are the guideposts learned during early abuse experiences. That is not to say that all abused children grow up to be either abusers or victims. Many abused children alter their interactions as a result of safe, corrective experiences or personality differences that allow them to fend off the negative impacts of abuse. Anthony and Cohler (1987) have studied "invulnerable" children who appear more stress resistant to the potential negative impact of abuse.

"Forgotten" Behaviors

Donovan and McIntyre (1990) did a great service when they emphasized the normative dissociative abilities in young children. "Any observant adult has seen normative dissociation in children, such as alterations in consciousness (daydreaming, tuning out) or sense of self: 'No, I didn't eat those cookies,' replies the adamant five-year-old whose face is still covered with crumbs. To appreciate the dissociative nature of the child's response, it must be understood that, at that very moment of denial, he neither remembers that he ate the cookie nor tastes the cookie still in his mouth." Although normative dissociative experiences in young children have not been routinely studied, Putnam (1989) has found that adolescents receive a "relatively high median total" using the Dissociative Experiences Scale developed by Bernstein and Putnam in 1986. (Putnam and his colleagues have recently developed a Child Dissociative Checklist.) Donovan and McIntyre discuss the fact that most children do not complain about dissociative responses and may be unaware they use them. In addition, they state that "It takes a certain affective and cognitive maturity to be able to experience depersonalization as unpleasant," and they can "forget entire episodes or periods," and "access memory or produce information at one time or in one setting, and not at another time or in another setting." These factors become germane in the treatment of children who molest, in that their denials of either prior victimization or current molesting behaviors may be less overt lies and more typical (normative) loss of memory from dissociative responses. Clinicians are advised therefore to offer children diversity and opportunity to access memory. Children who molest may be forthcoming about their molesting behaviors with an individual therapist and not within a group setting, or vice versa. Once children do access memory or provide information about molesting, the information should be documented and stored so that children can be reminded or helped to remember from time to time. In this way, fragmented pieces of information can be strongly assimilated into memory so clinicians can undertake the work of processing the associated feelings and thoughts.

Self-Injury

Most of the available literature on this subject discusses self-injury in adults and adolescents (Walsh & Rosen, 1988). However, in studying the histories of self-mutilators, Walsh and Rosen point out that "The profile that emerged was that the childhood experiences of the self-mutilators were replete with dysfunction and psychopathology. . . . Mutilators were significantly more likely to have experienced losses during childhood through placements outside the family and through divorce. . . . They were also found to have been victimized both physically and sexually, and to have repeatedly witnessed violence, impulsivity, and alcohol abuse" (p. 66). Children who molest may be victims of physical and sexual abuse and may come from dysfunctional families. They are susceptible to self-injury, which may be underdiagnosed in childhood because it is not often evaluated. Clinicians are much more likely to talk to adolescents than young children about self-injury. Likewise, the scars of adolescents may elicit inquiry, whereas the scars of young children may be relegated to the category of "normal" childhood accidents through activity.

As previously mentioned, children may be less likely to self-report discomfort with feelings of depersonalization. However, in my experience children may self-injure in an effort to recover from dissociative experience by feeling pain, or may inflict injury to attest to their humanity (thereby blocking feelings of derealization). Although young children may not approach self-injury with cognitive understanding, they may obtain affective relief that encourages repetition.

Assessment Issues

The first stage of effective treatment is rigorous assessment of the child. During assessment the clinician remains active, evaluating physical functioning, pattern of relationships, overall mood or tone, affect, anxieties and fears, and thematic expression (Greenspan, 1981). Assessment issues are addressed in Chapter nine and can also include the special issues preceding this section.

Goals of Individual Treatment

The treatment of children who molest needs to be abuse-focused. Berliner and Rawlings (1991) say that "Evidence suggests that generic victimization treatment approaches may not be effective for sexual behavior problems" (p. 4). Cunningham and MacFarlane find that "Because abuse-reactive children are often initially impulsive, angry, and highly anxious, traditional therapeutic methods are usually difficult to apply" (p. 17). The treatment of children who molest needs to be developmentally specific, individually tailored, and directed at both behavioral change and the relief of underlying concerns.

Once the initial assessment is complete, the clinician develops a treatment plan with clear behavioral goals, which is reviewed periodically. The clinician decides the treatment modality that best addresses the goals for each child. Children may be referred for individual and group therapy, or may enter individual therapy to prepare them to attend group therapy. As the treatment progresses, conjoint family therapy sessions with the children is useful. Family therapy sessions always precede the child's termination from therapy. The goals of individual therapy include primary (offense-related) and secondary (general) goals.

Primary Goals of Individual Therapy

Establishing a Working Therapeutic Relationship with Children

The first step in therapy is to make emotional contact with the child. Children do not seek therapy for themselves, and frequently view coming to therapy as disruptive to their schedules, frightening, or as a form of punishment. Parents may have threatened the children with therapy, warning them that if their behavior does not improve, visiting a therapist is inevitable. Children who come to see a therapist may feel resistant, fearful, ashamed, or defiant.

Therapists must convey interest in the child and offer the therapy hour as a nonthreatening, even pleasant, experience that children may grow to like or find helpful.

The most user-friendly environment is chosen. If the clinician has a separate child therapy office, the parents, child, and clinician can meet there. If the clinician keeps toys in the office or has a nook in the office for play therapy, the meeting can be held in that setting.

The therapist explains his or her role and the process of therapy, in a simple and clear fashion. Specifically, a therapist meeting with a child with sexual acting-out behavior must communicate that the problem behavior will be addressed in a variety of different ways. With the child present, the clinician asks the parent why the child has been brought to therapy, and what the child has been told about coming to the first visit. (This meeting occurs after a data-gathering session with parents or caretakers in which a complete psychosocial history is taken, as well as a comprehensive view of the child's sexual acting-out behavior, the settings in which it occurs, the children with whom it occurs, by whom it is observed, typical responses to the behavior, and any significant events occurring before the emergence of the observed problem behavior. (See Chapter nine.)

During this initial meeting with the parent and child, the clinician pinpoints language that will be used throughout the therapy to describe the child's sexual acting-out. For example, if the parent states that the child has been humping other children, it's important to ask the child what he or she calls what the parent describes. A child may use the word "rubbing" or "touching" to describe the sexual behavior. Then the clinician can set the stage: "When you come to therapy, you and I will talk together, and you can play with toys in the playroom. I talk to lots of children about their thoughts and feelings about mom and dad, brothers and sisters, teachers, baby-sitters, and all kinds of things. Something we'll be sure to talk about is your rubbing problem."

It's important to ask both the parent and child in what way the child's sexual acting-out is a problem to them. A child can be asked, "Tell me two things you don't like about the touching problem and two things you do like about it." If either parent or child gives any responses that imply confusion, the clinician can use this as an opportunity to do some gentle educating. One six-year-old child was referred to treatment because he regularly approached younger children and offered to suck their penises if they paid him. When I asked him the things he liked about sucking penises, he said, "I like sucking penis because I get $1.00 just for me." I said, "A whole dollar is a lot of money. I can see how you might like getting money. It's still not okay to suck someone's penis, even if you get money for doing it." The child persisted, "But Melvin says he likes it and it makes him feel real good." "Yeap," I responded, "sometimes kids will tell you it feels good to them, but even then it's still not okay to do. He is wrong to ask you to suck his penis and pay you to do it. You need to be real sure that you know that sucking penises is not okay to do." "How come it's not okay?" this child asked time and time again. "You can't suck penises," I would respond, "because it's a rule." The younger the child, the fewer explanations needed.

When I asked this child what he didn't like about sucking penises, he said, "When Melvin's friends hold me down so Melvin does it to me. That's gross, and I don't like it and they don't pay me nothing!" This child who was referred for his molesting behaviors had been physically forced down by three other boys and orally copulated himself. I called child protective services to report suspected abuse and their investigation revealed a small group of children who were sexually abusing younger children in the neighborhood.

Assessing Children's Readiness
and Preparing Them for Group Therapy

Clinicians must assess children's readiness for group, offering a context in which children can understand the group experience (see Chapter eleven). Most children are able to participate in a small group with peers; children frequently enjoy meeting with other children their own age. However, for some children the group experience may not be beneficial, or may be disruptive for the rest of the group members. In order to determine whether children are ready for referral to group therapy, clinicians must determine children's ability to do the following:

1. Follow group rules and respond to limits in an appropriate way
2. Moderate their own affect (some children become overstimulated by peers, and their affect becomes agitated and uncontrollable, blocking their ability to learn and distracting others from the tasks at hand)
3. Listen and understand
4. Follow directives
5. Relate to peers
6. Participate in group activities

These issues can be difficult for children with developmental disabilities, severe depression, learning disabilities (particularly Attention Deficit Disorder), conduct disorders, difficulties in attachment (Bowlby, 1973), or children with sociopathic tendencies. In addition, there are some children for whom the presence of other children is so anxiety provoking that they become unable to moderate their own affect or control their behavior. In these extreme and aroused states, children are not able to integrate the lessons being taught in group.

In addition to screening out children who cannot tolerate the group experience for a variety of reasons, clinicians must also be certain that children are sufficiently prepared to use the group process. Particularly because group therapy will focus on offending behaviors, sexuality, and possible victimization, children must be ready to acknowledge their problematic behaviors, and demonstrate at the very least a willingness to listen to, or participate in, group lessons and activities. Children who attend group benefit greatly from an opportunity to describe their offending behaviors or the ways in which they were victimized. This material is best addressed in a clear and specific manner in group, and it is highly useful if children understand the special focus of the group beforehand. The clinician can describe the group to the child and his family in the following way: "You'll be coming on Tuesday afternoons to meet with me, [the cotherapist], and five other boys [or girls][2] your age. You and the other children have some things in common—you're all boys, you're all about eight years old, and you've all had a problem with touching other children in a way that's not okay. We're going to meet together and talk about the [touching] problem and figure out ways to help you stop doing that." When applicable, the therapist adds, "When you come to group, your mom and/or dad will talk to other moms and dads who all have children with touching problems." Clinicians need to respond to any questions children may have about the group process.

Obtaining Specificity About the Problem Sexual Behaviors

The clinician first obtains a description of the problematic sexual behaviors from the child's parents; it is equally important to obtain the child's description of "what happened" in the child's own language.

Often, people who have done something others consider "wrong" find it difficult to admit to the problematic behavior. Adults who commit sexual offenses characteristically deny them; even young children may exhibit tenacious denial in the face of clear evidence. Young children may be afraid of getting in trouble, may have forgotten what they did, or may want to be seen in a positive light.

In the initial phase of individual therapy, clinicians create an environment of safety and trust; denial is allowed for a brief period to avoid early power struggles counterproductive to rapport building. At the same time, the clinician can take the opportunity to make positive statements to the child.

Clinicians must take great care to avoid colluding with persistent denial. It may help to say to children, "Lots of kids have a hard time talking about their [touching, hitting, etc.] problem at first. You may be able to talk about

---

2. In my experience, it is easier and more effective to have same-sex groups for young children. Material on sexuality can cause undue excitement and embarrassment (causing distractions) even among young children in a group with opposite-sex members.

it more later. I'll bring it up from time to time while we're getting to know each other."

Obviously, the offense-specific work must be undertaken as soon as possible. When children have molested other children, discussing the problem behavior is imperative to prevent recurrences. When children have sexualized behaviors that don't involve other children, and they are not hurting themselves physically, the individual therapist (if one becomes necessary) has less urgency and can approach questioning children about sexualized behaviors a little at a time, or simply watch for the behaviors to occur in the therapy hour.

Art work is a good diagnostic tool with children. Their drawings can elicit a great deal of information about their identity, self-image, and a host of underlying concerns (Kaufman & Wohl, 1992). The clinician asks the child to draw a self-portrait and then reviews the drawing with the child. This drawing can later serve to obtain the names of genitals from the child. Most children call their genitals their "privates," and others have specific names they've heard their parents use. The question about whether or not anyone has touched the child's genitals can wait. The important first step is to identify the child's language for genitals.

Clinicians can also ask children to draw a picture of themselves doing something they like to do, and something they don't like to do. Depending on their age, children can be asked to draw a picture of the best and worst thing that ever happened to them.

Clinicians are advised to employ a variety of techniques designed to get children to communicate, verbally or nonverbally. One useful technique was developed by Sandra Ballester and Frederique Pierre and is available in a book entitled *A Matter of Control.* This technique of externalizing the problem behavior away from the client is used successfully by Michael White (1985).[3] Children are given the concept that the problem behavior

3. Michael White is a gifted family therapist from South Australia who with his colleagues has developed some exciting concepts with application to the treatment of child sexual abuse (see in particular, *Ideas for Therapy with Sexual Abuse* by Michael White and Cheryl White). His works are available through the Dulwich Centre Publications, Hutt Street, P.O. Box 7192, Adelaide, South Australia 5000.

has become a monster that has gained control over them. Children label the monster (e.g., the hitting monster, the touching monster) and attempt to gain control of it by recognizing when and how the monster surfaces, how it affects them and what they can do to get help so they are not left alone to fight the monster. This technique gives children the explicit message that it is the problem (or monster) behavior and not the child, that is "bad." In this manner, children can be placed in a position of learning to control the problem. This approach is based on cognitive behavioral theory, since it focuses on how children think about the problem, behavioral alternatives to the problem behavior, and finally, it helps children expand their coping repertoires to deal with whatever precipitating feelings may be contributing to the sexual acting-out.

Children who molest or who develop compulsive sexual activity often report that the behavior feels out of their control. One nine-year-old boy who compulsively pulled other boys' pants down to touch their penises said to me, "I want to stop but my brain keeps telling me to do it." The strategies they learn will enable them to use alternative responses when they hear their "brains" telling them what to do.

Clinicians can also use a game developed by Johnson, called Let's Talk about Touching, a therapeutic game for sexualized children and children who molest (see the Resources section), which gives children a way to face difficult issues while playing a card game. Because it is a game, children approach it willingly and playfully. In addition, Cunningham and MacFarlane wrote a book entitled *Steps to Healthy Touching* (see the Resources section), which teaches children lessons about touching problems and alternatives. This book is loosely based on the twelve-step self-help programs and uses a football game metaphor in which children advance ten yards with each completed lesson. The tools mentioned here (*A Matter of Control*, Let's Talk About Touching, and *Steps to Healthy Touching*) are valuable resources specifically designed for children who molest that can facilitate the child's open discussion of molesting behaviors and underlying issues.

Other techniques can also be useful in getting children to communicate about their molesting behaviors. For example, the clinician can tell the child what is already known about the problem behavior, and encourage the child to fill in the details. The clinician can take a one-down position and ask the child to correct or add as needed. For example: "Today I want to make sure I understand what kind of a touching [rubbing, etc.] problem you have. I'm just not sure. You don't have to tell me anything new, just tell me if I'm right or wrong." The clinician then relates the story. It is common for the child to jump in with corrections, additions, or deletions. The clinician can even ask the child to keep doing what he or she is doing (drawing, sculpting, etc.); the child collaborates while the clinician talks and writes down the information. Frequently, children feel important when the clinician writes down what they say—they may also like being in a position where they can correct an adult; note-taking is discontinued if it distracts the clinician or child, or if it detracts from giving the child adequate attention. Once children can talk about the specifics of the sexual acting-out behavior, clinicians develop a clear picture of the precipitating factors, the specifics of the offense, and risk factors; this information facilitates the formulation of an individually tailored treatment plan. The primary focus of early individual treatment is to form a therapeutic relationship that can serve as the foundation for addressing the offense-related behavior, as well as underlying concerns. Clinicians need to obtain as much information as possible about the circumstances leading up to, and following, the offense-related behavior of the child in treatment, always noting risk factors.

Obtaining Information About Risk Factors Across Settings

Risk factors are those circumstances or situations that may contribute to the recurrence of offense-related behavior. In young children, a number of factors may indicate a high risk for reoffending (see Chapter nine for additional risk-factors). These factors include the following:

1. The use of force, threat, or violence
2. A history of impulsive aggressive behavior
3. A history of victimization, which has remained untreated
4. Predatory, compulsive, and repetitive behavior
5. An unresponsive family in denial
6. Selection of multiple victims
7. Pervasive sexual behaviors across settings
8. Lack of remorse and refusal to stop the behaviors (e.g., "I'll do it when I want. I don't care what you say" or "You can't make me stop and you can't watch me all the time.")

The younger the child, the more critical the involvement of the parents and/or caretakers. If the parents are unwilling or unable to monitor the child's behaviors, or set necessary limits, the therapist's efforts will be compromised.

After the therapist takes a complete history from parents, caretakers, and the child or other children in the family, a list of risk factors can be developed for each child. For example, one seven-year-old who molested many children in the neighborhood was more likely to act out sexually when any of the following risk factors came into play:

1. He was unsupervised.
2. He played with smaller, younger boys.
3. His mother punished him.
4. His mother had sexual intercourse in the adjacent room while he was awake.
5. His mother and her boyfriend were nude in the child's presence.
6. He went to the school bathroom with other children.
7. He played unsupervised behind the school yard.
8. He walked home from school.

This child had to be supervised round the clock. He could not play with other children unsupervised, and could not be in his room alone with another child with the door closed. His mother was asked to cooperate by being dressed in front of him and limiting her sexual contact with boyfriends to times when he was not in the house, or times when it was certain that he was asleep. Because he had previously molested children in the school bathroom, the teacher was asked to have an adult accompany this child to the bathroom (after several requests to go to the bathroom resulted in his being accompanied by a teacher assistant, he no longer requested visits to the bathroom). In addition, during recess, he was supervised and could not play out of view from the yard monitor. Finally, his mother made arrangements for someone to drop him off and pick him up from school, and he was not allowed to walk home alone. In three months his acting-out behaviors decreased significantly, and were replaced by more appropriate and effective interactions with peers. This change was a result of his participation in individual and group therapy, teacher and parental monitoring, and his mother's behavioral changes regarding her sexuality.

Stopping the Molesting Behaviors

Obviously, stopping the molesting behaviors is the overriding goal of abuse-specific work, and yet the goals discussed previously must be met in order to be fully equipped with the knowledge and understanding to fulfill this goal. Lane (1991) directs great efforts toward "discouraging any belief that exerting power over others, sexually or nonsexually, helps them cope with their victimization experience." In Lane's program, children are taught that sex does not equal love, and clinicians help the children with any confusion they may have related to the eroticization of affection. Lane believes that as children are held accountable for their behavior, they are empowered by learning that there are choices about behavior. Berliner and Rawlings provide psychoeducational training regarding sexuality, teaching children acceptable sexual behavior, providing developmentally consistent sex education, establishing a system of consequences for misbehavior, clarifying values about appropriate sexual behavior, and teaching strategies for anticipating and controlling the desire to sexually misbehave. In addition, they offer specific exercises regarding relapse prevention and structured outlets for sexual feelings. (These program goals are not mutually exclusive, since many of the treatment goals of the programs described here overlap.) The primary difference in these programs (Lane, 1991; Berliner & Rawlings, 1991) may exist in their philosophical differences concerning how children who molest should be categorized. Berliner and Rawlings state, "These children, generally, are not conceptualized as offenders. In most cases the behaviors are learned responses to abusive experiences and deficits in the family and community environment rather than intentional criminal conduct" (p. 17). Lane believes, "It is important, however, that the lack of legal accountability not be extended in definition or belief into clinical practice. Given what has been learned from adults and adolescents it is predictable that the child perpetrator will repeat their sexually abusive behaviors and may develop ingrained patterns that support the continuation of those behaviors without appropriate intervention" (p. 300). Lane succinctly defines the goals of treatment with the child perpetrator: "The primary goals continue to be the development of understanding, control, and elimination of the sexually abusive behavior and its immediate antecedents; interruption and correction of cognitive distortions that support compensatory, power-based behaviors, cycle progressions, and sexually abusive behaviors; reduction of arousal and sexual interest that supports the sexual abuse behavior; development of social and coping skills and abilities that may preclude the compensatory aspects; and the development of an understanding of the consequences of the behavior to victims [empathy] and the offender [deterrence]" (pp. 304–305). Johnson focuses on these issues and others in Chapter eleven. Regardless of philosophical differences about how to label children who molest, treatment goals appear to be duplicated from program to program. Clinicians resound in agreement on the difficulty of the work. "The more typical course of psychotherapy with sexually aggressive young children," states Friedrich (1991) "is marked by pitfalls, premature termination and wranglings with the legal and social service delivery systems."

Assessing a History of Victimization or
Other Relevant Issues

Since many children who molest have a history of prior victimization (Johnson, 1988) or come from dysfunctional families (see Chapter seven), clinicians must assess for histories of prior abuse, neglect, or dysfunctional family dynamics (e.g., domestic violence, substance abuse) and keep in mind the impact of these painful and confusing experiences for the children.

Entering into dialogue about the child's offending behavior naturally leads to asking about the child's prior experience with the behavior. For example, clinicians can ask the following:

1. How did you learn about this kind of touching/rubbing?
2. Did you ever see anyone touch/rub this way?
3. Who did you see rub/touch this way?
4. Has anyone ever touched/rubbed you this way?

The clinician can use the child's self-portrait to remind him or her what names were given (by the child) to the different parts of the body. The clinician can then ask if anyone touched the child's genitals, and if so, the circumstances. It is certainly not unusual for young children to have their genitals touched during normal hygiene, during toilet-training, or during medical examinations. In addition, if children have developed topical rashes, parents may apply ointments to their genitals. Parents may also be instructed by medical personnel to use thermometers, insert suppositories, or give enemas—children often describe these procedures as painful or uncomfortable. Clinicians need to be cautious not to over- or underreact to the answers provided by children, simply asking "what was going on?" when mom or dad was rubbing their genitals. Sometimes children can offer additional explanations such as "I had a fever" or "Daddy put cream on my boo-boo." In one memorable case, the child explained that her uncle, who frequently baby-sat had "hurt her pee-pee," which alarmed her schoolteacher. When asked additional questions, she added that her uncle had put the "stingy medicine" on her vagina. It turned out that the child was being treated for a skin problem with a medication that had an initial stinging effect. When the child reported that her uncle had hurt her vagina, she was being accurate. When allowed to explain further, she clarified her meaning. If children describe inappropriate sexual touching by an adult, clinicians are advised to proceed slowly, giving the children an opportunity to present the information in a narrative form, reviewing any points needing clarification. Material has been written describing interview processes with small children (Jones & McQuiston, 1989; Faller, 1990; Hoorwitz, 1992).

If children have been victimized or traumatized, an assessment is valuable in order to determine the level of damage. All children who are abused develop coping strategies, defensive mechanisms, and idiosyncratic explanations of the event (Gil, 1991). In addition, most children who are abused have a series of problems that can be symptomatic of the difficulty caused by the abuse.

When determining the level of damage, clinicians assess thought processes, affect, memory, self-esteem, sense of safety and vulnerability, affect and attachment disorders, dissociative processes, and behavioral problems. In addition, clinicians can observe physical functioning, pattern of relationships, overall mood or tone, affect, anxieties and fears, and thematic expression (Greenspan, 1981).

Understanding Children's Perceptions of Family Dynamics

Another important reason to engage children in individual therapy is to assess their perceptions about their family, specifically to understand whether the children's needs are being met in the family, as well as the children's perceptions of family conflicts, methods of discipline, and other relevant family issues. Children are least likely to camouflage what is going on in the family and may be in the best position to report family dynamics without hesitation. Particularly when children are living within a dysfunctional family, adults may be less likely to self-report problem areas. However, information from children cannot take the place of a full family assessment with all family members.

Process Material Generated in Group

Individual therapy gives the clinician an opportunity to address and process relevant clinical material that surfaces within group therapy sessions. For example, if a child seems particularly distressed in the group, the clinician may address this issue in individual therapy, or bring it to the attention of the individual therapist (if different from the group therapist). The group therapist must first discuss with the child if information will be shared with another therapist. Children must feel certain that their confidentiality will be maintained, unless specific circumstances arise (e.g., child discloses abuse by parents or others, self-abuse, or abuse of others). Clinicians must always discuss necessary information-sharing with children, before talking to others.

Secondary Goals of Individual Therapy

Improving Children's Self-Concept and Self-Esteem

Abused children or children living in a dysfunctional family can suffer from an undefined or negative sense of self, and frequently regard the abuse or lack of nurturing as something that happens to them because they are inherently bad, worthless, or unlovable. It stands to reason that abused and neglected children have difficulty with self-image or find it hard to develop positive self-regard. Children gain their sense of identity from the significant people around them. It is the task of parents and caretakers to instill positive regard to children, highlighting their children's strengths, and encouraging their efforts. When parents or caretakers belittle, criticize, and sabotage children's efforts, they develop a negative self-image. Children who are not given encouragement and validation will doubt their own abilities and worth and become self-critical. Eventually, abused or neglected children behave according to the input they receive: they are afraid to engage in normal activities, they are reluctant to make efforts on their own behalf, and they criticize themselves before others have the chance.

During therapy, abused or neglected children need exposure to new and consistent feedback about themselves. At the same time, the clinician must begin positive or encouraging statements slowly, allowing the child to become comfortable with the new ideas. Abused children may feel uncomfortable and frightened by sudden positive attention; many abused children find abusive behaviors expectable and familiar, often eliciting the negative attention. Clinicians seeking to challenge distorted self-concepts of abused children need to proceed with caution, understanding that children must develop the ability to tolerate positive statements or behaviors. A positive statement by a clinician is best followed by an inquiry about the child's thoughts, feelings, and reactions to the validating statement.

Abused or neglected children frequently integrate negative statements from parents or caretakers by engaging in critical self-talking. Clinicians can ask children to verbalize "What kinds of things do you say to yourself the most?" Sometimes children may actually make these negative or critical statements out loud. The clinician can offer an alternative statement. For example, a seven-year-old who said, "You're a total stupid" every time she dropped something, or colored outside the lines, or made any minor mistake was surprised when I said, "You're doing a good job. You're not stupid. Everyone makes mistakes. Mistakes are how we learn." After three months of weekly sessions, she stopped after she made a mistake and said, "Oh, oh,

I made a mistake again. That's okay, I'll try again." This intervention had been most effective because the foster parent also made the same intervention at home, and the child was no longer in an environment in which she was constantly criticized. All adults who are in caretaking positions with abused children have an opportunity to contribute to a repaired sense of positive regard by being consistent, respectful, and responsive rather than reactive. It is helpful to decode and depersonalize the behaviors of abused children because often they are behaving in ways that reveal their inner doubts, confusions, fear of attachment, and pain.

Decreasing Children's Feelings of Helplessness and Vulnerability

Abused and neglected children have experienced feelings of helplessness and a lack of control over their environment. They may have attempted to stop the abuse or neglect in a variety of ways, and yet their best efforts were usually overcome by the adults who hurt or ignored them. They may have learned that their power is very limited, and they cannot prevent or stop dominant adults. The feelings of helplessness can become generalized to other situations, and children may demonstrate persistent anxiety and fear, overcompliance, withdrawal, and decreased interactions with peers and adult caretakers. These children feel heightened vulnerability, which requires constant therapeutic attention.

Children have physical, cognitive, and emotional limitations. Their coping strategies are limited, and their ego strength is slowly evolving. In order to challenge their sense of vulnerability, clinicians can assist children to recognize their strengths in a realistic manner. For example, it is unrealistic to convey to young children that they are free, strong, and safe. These are abstract concepts that may apply to young adults. Young children are not free, strong, or safe. The statistics on child kidnapping, child murder, and physical and sexual abuse certainly prove that.

Children can feel powerful in some concrete ways, however. They can learn that they have their own thoughts and feelings, which no one can take from them, and that these thoughts and feelings make them powerful. They have the power of speech and the power of choice, and these things can make them powerful. They have the power to ask for help and trust chosen people with their thoughts and feelings.

Abused children can also benefit from knowing that power is used in both positive and negative ways, and that they can choose how to exert their power. For example, strength can be used to help or to hurt; children will readily understand these differences.

Therapists can create a multitude of situations in which children are presented with choices, which are then acknowledged and supported. Slowly but surely, children will regain a sense that they have some inherent powers and can control some of the situations they face on a daily basis.

Exploring Issues of Relatedness (Attachment, Dependency)

Children who are raised in dysfunctional homes do not receive the full range of parental nurturing behaviors designed to help them develop healthy dependency and attachment. The critical developmental process from full dependency to autonomy and shifting attachment from parents to others requires the guidance and direction of safe and loving parents. Without it, children suffer certain vulnerabilities. They will feel unable to trust others, lack the social skills to develop relationships, and will feel anxious and unable to engage in a full range of interactions with another.

These vulnerabilities are addressed in treatment. Therapists provide children with opportunities to experiment with attachment behaviors in the context of the therapy. Using the transference responses in the child (see Chapter fourteen) and/or by observing the symbolic use of play, therapists can encourage children's exploration of these issues.

One four-year-old girl who lived in foster care had a history of severe deprivation and neglect. Her mother, also severely neglected as a child, spent little time feeding, holding, nurturing, or caring for the child. Consequently, the child developed "failure to thrive." When the mother took the child to a physician at three years of age, the child was placed in a foster home after a period of hospitalization to stabilize her. The child was very lethargic in therapy. She did not play spontaneously and required stimulation to become interested in toys. She seemed disinterested and uninvolved for the first seven months of therapy. After this time, she became consumed with interest in a mother pig and seven piglets. At every session for about three months, she buried the mother pig in a corner of a sandtray. The piglets were brought over to the diagonal corner of the tray, and they took turns trying to find the mother pig. The child said nothing during this play, yet appeared to be absorbed in the play, frequently showing affective variance. The piglets would go looking for the mother and would alternately fall in a pool, climb and fall off a tree, fall off a bridge, and be unable to climb fences, mountains, or barricades of various kinds.

This play was repetitive and precise. There was no variation, and the piglets followed a similar course each time. Suddenly, there was a major difference in this child's play. One of the piglets overcame all the obstacles and unburied the mother. The play stopped abruptly, and the child did not respond to verbal inquiry about what had happened. The following session, the piglet who began the "search for mother" ritual found her immediately. This time the child put the piglet next to his mother and looked up at me and said, "Titty has no milk." She seemed genuinely sad and her eyes watered up. I said, "The baby has no milk from her mommy," and the child responded with tears, "The baby is sad." The rest of the session she alternately cried and took out a baby doll and rocked her and fed her with a plastic bottle.

The next session the child introduced an adult giraffe to the sandtray once the mother pig was buried. She then repeated the play in which the piglet sought out the mother, found her, and was saddened by her mother's lack of milk. The baby piglet then went to the mother giraffe and found that she had milk. She then brought a baby giraffe into the play, and the baby giraffe and piglet seemed to nestle together next to the mother giraffe. "This mommy has lots of milk for everyone," the child exclaimed.

This child was working on her feeling of abandonment by her mother, as well as her emerging sense of trust and attachment to her foster mother through symbolic play. Very little was verbalized by the child, but her working-through had a positive impact not only on her relationship with her foster mother but her relationship with me, her therapist. She was now making eye contact, asking me questions, relaxing her hand on mine, laughing, and making spontaneous remarks such as, "You're always here when I come" and "You have good toys." Symbolic play had been effective in helping her address the issues of dependency, abandonment, and attachment. The therapy with this child continued beyond this point, and many other issues surfaced. The stability of her placement, her positive attachment to foster mother and siblings, and the consistent availability of the therapy setting were major factors in her recovery.

Teaching Children Appropriate Social Skills

Abused and neglected children raised with inappropriate parental guidance and limits may not develop adequate social skills. Without these skills, children may find it difficult or impossible to negotiate peer interactions pivotal in the development of positive self-regard. Abused children may hit others to gain attention, or may use sexualized interactions to decrease their own anxiety or establish personal contact. Neglected children may attach indiscriminately, appearing clingy or needy. They may also appear frightened or withdrawn in spite of efforts by others to make them comfortable.

When peers avoid children because of their problematic antisocial behaviors, they can feel rejected, lonely, or angry. If they already feel bad, unacceptable, or unlovable these feelings may be exacerbated. As feelings of unacceptability grow, problem behaviors follow. This vicious cycle reinforces children's sense of victimization.

Therapists must consistently teach children safe and proper ways of meeting and befriending each other. This is best done within group therapy settings, in which therapists can intervene at the very moment that inappropriate interactions occur. As Johnson has specified in Chapter eleven, this ability to observe and take immediate action is one of the strongest reasons to refer children with problematic behaviors into group therapy.

Helping Children Identify and Get Needs Met

Another important task for therapists is to assist children to identify their own feelings. Unfamiliarity or discomfort with their feelings results from inadequate nurturing from parents or caretakers. Children can learn how to recognize, identify, and express their emotions, which will help them to get their needs met, whether in their immediate family setting or from others such as teachers, extended family members, friends, or therapists.

Clinicians working with children who live in dysfunctional homes must help the children deal with the realities of their environments. If therapy occurs in a vacuum, without a clear recognition of the parents' abilities or willingness to support the lessons of therapy, children are not well served. Therapists who instruct children to "tell someone" their feelings may put them in harm's way if they are unaware of parental or caretaker responses to children who verbalize their feelings. One eight-year-old child was encouraged and rewarded for sharing his angry feelings in the therapy hour. At home, he was slapped each time he verbalized his anger. When the therapist asked the parent how the child was doing at home, the parent complained about her child's "smart-ass" behaviors. The therapist was distressed to learn that what was valued and reinforced during therapy was far from valued in the home. In fact, the mother perceived the child's behavior as undesirable and punishable. The clinician apologized to the parent for inadvertently creating a problem between her and the child and discussed the kinds of behaviors that the mother could validate and reinforce and desired ways of expressing feelings. The clinician and parent worked as a team to develop rewarding situations for the child, which was much more effective than the clinician working in isolation.

Encouraging Children's Realistic View of Family and Family Roles

Clinicians help children recognize their family's strengths and weaknesses in a realistic way. Children need to understand how their family functions and the various roles assumed by family members. This process of helping children explore family roles, interactions, alliances, hierarchy, flexibility and/or rigidity, crises, methods of conflict resolution, and emotional connectedness, inevitably results in more realistic expectations of the family. This process allows therapists to both understand the context in which children live and to provide them with interventions tailored to their unique situation.

Helping Children Become Future-Oriented

Parents, caretakers, therapists, foster parents, or other alternative home personnel must redirect children to the future. Many traumatized children feel a sense of heightened vulnerability and futility, and may be unable to envision themselves growing older or having new (positive) experiences (Terr, 1990). Whenever possible, adults can ask children to imagine themselves older, and inquire what they foresee themselves doing, or what they anticipate with excitement. When children cannot look toward their own future, they can be asked about other people they know and how they will look or what they will be doing in the years to come.

Summary

Individual therapy can be helpful to children with a wide range of behavioral or emotional problems. Children with sexualized behaviors and children who molest can benefit from different treatment modalities. Children with sexualized behaviors (without molesting behaviors) are best served through individual therapy (especially if victims themselves) or education with their parents. Placing children with sexual preoccupations or behaviors that appear to be somewhat inappropriate to their age with children with similar problems may inadvertently exacerbate their interests.

Children who molest more often benefit from group therapy. However, groups are not always readily available, and even if they are, there are several reasons to engage children with sexualized or molesting behaviors in individual therapy either initially to establish a therapy alliance and set the context for group therapy, or later to gain a better understanding of the child's offense-related behavior. In addition, issues that emerge during group therapy sessions can be further reviewed and addressed in individual therapy. If sexualized children or children who molest have unresolved traumatic experiences, it is advisable to offer them an opportunity to recall traumatic incidences and process the material. In this way, children may be in a better position to integrate the lessons of group without feeling overwhelmed, confused, or frightened by unresolved traumatic material (e.g., through Post-Traumatic Stress Disorder symptoms).

Children who molest have problematic interactions with peers, and the most effective intervention consists of clear and prompt attention to the interactive behaviors of children, which are most likely to surface in group.

Individual therapy addresses both primary (abuse-specific) goals, and secondary (general) goals. Primary goals include establishing a working therapeutic relationship with children; assessing children's readiness and preparing them for group therapy; obtaining specificity about the problematic sexual behaviors and risk factors across settings; making efforts to stop the offending behavior; assessing a history of victimization or other relevant issues; understanding children's perceptions of family dynamics; and processing material generated in group.

The secondary goals include improving children's self-concept and self-esteem; decreasing children's feelings of helplessness and vulnerability; exploring issues of relatedness (attachment, dependency); teaching children appropriate social skills; helping children identify and get needs met; encouraging children's realistic view of family and family roles; and helping children to become future-oriented.

When individual therapy is provided, coordination between individual, group, and family therapists is critical to the success of the treatment.

References

American Psychiatric Association. (1987). *Diagnostic and statistical manual of mental disorders.* (3rd Ed.) Washington, DC: APA.

Anthony, E. J., & Cohler, B. J. (1987). *The invulnerable child.* New York: Guilford.

Berliner, L., & Rawlings, L. (1991). A treatment manual: Children's sexual behavior problems. Unpublished manuscript. Seattle, WA: Harborview Sexual Assault Center.

Bernstein, E., & Putnam, F. W. (1986). Development, reliability, and validity of a dissociation scale. *Journal of Nervous and Mental Diseases* 174:727–735.

Bowlby, J. (1973). *Attachment and loss: Volume II.* NY: Basic Books.

Cunningham, C., & MacFarlane, K. (1991). *When children molest children: Group treatment strategies for young sexual abusers,* no. 7. Orwell, VT: Safer Society Press.

Donovan, D. M., & McIntyre, D. (1990). *Healing the hurt child: A developmental-contextual approach.* New York: W. W. Norton.

Eth, S., & Pynoos, R. (1985). *Post-traumatic stress disorder in children.* Washington, DC: American Psychiatric Press.

Faller, K. C. (1990). *Understanding child sexual maltreatment.* Newbury Park, CA: Sage.

Figley, C. R. (Ed.) (1985). *Trauma and its wake: Volume 1.* New York: Brunner Mazel.

Figley, C. R. (Ed.) (1986) *Trauma and its wake: Volume 2.* New York: Brunner/Mazel.

Finkelhor, D., & Browne, A. (1986). Initial and long-term effects: A conceptual framework. In Finkelhor, D. (Ed.) *A sourcebook on child sexual abuse.* Newbury Park, CA: Sage.

Friedrich, W. N. (1990). *Psychotherapy of sexually abused children and their families.* New York: W. W. Norton.

Friedrich, W. N. (Ed.) (1991). *Casebook of sexual abuse treatment.* New York: W. W. Norton.

Friedrich, W. N., Beilke, R. L., & Urquiza, A. J. (1988). Behavior problems in young sexually abused boys: A comparison study. *Journal of Interpersonal Violence* 3:21–28.

Garbarino, J., Guttman, E., & Seeley, J. W. (1986). *The psychologically battered child.* San Francisco: Jossey-Bass.

Gil, E. (1991). *The healing power of play: Working with abused children.* New York: Guilford.

Greenspan, S. (1981). *The clinical interview.* New York: McGraw-Hill.

Hibbard, R. A., & Hartman, G. L. (1992). Behavioral problems of alleged sexual abuse victims. *Child Abuse and Neglect* 16:755-762.

Hoorwitz, A. N. (1992). *The clinical detective: Techniques in the evaluation of sexual abuse.* New York: W. W. Norton.

James, B. (1989). *Treating traumatized children: New insights and creative interventions.* Lexington, MA: Lexington.

Johnson, T. C. (1988). Child perpetrators: Children who molest other children: Preliminary findings. *Child Abuse & Neglect* 12:219-229.

Jones, D. P. H., & McQuiston, M. G. (1989). *Interviewing the sexually abused child.* Gaskell Psychiatric Series, Oxford. (Available from U. of Colorado School of Medicine, C.Henry Kempe Series, #6.)

Kaufman, B., & Wohl, A. (1992). *Casualties of childhood: A developmental perspective on sexual abuse using projective drawings.* New York: Brunner Mazel.

Kent, J. T. (1980). A follow up study of abused children. In G. J. Williams & J. Money (Eds.), *Traumatic abuse and neglect of young children at home.* Baltimore, MD: Johns Hopkins University Press.

Kernberg, P., & Chazan, S. E. (1991). *Children with conduct disorders.* New York: Basic.

Kluft, R. P. (1992). Editorial: Dissociative disorders in childhood and adolescence: New frontiers. *Dissociation* 5:2-3.

Lane, S. L. (1991). Special offender populations. In G. D. Ryan and S. L. Lane (Eds.), *Juvenile sexual offending: Causes, consequences and correction.* Lexington, MA: Lexington.

MacVicar, K. (1979). Psychotherapy of sexually abused girls. *Journal of American Academy of Child Psychiatry* 18:342-353.

Martin, H. P. (1976). *The abused child.* Cambridge, MA: Ballinger.

Marvasti, J. A. (1989). Play therapy with sexually abused children. In S. Sgroi (Ed.), *Vulnerable Populations: Volume II.* Lexington, MA: Lexington.

Peterson, G. (1990). Diagnosis of childhood multiple personality. *Dissociation* 3:3-9.

Peterson, G. (1991). Children coping with trauma: Diagnosis of "dissociation identity disorder." *Dissociation* 4:152-164.

Polansky, N. A., Chalmers, M. A., Williams, D. P., & Buttenweiser, E. W. (1981). *Damaged parents: An anatomy of child neglect.* Chicago: University of Chicago Press.

Putnam, F. W. (1989). *Diagnosis and treatment of multiple personality disorder.* New York: Guilford.

Reagor, P., Kasten, J. D., & Morelli, N. (1992). A checklist for screening dissociative disorders in children and adolescents. *Dissociation* 5:4-19.

Reidy, T. J. (1980). The aggressive characteristics of abused and neglected children. In G. J. Williams & J. Money (Eds.),*Traumatic abuse and neglect of children at home*. Baltimore, MD: Johns Hopkins.

Ryan, G. (1991). The juvenile sex offender's family. In G. D. Ryan & S. L. Lane (Eds.),*Juvenile sexual offending: Causes, consequences and correction*. Lexington, MA: Lexington.

Terr, L. (1990). *Too scared to cry*. New York: Harper & Row.

Thomas, J. (1991). The adolescent sex offender's family in treatment. In G. D. Ryan & S. L. Lane (Eds.), *Juvenile sexual offending: Causes, consequences and corrections*. Lexington, MA: Lexington.

Van der Kolk, B. (Ed.) (1984). *Post-traumatic stress disorder: Psychological and biological sequelae*. Washington, DC: American Psychiatric Press.

Walker, C. E., Bonner, B. L., Kaufman, K. L. (1988). The physically and sexually abused child. In C. E. Walker, B. L Bonner, & K. L. Kaufman. *The physically and sexually abused child: Evaluation and treatment*. New York: Pergamon.

Walsh, B. W., & Rosen, P. M. (1988). *Self-mutilation: Theory, research and treatment*. New York: Guilford.

White, M. (1985). Fear busting and monster taming: An approach to the fears of young children. In M. White (1989) *Selected papers*. Adelaide, So. Australia: Dulwich Centre Publications.

White, S., Halpin, B. M., Strom, G. A., & Santelli, G. (1988). Behavioral comparisons of young sexually abused, neglected, and nonreferred children. *Journal of Clinical Child Psychology* 17:53–61.

11

Group Therapy

Toni Cavanagh Johnson, Ph.D.

The Support Program for Abuse-Reactive Kids (SPARK) was developed by Kee MacFarlane in 1985, and was the first group therapy model for the treatment of children who molest other children (Johnson and Berry, 1989).[1] Since that time, many treatment programs have been implemented using a variety of treatment models.

Group therapy for children who molest is based on several key assumptions: (1) in treating the child it is essential to treat the whole family; (2) group therapy is the best approach with children who molest; and (3) treatment has to be specific and focused on the child's sexualized behaviors. Proceeding from these assumptions, treatment will have the following components: group therapy for the child; group therapy for the parents; group therapy for sibling-victims; and group work for nonabused siblings. These groups occur simultaneously, and the material is frequently similar across the groups.

A significant factor in the development of children's molesting behavior usually arises from experience in the family (see Chapters four and seven). These children cannot change their behavior unless the environment in which

---

1. I was Clinical Director of the Child Sexual Abuse Center at Children's Institute International from 1985 to 1990, and I supervised and ran groups in the SPARK program during that time. The treatment model described in this chapter was developed and implemented at SPARK, one of the programs of the Child Sexual Abuse Center.

they live changes, which necessitates behavioral change in the parents. Children also need help from significant people on a daily basis to provide positive reinforcement and negative consequences for molesting behaviors, help that parents have to be trained to provide. Finally, parents of these children have severe, ongoing psychological issues that hamper their ability to provide consistency, love, and nurturance.

Young children learn best with an interactive approach. Since the primary manifestation of the disorder is being sexual and aggressive with other children, the greatest learning comes from being with other children and learning other ways to interact with them. This approach provides immediate practice and feedback. Equally important is the discomfort many children feel when discussing sexual issues with adults one-to-one. Since most of these children live or have lived with adults who have very poor sexual boundaries, many feel uncomfortable in a closed room with an adult talking about sexual topics. This is often true of children who have been sexually abused, who may feel trapped or sexually threatened. Although these children all feel anxious when sexual topics are discussed, the anxiety is less when there are other children, a larger group, and more adults present. In this situation, the opportunity for abuse is diminished.

In order to be successful, treatment must be specific and focused on sexual issues. A large number of children are referred for treatment who have already been in therapy. Generally, their sexual behavior had been discussed once, perhaps twice, and then not again. The level of dysfunction and confusion in children who molest is pervasive. Many specific issues regarding the genesis, the immediate precipitants, the sustaining aspects of the behaviors, associated feelings, the targets of the behavior, situational risk factors, and many other concerns must be addressed, in many ways, at different times and from different perspectives. This must be done with the child in tandem with the parents. It is a process that takes time. Nonspecific play therapy is insufficient for children who molest.

Individual therapy is a very useful adjunct to group therapy for both children and parents, who can use individual time to deal with their intrapsychic issues and interpersonal family dynamics. Family therapy is an essential adjunct to bring members together to discuss issues arising in the family that may precipitate, maintain, or exacerbate the sexually aggressive behavior (see Chapter twelve).

Group Therapy for Children Who Molest

Group Format and Length of Meetings

There are many ways to structure group therapy with children (see for example, Mandell and Damon, 1989; Friedrich, 1990). With children who molest, it has been found useful to have several treatment cycles. In this way, parents and children get the feeling of completion and renewal. A cycle length is chosen, such as twelve or fourteen weeks. In between cycles, there can be vacation time, allowing for beginnings and endings.

In outpatient therapy, most groups meet once a week. In residential or inpatient treatment, greater frequency is possible and preferable.

Because of the need for concentrated effort on the issues, and time to socialize, one and a half hours is a good length for both the children's group and the parents' group. It is usually helpful to have a ritual (see the Group Structure section) that the group goes through every week. In this way, children know exactly what to expect and can learn to conform to expectations. This is often in direct contrast to their home life in which little remains constant or predictable.

Screening for Group

During the initial evaluation, it is important to assess the child's and parent's ability to benefit from group therapy. Many children who molest have special learning problems as well as Attention Deficit Disorder. Hyperactivity or hypermotility is also a frequent behavior for these children, as are anxiety, intense anger, impulsiveness, and low frustration tolerance. Children who cannot sit still and have difficulty processing information are not able to use group well and are too disruptive. Children with severe receptive or expressive language problems are not able to understand the material or interact effectively with the other children. Although it is positive for children to learn to interact with children with severe handicaps, therapy for molesting behaviors is too complex and anxiety producing to add this extra dimension. Children with low cognitive ability (IQ below 70 to 80) find it very difficult to function with children of average intelligence in a group situation in which learning is occurring using verbal interactions.

Because the population of children who molest extrafamilialy is usually fairly small in any particular locale, it is difficult to have separate groups, yet it is probably most beneficial for them to be treated separately from children who engage in sibling incest. The dynamic roots, parental issues, and safety issues are different enough that the single focus on sibling incest provides more intense work and support with the parents, children, and family.

Of the approximately nine subgroups of children who molest (see Chapter five), two subgroups, sociopathic children and violent children who molest, include children whose thought processes and ability to relate to others are severely disturbed. Although an adequate number of these children rarely appears in any one treatment program so they may be separated into their own group, it is generally better not to include them with less disturbed children who molest. Their thoughts are very violent, and they are fairly ruthless in attempting to get what they want. Sociopathic children and violent children who molest provide very poor role models for other children, and yet because they present themselves as powerful, other children may aspire to be like them. Two of these children can form their own group.

Group Configuration

Children who molest should be placed in fairly narrow age and developmental groupings. A maximum of a one-year age difference is optimal. For example, eleven-year-olds can be with twelve-year-olds or ten-year-olds. Generally a ten-year-old is significantly younger emotionally and interpersonally, less experienced, less worldly, and farther from puberty than a twelve-year-old. Prepubertal children are too emotionally immature to be included in groups with adolescents. Sexuality in adolescents becomes more erotic and genital than exploratory. Pleasure, orgasm, and genital satisfaction are relevant and appropriate subjects of concern for adolescents as they choose sexual partners for love and comfort. The discussion of these issues would be premature for most young children under twelve. Although children who molest have been prematurely sexualized, their emotional and psychological growth is generally regressed.

Children of five are too young to be grouped with eight-year-olds. Kindergarten is a far different place than second grade emotionally, socially, and in relation to independence and peer relatedness.

Because the dynamics of victim and victimizer are important to monitor and process during group therapy, the group configuration is important not only as it relates to age but also size, developmental and emotional level, and degree of pathology. Children who are too far from the group mean for any of these parameters should be carefully assessed before inclusion in the group.

Mixing boys and girls is generally not a good idea. In the best of circumstances, children get anxious when discussing sexuality, which only increases when boys and girls are together. One goal of group interaction is to teach children to act in a manner consistent with other children their own age. Sensitive topics concerning their bodies and sexuality are generally not shared between boys and girls at this age level.

Because of the volatility of these children both in the sexual and aggressive spheres, it is generally most beneficial to have four, perhaps six children in a group. With young children two therapists to four children, or three therapists to six children is a good ratio. With the eleven- and twelve-year-olds, two therapists to four or five children is effective. The low ratio allows therapists to control the behavior of the group and attend to the individual process of each child, while allowing children time to express themselves without having to compete for resources. Inadequate attention potentially recapitulates their experience at home and increases disruptive behavior in group. Since it is essential for each child to grasp the content of these groups, small numbers allow therapists to be more assured of what each child has assimilated. Two children form a group. This can often be more effective than one adult and one child when dealing specifically with the sexually aggressive behaviors.

Therapist Selection

Although initially it may be best for girls to have female cotherapists, it is valuable for both boys and girls to learn to relate to a mixed gender cotherapy team. In girls' groups, a male therapist may be integrated into the therapy after the initial phase of treatment. A male therapist too early in the group may increase the girls' anxiety and apprehension, restricting their ability to discuss issues such as victimization, sexual confusion, or general fears and conflicts. A male cotherapist can demonstrate the ability to talk about sexuality without acting on it; a nonsexist attitude toward sexuality; a balanced, respectful, and collegial relationship to the female cotherapist, with no ulterior motives; limit-setting in a nonabusive, caring manner; the ability to discuss feelings in a kind and considerate way; consistency; playfulness; and modulation of emotions. A female therapist is important because many children who molest are often raised by single-parent mothers who have significant problems with sexual, emotional, and physical boundaries, and ambivalent relationships with their children. A stable female figure who accepts them for who they are allows the children to define themselves apart from the rejection and projections they often feel at home. Because their mothers are often quite harsh and punitive with them, the kindness, caring, and objectivity of a female therapist is important. A female cotherapist can present a model to both boys and girls of an emotionally balanced, nonsexual, giving, consistent woman who maintains her role and boundaries regardless of what is occurring.

The selection of therapists to provide treatment to these children is very important. Because children who molest are young does not mitigate against very powerful negative reactions to them. Some clinicians who have worked with victims of sexual abuse do not want to work with children who molest. Clinicians must be aware of their limitations and respect them.

Individuals who have been victims of sexual abuse may find it very difficult to work with these children if they have not completed their own work in therapy. Therapists who have suffered emotional or physical abuse may also experience difficulty, since children who molest have often experienced this type of abuse, and their behaviors and psychological defenses may remind therapists of their own.

Working with parents may also be a powerful agent of discomfort. Parents can be highly defensive, aggressive, sexual, emotionally and physically abusive, and neglectful of their children. The parents of these children may trigger recollections of the therapists' own parents. Potential therapists for these children and their families must thoroughly examine their own transference and countertransference, because they provide a great therapeutic challenge (see Chapter fourteen).

The Setting

Although there are many suitable configurations, the easiest room to use is one large enough to have an adequate desk-height table and chairs, but not so large that there is a large open area that children may want to use for recreation. When they have a defined space with boundaries, children are more able to remain focused. This also mirrors the space boundaries they will learn in the course of treatment. In groups for younger children, it is nice to have an area with a comfortable rug on which they can sit to play board games or play with small toys when there is a break in the focused group work.

Another important feature of the room is that it does not have large numbers of accessible toys to distract children from their task. It is uncomfortable for all group members if the content and process of the group is on controlling the children's behavior. It is also important to have a room that is safe if the children become agitated. If the room is above the first floor, there should not be direct access to open windows. Objects that can be used to hurt others should be inaccessible as well. It helps focus the children's attention if only the materials needed for each group session are available. If there is play time during the group, those toys can be in the room also, which can be helpful in teaching the children impulse control and frustration tolerance.

Preparation of Children and Parents for Group Therapy

Consistent attendance in treatment is a major issue. The use of a signed contract that delineates attendance requirements is very useful. The ramifications of breaking the contract are specified and the contract can be made between the referring agency, the treatment staff, and the parents.

For children to be aware of the focused nature of group therapy, it is valuable to inform them that other children will tell them about their "touching problem" at the first meeting, and then they will be asked to tell the group about their touching problem. They should know that each session will have something to do with the touching problem, and that there will be work, fun, and food.

Parents benefit from group therapy given in tandem with treatment for their children (Damon and Waterman, 1986). Parents should be aware that modifications in the home environment and supervising their children's behavior is very important to help stop the problematic touching. Many parents of children who molest see no reason to attend therapy and want to send their children alone. This should be faced directly in a careful and sensitive manner, by stating that the child's behaviors arose in the context of the family and will need to be remedied with the help of the family. All members of the family may need to change to help the child. Parents should be supported in their struggle to help their children. Their own pain and need for therapeutic intervention should be identified and acknowledged. Families of children who molest are in crisis and need as much reassurance, guidance, and support as possible.

Confidentiality Issues

The limits of confidentiality must be explained to parents, not only in terms of the need to report suspected abuse, but also to alert them to the confidentiality of their children's communications with the therapist. Because parents hold the psychotherapist-client privilege for their young children, they have the legal right to know what happens in therapy. Parents can be given general information about their children's progress without specific communications being revealed. When this issue is presented in a positive manner, parents gain a better understanding of appropriate boundaries regarding their children's privacy. This assists the parents' understanding of roles, boundaries, and privacy. To stress the importance of parents in treatment process of the child, the parents' cooperation is sought in calling the therapists if a problem arises during the week. Parents should also be encouraged to make therapists aware of issues that can be raised in group to help the child. Some therapists ask parents to fill out a weekly written report on their child's positive and troublesome behavior and review it before group.

Group Structure

It is helpful for children and parents to meet in a waiting area. The children play for a short while as the therapists check in briefly with the parents or collect written materials from them for review. This time for parents to speak with one another and with therapists is an important part of the structure. Parents with emotionally impoverished backgrounds may feel that therapists are trying to usurp their children or feel they cannot compete with what the therapists have to offer. Some parents perceive therapists to be like their parents or other family members: critical, hostile, and punitive. Therapists can use this time to talk with parents, gain their trust, provide nurturance and acceptance, and decrease parents' feelings that therapists are superior and distant.

Children's groups begin with a snack. Food is especially important with children who have been deprived of consistent care and affection since it represents symbolic nourishment. Eating together simulates a family atmosphere. Since most of these children have a tense relationship with their caregivers and at school, it is helpful for them to feel comfortable in a group atmosphere.

During snack time, children talk about the good and not-so-good things that happened during their week, which offers them an opportunity to brag about something they did, and encourages them to share problems and disappointments. Because many children do not understand the purpose of therapy, therapists often select issues raised in an early part of the session to work on during group. Children soon realize that their joys and sorrows are the important content of therapy, and that some understanding and resolution in their lives can be gained through interactions with the other children and the therapists in the group. As during other parts of the group, children will encroach on other children's "space" (e.g., by overtalking the child who is speaking) and can be helped to understand that being a "space invader" can be verbal as well as physical, as in the touching problem.

After the snack and sharing time, the structured activity is introduced (see Skills and Therapeutic Interventions section), after which the group can relax while playing games, or playing with toys. After play time, the group comes together again to talk about the structured activity, what they learned, how the group went, and any homework. Unstructured activity time is specifically focused on helping children learn socialization skills in which they are painfully deficient.

After group it is helpful for children to have time to play together again in the waiting area while the parents talk together or with therapists. During the pre- and post-group time, valuable information regarding the parents' parenting skills and interactional style can be gleaned.

Reinforcement Systems

An important aspect in treatment of children who molest is the balance between managing children's behavior and having children learn to manage their own behavior. Most children who molest have significant behavioral problems. Many have more physiologically based problems such as Attention Deficit Disorder and hyperactivity, making it very difficult for them to sit and concentrate in group sessions. Clinicians need to implement behavioral control methods consistently from the beginning. Children who molest have not experienced consistent behavioral management in their lives and doubt that it is possible.

Behavioral systems can be more or less rigorous. For groups of children in which the behavior is less problematic, reinforcement can occur after every group. When the behavior is very difficult to manage, the reinforcement can be every ten minutes during the group period or after each section of the group (i.e. after snack, after structured activity). The length of time between reinforcements can be modulated throughout the life of the group. When the behavioral system is being implemented, therapists should assess behavior and manage the reinforcers. As the group becomes more functional, reinforcement can be after every two or three groups.

As the group coalesces, the behavioral system can be modified so that group members themselves give input on the behavior of other group members. With older children, scoring sheets can be developed for them to rate one another on different behavioral and performance objectives. This can be very helpful for children's personal development in that they hone their ability to observe another's behavior and be objective in rating it. This skill is one their parents have not generally had and of which the children have been victims. The group can develop goals that all members need to meet to be reinforced. In this way, members become responsible for one another. Each child can learn how to help and encourage others to meet group goals. This should be monitored carefully. Whereas in some groups it can bring group cohesion, it can also create a very divisive atmosphere. This step should not be considered if there are children present who are likely to become scapegoats for not meeting the group goals. Children who have been victimized can be severely retraumatized in this situation if they become the focus of the group's disappointment and anger.

The use of behavioral systems can have a potentially negative effect on the development of self-esteem and positive coping. When children are always being reinforced for their performance from an external source, it does not lead to the development of internal self-regulation. When a child behaves only in order to receive a reward, it can have a negative rather than positive effect. With this awareness, it is valuable to move toward elongating the reinforcement schedule toward the end of the life of the group. As the group becomes more manageable, therapists can focus on decreasing the rigor of the reinforcement system and increasing children's awareness of their own ability to self-regulate. Reinforcement for good behavior becomes praise from the therapist and self-congratulations, rather than material objects.

Fee for Services

Therapy costs will vary according to the provider and setting. Programs that receive state or federal funding provide services at no cost to the client or use a sliding-scale fee. Private agencies will often use a fee schedule that considers the family's ability to pay. Children who are victims of crime may qualify to receive financial help from special funds available through most district attorney's offices (Victim Assistance Programs). Clinicians providing the full compliment of individual, group, and family therapy will need to establish a reasonable fee for services.

Goals of Group Treatment

A number of important abuse-specific and general goals are associated with group therapy. After each goal some of the significant issues related to the goal are listed. The issues can be used to develop structured activities. Additional important issues for each goal are provided in Appendix E. Examples of structured activities are given in the Skills Training and Techniques sections in this chapter. Other activities can be found in books listed in the Resources section, for example Cunningham & MacFarlane, 1991.

GOAL: Decreasing children's molesting behavior.

This first goal should be the focus of treatment until the major issues have been covered and molesting behaviors begin to wane. It takes a long time to address general issues of sexuality; it is of more immediate importance to decrease the molesting behaviors. All group sessions must deal with some aspect of the touching problem even after it is no longer the major focus of the group sessions.

All children and parents need a clear understanding of abusive and all other sexual behaviors in which the child engages. Abusive behaviors are worked on first, and agreement is reached concerning other behaviors that elicit concern. Events, people, or environments that precipitate sexual or aggressive feelings need to be identified and then changed or eliminated. This is often difficult, because family atmosphere and behaviors are frequently an important part of the problem. Firm and consistent boundaries related to sexual, emotional, and behavioral issues are a constant theme in treatment and are a large and ongoing part of parents' treatment as well.

The child's sexual behavior patterns need to be identified through careful observation and charting to determine what triggers precede the molesting behaviors. Different methods have been described to detail the steps children go through in sexually abusive behaviors (Lane, 1991). It is helpful to use a graphic to make children aware of how they start with a feeling, thought, or environmental stimulus and progress to the sexual molesting (see Cartoons in the Techniques section).

A specific and detailed plan is tailored to each child's sexual behavior pattern. Children learn what they can do at each juncture to stop the pattern. An essential element of the plan is the use of substitute behaviors and distracters. Children need to know to whom to go to for help when they feel like touching. At that time, they can be distracted to another activity at random or by an agreed-upon substitute behavior. It is paramount that the child be the active person who seeks help and uses distracters to control his or her own behavior. Substitute behaviors share the following characteristics: (1) Things children like to do and find pleasurable. Children are asked to determine what these are. (2) Activities that expend energy, for example, riding a bicycle, skateboard, or tricycle; and playing kickball, or handball. Activities involving aggression or bodily contact are best avoided. (3) Activities that redirect attention from the sexual focus. Playing video games, particularly handheld games, works well for some children. Although they do not require children to expend physical energy, they require concentration and distract children from sexual feelings or thoughts. Other possibilities are jacks, crossword puzzles, and jigsaw puzzles. (4) Activities may be solitary or require parental participation. Doing something with parents is a positive motivator not to engage in sexual behaviors. If, however, parents feel that children are fabricating sexual feelings to spend time with them, they must determine why this is so. Parents may increase the amount of "special" time spent with children to try to decrease the fabrication. As meaningful attachment to others is a major issue for children who molest, teaching them to turn to others to help reduce their anxiety or anger is highly beneficial.

Clinicians and parents need to agree on consequences for sexual behaviors. Which behaviors will receive a reprimand? The exact words and actions to be used should be explicitly discussed. Will only coercive sexual behaviors receive a consequence? Is masturbation all right in private? Will children be rewarded if they do not engage in coercive sexual behaviors? Who will give the consequences? What are they? Who will give rewards and on what schedule?

Planning consequences is best done with the children, so children and parents have the same understanding. It is helpful for the plan to be written. If children participate in establishing consequences for their own behavior and agree which behaviors require consequences, this is far superior to parents establishing consequences independently. Children are more invested in stopping the molesting behaviors when they are in control of the process. Control is an important issue with abused children—the more positive control they can exercise, the less powerlessness they feel. Children can be helped to understand that the purpose of consequences is to help them think before acting. They need to be encouraged to pick a consequence they genuinely do not want to receive.

Other family members need to be aware of the problem so they too can let parents know if children engage in molesting behaviors. Children should be aware that this is to help them. If everyone knows, children can use other family members as reminders not to engage in molesting behaviors. Ultimately, treatment provides other reasons not to engage in them, such as empathy for the victim.

Once the plan has been set in motion, it requires frequent follow-up with both parents and child. This can be done in parallel parent and child groups and in family therapy. No assumptions can be made that the plan is being followed. It is hard for these children and families to be consistent, and therapists must model consistency for them.

Generally, these children abrogate the rights of children and adults in other, nonsexual ways. Physical and emotional aggression is not uncommon, nor are stealing, lying, cheating, fire-setting, abusing animals, and using scatological language. Molesting behaviors are a primary focus at the beginning of treatment, but related issues can be integrated into the discussions. When a child has bullied another child on the playground, this can be addressed and the similarities to sexual abuse mentioned. The victim-victimizer dynamic is a constant theme throughout the group sessions.

It is important to attend to the immediate aspects of sexually abusive behavior while keeping in mind that sex and sexuality must not be portrayed as bad, dirty, or frightening.

Coordination of this goal with appropriate school personnel is important.

<u>Issues</u>

Making a clear plan for children in the event the touching feeling starts

Identifying and discussing children's sexual behaviors (CSBCL)

Identifying and discussing molesting behaviors (CSBCL)

Identifying substitute behaviors and how they work

Identifying adults who can help children when the touching feelings begin

Sexual behavior patterns of each child

Which things or people in my environment make me feel like touching?

What do I think about before I feel like touching?

What emotional feelings do I have before I touch someone?

How does my body feel before I touch?

Where on my body do I get the feelings?

How do I feel when I am touching a child?

How do I feel after I touch a child?

Who are the children I want to touch? Why them?

When I get the feelings or thoughts, *Stop and Think*. Think of the consequences, for me and the victim, before I touch.

Mutual sex play versus coercive sexual behavior

GOAL: Increasing children's understanding of their unhealthy associations and beliefs regarding sex and sexuality

A complex relationship exists in the minds of children who molest regarding sex and sexuality. The most fundamental association is usually between sex and aggression. This basic association is then paired with others that precipitate sexual behaviors. Some children experience a chain of associations that precipitate sexual aggression. It is essential that these be clarified and understood.

Issues

Sex equals anxiety.   The need to reduce anxiety precipitates sexual expression.

Feelings of jealousy, loneliness, powerlessness, hopelessness, or anger precipitate sexual aggression.

Sex equals pleasure at another's expense.

Emotional neediness precipitates sexual neediness, which precipitates sexual aggression.

Unmet or blocked needs precipitate the desire to hurt someone.

Sex and aggression can become fused.   Sex equals rage.

Revenge and revenge fantasies

"Since I was a victim, I victimize."   "They did it to me."

Confusion about sexual intercourse, touching, caring, love, and nurturing

Cognitive distortions regarding sex and sexuality—Stinking thinking. (Rasmussen, Burton, & Christopherson, 1992).

Earliest sexual experiences

GOAL: Increasing children's understanding of natural and healthy sexuality

Virtually all children who molest were born into families with significant sexual problems. Many never experienced natural, healthy exploration and curiosity about sex unfettered by confusion and anxiety. They do not understand age-appropriate sexual behaviors. Early in their lives, they were prematurely overexposed to inappropriate sexuality, which overwhelmed their ability to make sense of what they saw, heard, or experienced. Whereas other children gaily explore the sexual universe, these children feel confused, angry, and anxious. Some have experienced deep shame and guilt about sex early in their lives.

Issues

Age-appropriate sexual behavior versus problematic sexual behavior

What is sexuality? Are male and female sexuality the same?

Values, attitudes, and feelings about sex and sexuality

Myths about sexuality, sexual stereotypes

How to talk about sex with your parents

Sexuality curriculum (Johnson, 1989)

GOAL: Increasing children's awareness of their own and family patterns that precipitate, sustain, or increase sexually abusive and other nonadaptive behaviors

Many maladaptive patterns are related to sexual or aggressive themes in families of children who molest. Of particular importance are issues related to physical, sexual, and emotional boundaries. Questions can be addressed to children and their parents concerning rules about privacy. Who decides who touches another person's body? If children do not want to be kissed by a relative, are children forced? Who sleeps where, and who makes the decisions? Do children bathe and clean themselves? What do children know about the parents' personal life, its sexual and emotional aspects? Who is the mother's and father's confidant? Does anyone come to the house who makes them uncomfortable? How is anger shown at home? Do adults express their anger or rage in front of children? Do people hit others in the home? Do the children feel physically safe?

Family therapy and joint exercises with parents' and children's groups can help meet this goal. Boundary issues should be explored early, and throughout treatment. Frequently, children are more consistently aware than parents of nonadaptive family boundaries. Children bring these to the therapists' attention, often to the parents' chagrin.

Issues

Boundary issues: sexual, physical, and emotional

How information is transmitted in the family

Sexual behavior patterns of family members

Aggressive behavior patterns in the family

House rules regarding privacy

When I grow up will I use the same rules and punishments with my children as my parents?

GOAL: Understanding and integrating feelings and thoughts associated with prior victimization including physical, sexual, and emotional abuse, abandonment, neglect, family breakups, and deaths

The vast majority of these children and their parents have been sexually, physically, and emotionally abused. Their lives have been a series of debilitating events. Many want to forget everything that has happened;

however, it is likely they need to recall traumatic and abusive events and associated conscious and unconscious feelings and thoughts to come to some understanding about them. These thoughts and feelings often overwhelm children's ability to integrate their experiences, make meaning of them, and move on. Past experiences frequently drive current behaviors in negative and self-defeating ways. Parents' lives may also be guided by unfinished business related to abuse. They may need additional therapy of their own to work on these issues.

Children's experience of trauma is idiosyncratic. Clinicians should not assume which abusive or traumatic events have had the most effect. They must observe and listen carefully to the children.

Issues

How has the abuse affected me?

Physiological arousal associated with abuse (e.g., tension, fear, anxiety, hypervigilance, anger, sexual arousal)

Trust/betrayal. Trusting is okay. Whom can I trust?

Feelings of abandonment and loss. What have I lost that matters the most?

Victimization, helplessness, hopelessness

Prevention skills. What would I do if someone tried to abuse me again?

GOAL: Helping children observe and assess their own behavior, be aware of the circumstances preceding their behavior, and think of the consequences of their behaviors before they act

Molesting behaviors and other maladaptive behaviors such as fire-setting, property destruction, insulting others, lying, and stealing can be analyzed using a similar methodology. Children are taught to become aware of what precedes their behavior and then to *Stop and Think* before engaging in any behavior. When they stop and think about the consequences, they can decide what to do.

Some children need to understand their feelings and thoughts. In other cases, they need to attend to what is occurring around them. By focusing on the behavior step by step, they come to realize there are many parts to their actions and many opportunities to abort what they thought was inevitable. Many believe their behavior is so spontaneous they cannot control it, they just do it.

Parents have similar problems, and it is often beneficial to do parallel exercises in parents' and children's groups. In joint groups, parents and children can work on problems arising at home. Parents can become aware of antecedents of their children's behavior and help modify it. Parents can learn how to help their child *Stop and Think* and immediately reinforce positive behavior. Role-plays are helpful. Both parents and children learn better in vivo than in the abstract.

Issues

What are my self-defeating behavior patterns?

What are the things that make me hit, lie, steal, destroy things?

What are the things I can do to stop myself from negative behavior?

Feelings and thoughts can precipitate actions, but they don't have to.

Stop and Think.

Natural and logical consequences: name ten misbehaviors and ten logical consequences.

GOAL: Increasing children's ability to observe and appreciate other people's feelings, needs, and rights

Children who molest often are centered on their own pain and are unavailable to attend to others. This results in a lack of appreciation of the feelings, needs, and rights of others and may result in violations of others' emotional and physical space.

Because parents of children who molest also lack these qualities, these children may never have received warm, empathic, caring responses when they felt emotional and physical distress. Some children who have been removed from their homes for severe abuse or neglect may feel they must subjugate their own welfare to respond to their parents' narcissistic needs. Children who molest have not had good role models for responding to others' pain. It is hard for them to give what they did not receive.

To stop molesting behaviors, it is important to help children see the effect of their behavior on others. This can be done in part by helping them understand from their own pain how others experience pain. Children who have been victimized, and who understand their feelings in relation to their victimization, can translate their experience of pain to someone else. This can be facilitated in group using plays (see Plays in the Techniques section).

Issues

Who do I care about? How do I show it? Who cares about me? How do they show it?

How do I feel when I do something wrong? How do I feel when someone hurts me?

Whom do I hurt when I do something wrong? What does it feel like to them?

When someone I know gets hurt, what do they expect me to do? What would they want me to do?

Can people have hurt feelings or just hurt bodies?

How do my actions affect the actions of others?

How do others see me?

GOAL: Helping children understand their needs and values and develop their own goals and internal resources

In general, children who molest lack goals, their values are unformulated, their moral development is arrested, their internal sense of self is undeveloped, and they feel incapable of positive and consistent action. The same is often true of their parents. Because of the intensity of parental needs and feelings, there may be massive projections onto the children and harmful displacements. Children must learn to separate their needs, desires, and feelings from these projections.

Few of these children have a positive sense of self. Their daily lives are spent in misbehavior, and most people respond negatively to them. This occurs at school, at home, and on the playground. Group therapy can help them learn new ways to act and react. By getting positive attention from others, and learning how to interact with peers, they can begin gradually to build self-esteem. Positive self-regard is their best resource to meet life's challenges.

Joint exercises with parents' and children's groups can help parents develop self-esteem in their children. Parents are taught how to encourage self-esteem before bringing the groups together.

Issues

Who am I? What do I value? What do I like to do? How can I get to do it?

Who are my parents?

Do my parents and I want and need the same or different things?

Who do my parents say I am? Are they correct?

Whom do I want to be like when I grow up? What type of person do I want to be? How can I achieve this?

Moral development exercises

Values clarification

GOAL: Increasing children's ability to meet their needs in socially appropriate ways

Children who molest usually have problems in every sphere of their lives. Because their needs are intense, and they have limited understanding of how to fulfill them, they become frustrated. As their frustration mounts so does their aggression, and people turn away from them. Feeling isolated and shunned, they strike out to take what they want.

The group process lends itself to identifying what children want and learning how to get it, if it is acceptable. The group milieu can also serve to point out children's socially inappropriate actions. This can be invaluable, because these children frequently do not understand the specifics of their problems, only that they have problems and make everyone angry. In group therapy, children can learn how to approach another child to make a friend. They can learn how to express their negative feelings to other children without making them angry. The therapist can stop the group process to help a particular child, thereby showing everyone where an interaction has gone awry and how it can be handled differently. When this is sensitively done, it is of great benefit. Coordinating this work with the child's parents and teacher is helpful.

Issues

What do I really want? How can I get it without hurting someone else?

How do I hurt other people?

Do I make people go away from me? When and how do I do this?

List all the things I do when I'm angry. How many hurt someone else?

What is right and what is wrong to do? How can I figure this out?

Assertion versus aggression

GOAL: Increasing children's connectedness to positive others and building internal objects that support future growth

Frequently, children who molest have withdrawn emotionally and do not seek out others for consolation, assistance, or emotional support. They feel alone. They did not develop solid attachments to positive others in their early development, and they generally do not trust adults. They attempt to rely on themselves, creating basic fear and insecurity.

Children who are raised in healthy homes develop ego structures that are emotionally sustaining. They have a basic trust that they will be cared for and safe. When lonely, fearful, or hungry, they can rely on an internal feeling of a kind, benevolent parent who attends to their feelings and comes to their aid. The internal objects of children who molest are often hostile, rejecting, and aggressive rather than benevolent, kind, attentive, or stable. Superego development is minimal.

Although some work can be done in group, family and individual therapy are also suited to meeting this goal. In their groups, parents can learn how to meet their children's needs, and this knowledge can be fostered through family work. If children are in residential care and do not have a relationship with family members, a closer relationship can be fostered with someone who can be consistent and caring. This may be through the facility or an outside agency such as Big Brothers or Big Sisters.

Issues

Who do I want to be when I grow up? Who can help me reach my goals?

What are the characteristics of the people I want to be like?

What values do I hold? Who holds the same values? How did I decide on these values?

Who can I turn to when I am hurting?

Who can I trust? Who trusts me?

Skills Training

Skill deficits are virtually universal in children who molest. In order to meet the group goals, skill building is essential. Skills are worked on during group time, yet a lockstep approach to teaching them is not advised. In fact, if well integrated in the group process, children may not be aware of the specific skills training. Games may be used, as well as books, plays, creative materials, and the group process itself. Paper and pencil tasks or highly structured educational situations need to be minimized due to the learning difficulties of many children who molest.

Identifying and Expressing a Range of Feelings

Children who molest have a very limited ability to identify feelings other than anger. When a parent says to a two-year-old, "You look sad" or "What a happy face you have today," the parent is teaching the child to identify his or her feeling state. Unfortunately, many parents of children who molest are absorbed with their own conflicts and do not have the emotional resources to attend to their child's development.

Identifying and expressing feelings can be facilitated in the group. Whereas therapists must be careful about identifying feelings for a child, they can at times say, for example, "When you sit with your shoulders slumped, does that say anything about how you feel?" or "When you look that way I think you are mad. Is that correct?" Therapists must be careful not to label feelings, but to let children learn to label their own. Other children in the group can help by asking questions to understand more about what the child is feeling. As children learn to ask other children questions to elicit their feelings, they learn which questions to ask themselves. This process can be helpful in developing empathy.

If a child is hitting another, the therapist should be careful about labeling the feeling as "anger," because anger is overutilized. Children who have intense emotions frequently label all emotions anger. Feelings such as arousal, loneliness, fear, and many others may be lumped under the feeling of anger.

A feeling can be more fine-tuned than anger. It may be useful to help the child identify the feeling that preceded the hitting response. If the child was jealous or afraid, the feeling is best labeled this way, and the behavior understood as an outgrowth of jealousy or fear. Only by understanding true derivatives and feelings can they be understood and overcome.

It is useful to use a picture of a thermometer with four to eight gradations as a method of teaching children about a range of feelings (fewer gradations are used for younger groups of children). The therapists explain that thermometers are used to measure the temperature of the body. The higher the mercury goes, the bigger the temperature. Using a feeling such as anger, children are asked to find a word they use to describe just a little bit of anger, a little bit more anger, and so on, for example, enraged, furious, pissed, annoyed, peeved. Children can describe something that has happened in their own lives to illustrate a particular word and feeling. This helps fine-tune feelings to situations. As with all skills they learn in group, children are periodically reminded how these can help them control their touching problem.

Impulse Control/Self-Monitoring

Impulse control is an important area for children who molest because they are used to reacting instantly to feelings of the moment. When they molest, they have feelings that are uncomfortable and impel them to act. Although children have different ways of describing their molestation behavior, it is common to hear a child say, "I felt bad [sad, mad, lonely], and I thought if I touched someone I would feel better." The direct link between feeling and action has to be broken. Some children say, "I feel better when I am hurting somebody. Even if the good feeling doesn't last, I feel better for a little bit."

Children need to identify their impulses and give them names. Opportunities arise endlessly in group—children have impulses to yell, hit, cry, spit, make noises from various orifices, and so on. Children can be playfully stopped when they begin to act on impulse: "It looks like you want to kick John" or "Fred is screaming and you are not. Congratulations. Do you feel like screaming?" This encourages them to be self-observant.

Stop and Think is a motto children learn. To mediate between impulse and action, children are encouraged to stop as soon as they feel the impulse to act. When therapists see restraint, they congratulate the child: "Wow, you looked like you wanted to kick John and you stopped." Children are encouraged to think of the consequences of their actions when they stop. "What will happen if you kick John? Do you want this to happen?"

The connection between not acting on the impulse to kick is directly relevant to not giving in to the impulse to touch. If the consequence of kicking is a school suspension, the consequence of touching would be decided on by parent and child (e.g., being supervised with other children). Children should be aware of the consequences of molesting another child. It is useful to understand the consequences to the victim-child, not only the consequences that affect the child who molests.

Children are encouraged to feel proud of themselves for moderating their impulses and thinking of the consequences. They are encouraged to see that being successful is a matter of learning control and choosing to exercise it. Many are so accustomed to acting on impulse and watching their parents do the same, they do not believe they can succeed. A very high percentage of parents of children who molest have impulse disorders such as alcohol and drug abuse, poor money management, temper outbursts, and physically aggressive behaviors toward others.

Children who molest have an exceptionally difficult time tolerating disappointment. They are sensitive to criticism and being called on their mistakes. This is an area in which they must practice monitoring the impulse to react explosively.

Playing *Mother May I?* and *Simon Says* with younger children is great fun and gives them practice controlling their bodies. A wonderful exercise for young children to practice impulse control is to sit with a snack in front of them, but not eat it right away. The therapist asks how long they want to let the snack sit without eating it. Children enjoy "proving" how long they can do it. They can gain more self-pride by extending the time, little by little.

Another exercise is having children sit one by one in a swivel chair without moving it an inch in either direction. Again, children take pride in proving how long they can do it. Even children with extreme impulse problems can keep the chair still for ten to fifteen minutes. The other children watch, congratulate, and encourage the child showing the self-discipline, as they monitor the time. These exercises are referred to throughout the life of the group to help children feel pride in themselves. Parents are taught to congratulate their children and encourage restraint at home.

Seeking Alternatives/Substitute Behaviors

In group, many opportunities arise to teach children to stop and do something else (i.e., substitute another behavior). This can be done in a playful way. When a child succeeds, he or she is positively reinforced. The group is also reminded that stopping and doing something else is just like distracting themselves to avoid molesting.

Opportunities in group arise when one child gets mad at another and instead of doing something hurtful, says, "I am angry at you." Another occasion would be when one child has the attention of the therapist and another feels jealous but does not throw a tantrum. Therapists should always look for opportunities to reinforce children for modifying their behavior. Finding alternative behaviors to acting-out is a big step, and is particularly relevant to molesting behaviors. Alternatives to yelling can be sitting down, relaxing, and controlling the impulse. Alternatives to the touching problem should be something the child picks and likes, something that expends energy and refocuses the mind. As children learn to control nonsexual impulses, the restraint they learn can be transferred to the touching problem.

Problem Solving

Children who molest have not been taught to identify and solve problems, nor have adults in their environment modeled this behavior for them. They need to learn to define the problem, identify the alternatives, evaluate each alternative and its consequences, select the best alternative, and evaluate the outcome. This process can be followed in many situations in group. When conflicts arise, the therapist moves in and instead of solving the problem, tries to figure out what it is. The children then try to describe it. It is imperative that the children generate alternatives themselves. It is not easy at first, because they are used to being parented by fiat. Most do not share in decision making in their homes and are surprised by a democratic approach.

After the alternatives are delineated, each child's perception of the best alternative is requested. Their first reaction is to select the alternative that they want without regard to the other children. Although this is characteristic of young children, it is exacerbated in these children who have experienced their parents reacting in the same way. The egocentric response takes time to alter.

Consensus must be sought in determining an alternative. If consensus cannot be reached, the group moves to a different alternative. After putting the alternative into practice, everyone decides how it turned out. Group members may want to remember those who agreed to compromise the most, and reward them the next time an opportunity arises.

Every opportunity for positive reinforcement should be used. If children are particularly gracious in compromising, they need to be praised. Children learn to absorb comments and build an image of themselves based on positive rather than negative statements.

Cognitive Strategies: Thought Stopping, Self-Talk

In group there are many fun and practical cognitive strategies to teach children. Children who have intrusive or persistently troubling thoughts can learn thought stopping. In its simple form, children find something to distract them from these thoughts whenever they occur such as reciting nursery rhymes or singing a popular song. Thought stopping procedures that include visual scenes are useful, for example, children can practice singing a song and forming a mental picture of the action. An excellent group activity and empathic gesture for the group is to work with one child to develop a tune and visualization especially suited to him or her.

Self-talk is a skill children can use when there is the possibility of anger, anxiety, fear, or other overwhelming emotions. Self-talk is memorized to help children talk their way through problems or emotions or the desire to touch someone. Self-talk can be any statements children find helpful. Specialized statements can be prepared for each child, for example, "I can do it" or "I can leave" or "I don't want to hurt anyone" or "I will get in trouble." Children are taught to repeat these statements over and over while they leave the situation and seek help.

Self-talk can also be in the form of longer monologues: "I am really mad. I want to hurt someone. If I hurt someone, I will get in trouble. I don't want to get in trouble. I can go away now and do something else. I can make my angry feelings change. My bad feelings will go away if I distract myself.

It is working, I am feeling better. I am proud of myself. I didn't hurt anyone. Everything will be fine. I am a good person. I am proud of myself."

Therapists can model this for the children. In a group session, therapists can recount incidents in which they used self-talk, for example, after getting cut off on the freeway. They can illustrate the use of an inner dialogue that prevented them from acting in an unsafe manner. Therapists can demonstrate how focusing on negative feelings can lead to thoughts that encourage negative actions.

Self-Observation/Self-Monitoring

Although young children are generally not self-aware, it is helpful for children who molest to become cognizant of their thoughts, feelings, and actions in order to stop the molesting behavior. Role-plays, plays, cartoons, and "stop the action" are techniques that encourage self-observation (see the Techniques section).

Boundaries are also an important issue in self-monitoring. Generally, the children's parents do not have good boundaries themselves and have therefore not taught this to their children. A metaphor for a person who is encroaching on someone else's boundaries is a "space invader." Different exercises can be made up using this theme. Without announcing what the activity is about, each child can be asked to approach another child and begin to tell a story. The therapist uses a tape measure to measure the distance between the two people. Children can then find a way, using their own body, (e.g., the length of an arm) to measure the comfortable distance between adults, between adults and children, and the comfortable distance between children. Raising the consciousness of parents and children by measuring is a concrete way for them to think about the issue. Space invasion occurs frequently in the homes of these children. Games can be made about space invasion regarding hugs, other types of physical contact, bathroom and bedroom privacy.

Additional exercises can be fashioned regarding emotional boundaries. Children can be asked about subjects they don't like others to ask them about. What are the subjects that therapists like to discuss and that children don't like? Are the therapists (emotional) space invaders? Is there a difference between the reason the therapists ask these questions and why others might ask them? Are there subjects their parents talk about or ask them about that invades their emotional space? Do they ask other people about things that invade their emotional space?

Perspective Taking/Empathy

Frequently, children who molest misread cues from others. They believe someone may be angry when they are not, or they do not attend to the feeling state of another person. Misreading cues often causes them to act out aggressively when the situation does not call for it. A quick, aggressive response is associated with their defensive posture in the world and their lack of perspective taking.

Children can best understand perspective taking through plays, during which they can play a role, indicate how they feel in the role, and describe how they think persons in other roles feel. They can check their perceptions by asking children in other roles. Children can also switch roles to see the problem from a different perspective. Perspective taking is also effective when a conflict arises in the group. The children can use real situations to see if they inferred people's feelings and thoughts properly from the cues given.

Attention to others' pain is not characteristic of children who molest. They tend to be engrossed in their own tumultuous feelings and anxieties. Although this is understandable given the chaos and pain of their lives, it is important to help them see others' pain.

Empathy is an important aspect of treatment, although difficult to achieve with many children. Throughout the life of the group, situations arise in which empathy for another is warranted, and therapists will need to model the proper responses.

When children are working on their own history of abuse, they can be encouraged to feel empathy for each other. They can discuss their ability to understand someone else's pain. Often children can understand their own pain as a victim and begin to understand how others feel when they are victimized. The concept of empathy is used for all occasions when children victimize someone else, not just for sexual victimization. Children who molest often physically or verbally abuse others, both adults and children.

A few children have been so badly emotionally damaged that little progress can be made in teaching them empathy—empathy never becomes a heart-felt response.

If children who molest are asked to write a list of all the things they do when they are mad, they are often surprised to see how many of their actions victimize others. Children can learn that being angry is fine; the problem is what they do to express their anger. Expressions of anger are positive unless they are destructive or there is a victim.

Anger Management/Frustration Tolerance

Virtually all children who molest have problems managing their anger. Teaching them to manage anger incorporates many of the same skills they are learning to control touching. Children learn what their body feelings, emotional feelings, and thoughts are before getting angry. They learn the major precipitants of their outbursts. They learn to short circuit anger by *Stopping and Thinking*. They then think of the consequences if they were to act.

Children are encouraged to talk themselves through anger. Self-talk such as "I can control myself. I have gotten good at stopping myself from getting angry. I am doing great" is very helpful. Each child can have individualized self-talk. Children learn to count to ten as they gain control.

Some children profit from a physical rather than a cognitive approach, such as punching a pillow to release feelings. Children can draw someone or something they dislike on a huge piece of paper and write things on it they would like to say, or have the therapist write on it. Afterward they can step all over it, tear it up, and stuff it in a trash can. Children get a visceral release from this type of exercise.

Metaphors are also helpful and educational, for example, having children think of a tea pot. At first the water simmers, then it steams and then it boils. If the tea pot is pulled away from the fire, the water will cool. Children are encouraged to talk themselves out of boiling over or exploding by moving away from the source of anger or heat.

Children who molest have little tolerance for the frustration of their needs and wishes. They are not very different from their parents in this respect. This is caused by impulsiveness, hyperactivity, and the inability to modulate needs and emotional states. Additionally, the limits that have been set for these children have often been overly rigid or unfair. They have often been asked to disregard their own needs so the needs of others can be met. Practicing and identifying the need to tolerate limits and recognizing the similarity to respecting another's right to privacy and not victimizing is helpful. When children are able to follow the rules of the game, wait for their turn, or respect the limits placed on their behavior, their restraint should be praised.

Planning

Parents of these children rarely engage in systematic planning to make things happen. In fact, most frequently they do not follow through on their promises. Not having role models for short- or long-term planning, these children have great difficulty completing their school assignments, getting their books to and from school, and acting responsibly.

In group, therapists can suggest planning an activity, such as a kickball game. Children are asked to figure out what needs to be done to make it happen. Therapists guide children through the planning stages, asking where the game could be played, how they get permission to use the location, where they would get the ball, how long they plan to play, when they would leave group to do it, how they would finish their group work so they could go play, and so on.

Therapists can also model consistency and follow-through in group. If an exercise, ballgame, or birthday party is planned it must be completed. The behavioral system must be carried out consistently. Therapists do not want to further the child's world view that things happen randomly.

Mastery

Children who molest have few instances in which they feel proud of themselves. Because their home lives are characterized by unplanned change, they do not generally follow through and complete tasks. In planning, it is important to know all the steps necessary to approach a task. For mastery the child must get a sense of accomplishment. Tasks performed well provide satisfaction, and help children build an internal image of themselves of which they feel proud.

Group activities can provide these kinds of experiences. A sense of mastery can be achieved at the individual and group levels. Individually, a child can feel completion by finishing a drawing or jigsaw puzzle. As a group children can feel proud by planning and having a birthday party for a group member. The opportunities are endless.

As children begin to feel proud of themselves, they naturally want to get congratulations from their parents. This is not always forthcoming. Therapists working with parents must help them understand the need to extend themselves to offer praise to their children. Therapists can encourage parents to provide children with opportunities to complete tasks and feel successful. If children can draw well, they should have drawing materials. If children can sing, the parents should listen to them regularly. If children are athletic, they should be encouraged to participate in sports after school or on the weekend. (Most children who molest have to substantially modify their behavior before they can participate in group activities such as scouting or team sports. Future participation may encourage children to control their behavior.) Parents may feel they do not have the energy, time, or enthusiasm to provide these opportunities for their children and may need encouragement.

Seeking Help from Adults

In families of children who molest, parental and child roles may be reversed, with the child feeling the need to take care of the adult. It may be that the parent and child behave at the same developmental level, both acting like young children, preadolescents or adolescents. This leads to children who do not rely on adults, or who have come to doubt that adults are trustworthy or consistent. To fill the vacuum, these children attempt to care for themselves. Similarly in school, they do not seek out adults for help with their schoolwork or social conflicts.

Working on family roles is done in the parents' group and in family sessions. Role reversals are reversed, placing the parents and children in proper roles. In children's sessions, they can be encouraged to see therapists as helpful resources, to learn that adults can give them emotional and physical support.

Children in residential placements may be unsure of how much faith to put in adults. They are often faced with ten or more adults (with different behavior management styles) who take care of them on different shifts throughout the week. Children often feel little appreciation for the staff, because they think of them as paid caretakers who do not care about their welfare. When a child lives in residential care and is in treatment for molesting other children in an outpatient setting, it is beneficial to have the same staff person take the child to therapy every time. The staff person should be someone who lives with the child and knows everything about him or her. The child can rely on that person to be proud of his or her progress in treatment. That person becomes a stable, caring adult in the child's life. Children who are unattached need a reason to stop negative behavior—pleasing a caring adult can be a powerful motivator.

Social Skills

Virtually all children who molest are deficient in social skills. They alienate potential companions because of their aggressive manner. Many are hyperactive and have poor attention skills. As a result, they appear bossy and unruly, and have difficulty taking turns and sharing toys. Some part of their molesting children emanates from difficulty in knowing how to engage with children in a positive and mutually satisfying manner.

Group therapy is an excellent arena in which to teach children social skills. Virtually every aspect of the group provides an opportunity for children to be aware of themselves and how they interact with their peers.

Children need to learn how to make friends and how not to alienate other children. In group, when therapists see an interaction that could foster or deter a friendship, they can stop the group and comment on it. In this way, the children learn specific behaviors. "Go make a friend" does not work, because these children do not know how to do it.

Discriminating Right from Wrong

We expect children to have a sense of right and wrong consistent with their cultural experience. Children who molest have generally integrated a set of beliefs about themselves and the world based on an environment that may be characterized by drugs, alcohol, and persons who looked out for themselves, often at the expense of others. Stealing, lying, cheating, hoarding, overt and covert sexuality, sexually abusive behaviors, swearing, impulsive acting-out, explosive rage, physical abuse, and victimizing others may be more normative than deviant. Children's beliefs developed in this atmosphere are generally maladaptive in a more socialized environment.

On the surface, children who molest may say things that seem consistent with a culturally normative view of right and wrong, however, what they say is not always consistent with what they think and how they behave. Therapists must listen carefully to children's basic assumptions. Whereas a child may say it is wrong to molest his or her sister, it may be all right to hurt her physically. The reason it is not all right to molest her may have something to do with being punished and nothing to do with a violation of her rights. Physically hurting his or her sister may be covertly accepted at home and not bring much retribution.

Is stealing wrong? The answer may be yes, but in practice the child may steal, and the behavior feels ego syntonic. It is not uncommon for parents to be engaged in activities that are wrong, but to which the family has accommodated in practice and accept.

If someone hurts you, can you hurt them? Whereas the answer may be yes for many persons, children who molest may not think in terms of an eye for an eye. They may want to run someone down with their bicycle and make them fall down a steep hill in retribution for having taken their ball on the playground.

Taking Responsibility for One's Actions

The attributions of these children are often askew. Many children who molest blame their behavior on anything besides themselves. One eleven-year-old boy said that it was not his fault he molested his sister. When asked whose fault it was, he said seriously, "My penis just did it."

In sibling incest cases, children frequently blame the sibling-victim: "She was such a pest, she wouldn't stay out of my room," or "She was always bossing me around" or "It was his idea" or "She asked for it."

Often the mother is blamed. "If mom hadn't made me baby-sit for her I wouldn't have done it" or "Every time mom changed his diaper, she let me look at his penis—that's what made me do it" or "Mom always gave her everything, and she hated me. I showed her." In group, children can be encouraged to catch each other in this type of thinking.

Some of the major defenses used by children are externalizing the problem, projecting blame onto someone else, denying the problem completely, minimizing the seriousness of the offense, and rationalizing.

Some parents and children are aware of the phrase "victim to victimizer." This may create self-fulfilling prophecies for victims if they feel they are destined to molest others, just as they were molested. When parents believe this it makes them feel less able to stop their children's behavior. It is useful to help parents and children understand that not every abuse victim becomes a perpetrator. A history of victimization alone does not cause molesting behavior in young children.

Although it is sometimes very clear how adults in the family were responsible for modeling sexual and aggressive behavior, providing an atmosphere conducive to the development of deviant behavior, it is not helpful to portray this as a focal reason for children's molesting behaviors. Children must take responsibility for their actions. They need to learn to accept that although the touching problem is only one part of them (and they are made up of many, many parts), it is still their responsibility. They are the only ones who can stop it. They must learn to control it with the help of people around them.

Some children may not have internalized the concepts of right and wrong and may view it as external to themselves. Some children believe something is wrong only if they are caught.

Therapeutic Techniques

Many techniques can be used with children in group therapy. The following methods have been found successful with these and other children. Every therapist has his or her own favorite techniques to use with children. To create a structured activity, select a goal, the skills you want to stress, and a salient issue. Then select a technique or a pen and paper task and create your own structured activity.

Plays

Children enjoy putting on plays during group. A child is chosen to be the director. It may be that this child has gotten in trouble at school, but insists it was someone else's fault. The therapists may suggest that this child be the director, and coach the children in how to act out the situation. Alternatively, the director can be selected because he or she was the most controlled, most helpful, stopped and thought the most, or displayed some other positive characteristic. The director decides what the play is about, or the therapists may direct the children to act out a story that includes an important theme the children can explore using the play format. The director selects which roles group members will play. Clinicians must stay aware of transference issues. Children can rehearse the play or simply learn the story line, with each child acting the way he or she conceptualizes the role. If the director says the roles are not being played correctly, this provides an excellent opportunity for children to see that there are many ways to act in a given situation, and that different people make different choices about how to act and react to what happens to them.

After the first version of the play, the director can reassign the roles. When the play has been done with children in different roles, they can be questioned about which role they liked best and how it felt to be in different roles. Taking different roles helps children understand how it feels to be in someone else's situation.

In most plays, there are strong characters and weaker ones. Often someone takes advantage of another. The perspective gained from playing each role can help children understand how it feels to be victimized and how it feels to be the victimizer. Therapists can highlight how the theme in the play parallels the children's touching problem in that one person takes advantage of and harms another, and the victim does not feel good. At other times, this theme can be used to talk about how children felt when they were victimized.

When a touching incident has occurred, a play can be used to help a child describe what happened. Explicit sexual behaviors should not be portrayed. If warranted, an inanimate object may be used as the victim to emphasize that no one should have to play the role of a victim of sexual abuse. A play is often good to break down the sexually aggressive child's attempts to minimize the effect on the victim. If the play enactments seem to cause unhealthy arousal, the play is best stopped and discussed with the group members.

Stop the Action (Hollywood Style)

This technique can be used in a variety of ways: in group, after group, and in family or individual sessions. Everyone freezes when "stop the action" is said. Whatever has been going on stops instantaneously, and everyone thinks about what has occurred.

When the concept is being introduced to group members, the therapists are the only ones who can call "stop the action." After the therapist has called "stop the action," he or she describes what was going on and asks the group to reflect on it. This is one more way of slowing down life for children and having them look at actions, reactions, and themes.

After children are more comfortable as a group and the concept of stop the action is clear, the therapist can announce a theme that the group will be looking for during group time, for example, anything that represents sadness, anger, guilt, victimizing behavior, empathic behavior, or cognitive distortions. The theme can be selected from the issues listed after the goals and should be selected for its relevance to individuals in the group. "Stop the action" is called not when the actual words are said, but when the theme is occurring in the behavior of the children or therapists.

Therapists can assign all children the right to stop the action or select one child to call "stop the action" when the theme occurs. This increases children's observation skills, sense of mastery, and self-importance.

Looking for "space invaders" is a good metaphor to use with stop the action (see the Metaphors, Self-Observation, and Self-Monitoring sections in this chapter).

Therapists may use stop the action to ask children what they are thinking and feeling at times when strong affect is registered in their bodies or facial expressions. It can help children to key in on the emotions that accompany their body feelings. Somatic feelings almost always precede touching behaviors. Children need to learn these associations.

Cartoons

Children like to look at cartoons, the funny papers, and comic books. Even children who cannot read enjoy cartoons. To teach self-observation, children can be asked to draw pictures of themselves in cartoon fashion. They can be interacting with others or be by themselves. Children can use cartoon symbols to signify thinking or speaking. The clinician can ask children to explain what is going on in each frame. Children learn to describe the progression of events through the cartoon sequence. They can learn to identify the precipitants and aftermath of their behavior using this technique. Therapists can write in words or help children spell, when needed. When children have built a behavioral sequence with at least three frames, they can cut the frames apart and put them back together in the correct order. The aim is for children to understand the antecedents and consequences of behavior.

After children understand behavioral sequences, therapists can have them take out one frame and insert another. Children can see if subsequent frames can stay the same, or if they need to be changed. They learn that different actions get different reactions, that if they say or do something different, it changes the course of events. This concept can be reinforced in the group in interactions among children.

After children have used the technique successfully in other situations, cartoons can be used to describe when children molest. They can draw frames identifying what was going on beforehand, what their feelings and thoughts were before they molested, and then how they engaged the children in the sexual behaviors. Frames should be included showing the aftermath of the molestation. Children should be asked to show the thoughts and feelings of the child who was victimized and anyone else involved in the sequence. Depending on how much they understand about their molesting behaviors, cartoons can be three to ten or twelve frames long. The more knowledgeable children become about the precursors, events, and aftermath, the more opportunities they have to stop the behavior.

When children have understood their molesting behaviors using cartoon frames, they can draw a frame or frames representing the substitute behaviors they use to short-circuit the molesting behavior. The frames portraying the molesting behaviors can be cut apart and the substitute behavior placed where it would go in the sequence. Children can then draw frames illustrating how the sequence would look after the substitute behavior occurs. They can simply tape one end of the substitute behavior sequence over the molesting behaviors. In this way, children can look at the differences by lifting the substitution behavior sequence to see the sequence of molesting behaviors underneath. They can build several substitute behavior sequences and keep taping them over the others. They then have something like a book of ideas.

Materials are shared by each child with other group members. The other children can ask questions and help the child elaborate the sequences or particular frames in the sequence. As children see what can be added to another child's sequence, they see how they can extend or be more clear about what they are thinking or feeling in the frames of their own sequences.

If there are no adults rewarding the child, or no signs of positive reinforcers for using substitute behaviors in the cartoon sequences, this can be discussed with the child's parents-caretakers to ensure that the child is being reinforced for diverting from the molesting behaviors. Eventually, children should feel internal reinforcement for their positive behaviors, but in the early stages, reinforcement comes from parents-caretakers and other external reinforcers.

The cartoon sequences are valuable to help parents understand their children's problems. Children generally feel proud of what they have done and enjoy sharing it with their parents. This can take place, with the child's agreement, in mixed parent-child groups or in family sessions.

Another way to use cartoons is to have children draw just one frame at a time. Therapists may want to learn about the thoughts and feelings of children on a particular issue. If the theme is nudity or body image, they can ask children to draw a picture of themselves washing up after a hot, sweaty, running game; a girl getting ready to go swimming; a boy at the doctor's office; and a boy in his room. Nothing is said about nudity or body image. The directions specify only which scenes to depict. Children are instructed to put any number of people they choose in the scenes. The main character must be thinking something and may be saying something. Cartoon balloons should be used. After children have drawn their pictures, they are shared with the others, who are encouraged to ask questions and think about the drawings.

The cartoons can be done in any way the therapists choose. There are an infinite number of ways to make this idea conform to children's needs. As a projective device cartoons have far-reaching benefits.

Progressive Stories

With this technique, children take turns adding on to a story the therapist starts. The clinician may want to focus the story on one of the issues listed under the goals. The children sit in a circle or around a table so each knows when it is their turn, and therapists place themselves at intervals between the children so they can redirect the story if it gets too far from the theme. Each child talks for a while or until the therapists ask another child to take a turn. After children have practiced, they learn not to monopolize the time and give the next child a turn without being prompted.

This technique gives therapists important information about the connections children make to the theme. Attending carefully to the transitions they make as they take their turns provides information about their associations to the theme. Where children move the story on their turn often provides insight into their thought processes, anxieties, and conflicts.

The quality of the story generally indicates how well group members are working together. When a group is a real working group, the story can continue for 15 to 20 minutes or longer. The content of the story also reveals the level of trust that exists in the group. Some groups make very safe stories, revealing none of the concerns of group members or the group as a whole. Other groups move the stories directly to touching problems or problems with aggression.

Making Videos

After a theme is selected, children decide whether to make a play about it, give a "speech" on camera, mime, or do a television talk show. There are infinite possibilities.

One topic children like to do on camera is abuse prevention. They can imagine they are making a television commercial for Saturday morning cartoons. They then decide how it is best to teach children not to get sexually abused or touched by someone else. This is generally first done as a commercial to protect children from being abused by adults. At a later time, a commercial can be made teaching children about sexual abuse by other children. This forces them to face their own molesting issues directly.

Making Pamphlets

Many themes lend themselves to the writing of a pamphlet, for example, the effects of being abused, living in a foster home, group home, or residential center, how children need to protect themselves from being sexually abused, all the different types of mothers in the world, and so on. Children can do the writing and drawing for pamphlets, or the therapist can type it after the children have created the content, and the children can illustrate it. If an 8.5 x 11 inch piece of paper is folded in three and the different surfaces used, it will look like the flyers and pamphlets put out by professional organizations. The pamphlets can be copied and distributed to the other parents and children in the program. Children's first names can be used so they become authors, and their confidentiality is respected.

Relaxation Techniques

Children who molest are often anxious and tense and suffer from hyperactivity. The amount of motor activity in a group situation is often very high. Relaxation exercises allow children to experience a feeling of control over their bodies and emotional state.

Before teaching relaxation exercises, the therapist should assess whether children will benefit from learning to relax. Whenever therapists use an activity focusing on the body, they should be aware that children can eroticize the exercise. If this happens, therapists need to stop and discuss what is happening. This exercise is best done after the bulk of the abuse-focused work has occurred.

Often children who have been abused do not feel safe to close their eyes. It is not important for them to do so, but they can if they want. The children should get in a relaxed position in their own chairs with their arms and legs supported. The various muscle groups are reviewed. Once the exercise begins, you do not want children to ask you what part of the body you are talking about.

Tell the children they are going to learn how to relax by tensing and releasing various muscles in their bodies. Give them an example and practice before starting.

Some people like to begin with the feet, some with the hands, face, or neck. It is easiest to use only large groups of muscles and progress in some pattern through the body. Your voice should be calm, soothing, slow, and almost monotonous. Each muscle group should be tensed for approximately five to seven seconds. The amount of time can be modulated depending on the children.

An example is: "Tense your fists. Make your fists feel very tight. Hold that tightness. Hold it so you can feel it tight. Now relax your fists. Feel the tightness going out of your fists. Feel the relaxation begin. Relax your fists."

Progress through the muscle groups as long as you can hold the children's attention. It may be that in an initial session you do only three muscle groups and later progress to more. After you complete the exercise, discuss with children how it felt. As they begin to differentiate the muscle groups, children will become more aware of these muscles and how they can control how they feel. The aim is to encourage them to feel in control of their bodies and increase their ability to make things happen in their world.

When children have learned the process of relaxation, they can take a larger part in the exercise by choosing the next muscle group or learning to give directions, which gives them a positive sense of control and leadership.

Children should be encouraged to practice relaxation outside of group. There are many times in their lives when it would be beneficial for them to relax. As they learn the precursors to their feelings of molesting, they can use relaxation skills to help intervene. Most children become aware of the build up of their emotions before problematic behaviors, whether sexual or otherwise. Although it is difficult for them to want to stop the behaviors, they need to have resources available to help themselves.

Guided Imagery

Some children have a wide range of active fantasies, some of which are sexual and many of which are aggressive. Children also daydream. Many of the fantasies or daydreams are maladaptive. Guided imagery exercises can help them understand the power of fantasies and introduce positive ways to use fantasies and daydreams. Asking what kind of thoughts, fantasies, or daydreams they have is a relevant question with children who molest, because sexual and aggressive fantasies can be precursors of negative behaviors. Fantasies can also be the substitute for negative behavior. Clinicians and children need to understand how the fantasies are being used. If children use them in a maladaptive fashion, it is important to help modify the behavior.

Sometimes children describe dreams when asked about fantasies. Although it is clinically relevant to hear and understand children's dreams, they need to distinguish between dreams that take place when they are asleep and daydreams or fantasies that happen in awake states.

One of the main purposes of guided imagery is to provide children with a technique for relaxation. To start a guided imagery exercise ask children to get in a comfortable position, usually resting their arms on the table, and stretching their legs in front of them. They may close their eyes if this is comfortable. Children can do breathing exercises, by breathing in slowly and deeply through the nose and gently exhaling through the mouth. They do this three or four times slowly and methodically until the tension goes away.

Children should focus on the story the therapist tells. They are to imagine the scene being described, experiencing all the smells, sounds, and movements as closely as possible. Stories can be about walks on the beach, by the side of a lake, in the mountains, or any other location. Scenes can have any number of people, can describe loving and respectful relationships between people, can describe a child being successful, or other positive representations of the world.

Negative scenes can be depicted using guided imagery if the therapist wants to describe a scene in which a child is caught touching another child or otherwise victimizing a child. The imagery can depict the child getting caught and suffering the consequences. The child's feelings should be described in detail. If the therapist is going to do a negative guided imagery scene, the children should know in advance. They should be told to rehearse this in their minds and bring it back to mind if they feel they might act-out.

Children can reuse the images given them in stories. With negative imagery they can reimagine the scene and enter into the feelings of the child when he or she is punished. This image can be used as a deterrent. The scene should be quite elaborate so the child can use it and become emotionally involved with it.

Children can also lead the guided imagery session. Some children make up wonderful stories about happy families going on outings together or doing other family activities. Most of these scenes are full of unfulfilled wishes.

Metaphors

Every child can have a metaphor for their touching problem. Some of the metaphors children have used are the "uh-oh" feeling, the "tingly" feeling, the "scary" feeling, the "watch out" feeling, the "wiggly" feeling.

When children have a name that represents the way they feel, the feeling and the name take on a stronger association and become more alive and understandable. They can then use the metaphor to describe their feeling to others. This name can be their catchword when they need to ask for help. This shorthand also makes feelings less frightening and foreign and more manageable.

Metaphors are useful for other aspects of children's lives. Children who are hyperactive, have explosive tempers, and learning problems often have metaphors for the way they perceive themselves or others.

Because these children have a difficult time respecting others' space, a focus of treatment is physical and emotional boundaries. The term space invader can be used when a child wants to talk about someone encroaching on him or her. Parents of these children are both physically and emotionally invasive. The term space invader has an aspect of comic relief, and can be used to alert others and themselves that they are not respecting boundaries.

Metaphorical Stories

Nancy Davis (1990) wrote a helpful book of metaphorical stories entitled *Once upon a time—Therapeutic Stories to Heal Abused Children.* In this book are stories for children with touching problems, as well as many other stories pertinent to children who have been abused. Another book entitled *Therapeutic Metaphors for Children and the Child Within* by Joyce Mills and Richard Crowley (1986) also provides useful therapeutic metaphors.

Clinicians can read some of the stories to the children and discuss them together. Children can be asked to make up their own stories. Gardner (1971) developed a technique called Mutual Storytelling, in which the child tells a story and the therapist repeats it back using the same characters and themes, but proposing a healthy resolution to the conflict identified within the child's story. Children can be asked to choose animals or other characters and create a tale. The morals children derive from the stories they create can be very diagnostic.

Role-Plays

Role-plays are like miniature versions of plays. There are only two people involved, and there is no director. Role-plays are generally used to solve problems. In a role-play, two children act out something that has been a problem for one of them in the previous week. If a child has had a problem in an interaction with his teacher, the child can tell a group member how the teacher acted and how the child responded. Someone else acts out the teacher's role as the child acts out his or her part. The group members can then assess the interaction and suggest alternate ways for the child to act. The child can change the way he acts and see if it alters the way the teacher reacts. Children can then reverse roles to understand how it feels to be in each person's shoes.

Role-plays can be reenactments of something that just occurred in the group. If there is an altercation between two children, or a problematic interaction between a child and therapist, it can be reenacted. In the reenactment, each part of the interaction can be studied. Action and reaction can be studied. Elements can be changed and the reaction to the change can be studied. Examining interactions gives children the opportunity to observe others' behavior and begin to observe their own behavior.

A variation is to have a child do a role-play with a group member standing in for the person the child would like to address but is afraid to speak to. This is similar to the Gestalt method of talking to an "empty chair."

Children often find it hard (silly) to talk to the empty chair, but can profit by having a child or therapist sit in for another person. Sometimes they want to speak to the person who physically, sexually or emotionally abused them. This technique is often very powerful for children who have been abandoned by their parents. They can tell the group what they think the other person would say, or what they hope the other person would say. It may be the child wants the person just to listen. Sometimes other children want to join in and say things to that person also. If a child wants to speak to someone who abused him or her, the other children may want to add their voices to express their feelings about their friend being abused. Support from other children not only encourages empathy, it also can be very comforting to the child.

Art Materials

The use of art materials is universal in group work with children. Many authors have described its general use (Kramer 1971, Lark-Horovitz 1976, DiLeo 1983, Nickerson 1983, Oster and Gould 1987) and recent works have focused on the use of art with abused children and children from violent homes (Wohl and Kaufman, 1985; Kaufman and Wohl, 1992). With children who molest, a useful exercise is the family drawing (Kwiatkowska, 1967). Every few months children can be asked to draw a picture of their family doing something together. Often children want to know if all family members have to be doing the same thing. They may be expressing the idea that the whole family never does anything together, and it would be a complete fantasy to draw that scenario. They can draw the family any way they want.

One of the primary indicators of progress for a child who molests is the health and support of the family; therefore the family drawing is an important indicator of progress. What each person in the family is doing in the drawing and the relationship between the members provides one more piece of information about family functioning. Children can be asked to describe what each person is doing in the picture, along with their feelings and other pertinent questions. Children sometimes use family drawings "to tell on" a family member. Family drawings can be done in family sessions, in group therapy, or in individual therapy.

Music and Dance

Music and dance are excellent tools for group activities. Therapists who play the guitar, piano, or any other instrument can help children think about an issue, listen to the music, and create a song. Children can sing it in their heads as a prevention tool, if appropriate. Performing for the other groups is a very rewarding thing for children to do. They can write the words, perform the song, and teach parents and other children the song. This type of exercise brings great pride and accomplishment to everyone.

Movement can be quite beneficial to abused children whose bodies may be full of tension and anxiety. Music and dance can allow children to engage in physical activity to free up physical and psychic energy.

Letter Writing

Some children want to communicate with the people who have hurt them. (If children cannot write yet, the therapists can take dictation.) In a letter, children can say all the things they never got to say directly or the things they are reluctant to say. The letters can be mailed or not. For some children, the effect is the same whether or not they mail the letter. If the letter is to be mailed, the repercussions should be thought through first.

Some children like to write letters to people to whom they have had a special attachment, but who are no longer available to them. In their letters, children can often express feelings they cannot express out loud, which often help therapists and children understand their deep emotions. It is not uncommon for children to express in letters positive feelings toward people who have abused them. Children must feel free to express their feelings as they feel them and not as others want or think they should feel.

Phases of Group Treatment

Phase 1: Becoming a Group Member

The first phase of the group is for children to identify all they can about their touching problem. Each child should begin to get as clear an understanding as possible about when their touching problem starts; how it starts; and what things, people, or times precipitate it. Are there particular feelings or thoughts they get before they feel like touching? Whom do they want to touch? Where on the child's body do they want to touch? Are there places such as their bedroom, or bathroom, that are more likely to make them feel like touching? Are there any thoughts or feelings they get from their earlier years that make them want to touch?

Although understanding the precipitants is an important step, it is also essential that children have a plan to short-circuit the touching. The group can help in this process, but the work must be done in conjunction with parents or caregivers, as they need to lend support to the child's struggle. Children must have a plan to move to if the touching feelings start. The parents-caretakers of the child should work together and, with the help of the therapist, devise a plan. Implementation of the plan must be carefully monitored by the therapist. Without help, it will be neglected. Modification of the plan may be necessary as different circumstances develop.

During this initial phase, children learn that they are important, knowledgeable, and can be the masters of their own fate. They begin to understand who they are and what they want to be. Therapists encourage them to think for themselves and to understand how they act and react. A sense of personal pride is encouraged.

Therapists teach children they are essential in helping one another to get over the touching problem because they have similar experiences. After the initial sessions, children are encouraged to ask each other questions to elicit information. If a child has had a problem on the playground with parents or teacher, the other children in group are encouraged to help the child understand the problem and look for solutions. If a child has remolested, the children are to ask questions to help the child understand the problem. As the children learn to help group mates, they understand their problems better. If the child is not acknowledging the behavior, the other children challenge his or her denial or minimization.

In phase 1, children learn to trust one another and the therapists. These children will learn communication, coping, and problem-solving skills as well as how to listen and play with others. The molesting behavior may develop from a variety of factors, including not knowing how to play and relate to children. The structure of the group must lend itself to the development of positive peer relationships.

If there has been sibling incest, the children are not brought together for therapy during this phase. The sexually aggressive child should be living separately, with the victim remaining in the home. Hopefully, family members with no young children are available to help take care of the child with the touching problem. If it is unsafe to allow the child to remain in the community, then the child must be placed in a more secure environment.

Phase 2: Working as a Group

By phase 2, the children have become a working group. The level of disruption is less. Children seek reassurance and praise from the group. The group becomes a source of nourishment for them: if a child does not come, the other children ask where he or she is. The group is less complete and satisfying without each member present. Children experience the group as they wish to experience their family—they want it to stay together and work toward its goals cooperatively.

They are now aware that they are the experts on their touching problem. It is their group, and accordingly, their job is to help each other when there is a problem. Encouraging children to ask each other clarifying questions when a child has a problem helps them think about the genesis of their own problems and to ask themselves the right questions about their actions and thoughts. Children begin to be keenly aware of each others' denial, manipulation, minimization, and cognitive distortions. The effect of a six-year-old addressing the denial and minimization of a fellow group member is far more powerful than an adult intervention. If a child remolests a child, there is a sense of sadness and disappointment on the part of the other group members. The group becomes a powerful tool in deterring children from remolesting.

Children begin to approach other children's parents and become acquainted. Often they want to visit outside the group. This is not discouraged, but the parents are advised to provide diligent, vigilant supervision. This can become difficult if two children become a unit and exclude other children in the group situation. This can be dealt with as a part of the victim-victimizer dynamic. Children should be helped to see that when they gang up or exclude another, they are being unfair and potentially emotionally abusive.

By phase 2, children's social skills are improving and cooperative games are easier to sustain. As they develop cohesiveness, the therapists can provide more opportunities for group problem solving. Whereas in the first phase, the group cannot generally function cooperatively in problem solving, this skill has increased by this time. The therapist may want to bring in five pieces of fruit for four children or three pencils and three markers for the four. These kinds of problems require the group to work together.

Phase 3: Integration and Consolidation of the Work

During this phase there is an integration and consolidation of all that has been learned. Most of the goals and skills are addressed in the first two phases. Previously, children focused on themselves, their behaviors, and their interior life. As they move to this phase, they look outward at who their role models are, how they choose friends, how they operate in their homes, and who they want to be. Their future goals are explored.

Many sessions are planned with the parents and children together. Multifamily groups are a very useful and practical way for interpersonal skills to be practiced. Sharing knowledge, laughing, and enjoying the company of other families is stressed. Most of the families do not have a supportive network of friends and family. This may be the first group they have tried to relate to outside their family.

Phase 4: Termination

Generally, if children have been in therapy for a year or a year and a half, six sessions before termination they should be made aware of their graduation from group. All six sessions will not necessarily be used to terminate, but children will have adequate time to work through feelings about termination.

Children frequently are very distraught about terminating. The containing function of the groups is experienced as a great loss. Many fear they will revert to their previous behaviors without the group's help. They also may feel their parents will revert to their behaviors.

Children generally talk about missing one another. The group mates are often their closest and sometimes first real friends. Some children regress rather dramatically when termination is announced. The six-week period gives them time to pull themselves back together before graduation.

An important message for parents and children to receive at termination is that they are doing well, but must remain aware that the problem may arise again. Children should remain aware of their sexuality and how they interact with others in relation to both their sexual and aggressive drives. They must have a clear understanding of their problematic sexual behaviors and a specific plan for what to do if danger signs arise. Parents must also be aware of the danger signs for the child, and any contribution they make to elevate the child's feelings, which may result in molestation. Parents and children must both be aware of what to do when they need help in the future.

If the school has been a part of the treatment plan, the plans for termination should be made clear to school personnel. Communication between the school and the treatment program should remain open in case the child has problems. Any signs of overly sexualized behavior should be evaluated quickly.

Phase 5: Graduation

It is generally very clear when children are ready to graduate from group. The unsettled, anxious, angry acting-out is gone and they are more comfortable with themselves and with others. The children's behaviors across the board have stabilized, and they have developed a working relationship with their parents or caretakers.

Children who are ready to graduate have an understanding of the abuse they have suffered. They do not refuse to talk about the abuse or break down when thinking about it. The abuse has been placed in a perspective that is meaningful and acceptable to them.

Sex and sexuality no longer draw feelings of anger, rage, loneliness, fear, anxiety, or other intense emotions. The child has not molested another child for at least six months and has been able to develop friendships with peers. Children's thinking about sex is not confused or distorted, and they have developed a sense of right and wrong related to sex, relationships, boundaries, privacy, and others' rights. They know that sex is a natural behavior in which adults engage for pleasure and to bring children into the world. They also know that children are naturally sexual beings, and they are aware of age-appropriate sexual behaviors and problematic sexual behaviors.

If children are preadolescent, or reaching puberty, there may be an upsurge of interest in sexual activity with peers which is normal and expectable. This should be analyzed by the therapists for any problematic thoughts, feelings, or fantasies, but responses may well be age-appropriate. Because these children are more advanced in their sexual experiences, they may want to move into sexual behaviors more rapidly than other children, but the most important aspect for a child who has previously molested other children is that the sexual behavior is mutually agreed upon, without malice, mutually terminated, safe, respectful, and that the other child is a friend, age-mate, and at the same developmental level.

An essential aspect of the readiness of children to graduate is the readiness of the parents to provide an environment that does not stimulate the child to molest other children. If the child has molested a sibling, a substantial amount of work is necessary to ensure that the victim feels safe with the child returning home, is prepared to tell the parents if any further advances are made, and the parents are prepared to listen and react appropriately. Children should be home and closely monitored for at least three months before being graduated from the group. The family should remain in weekly family therapy for at least another three months to monitor the safety of the children while living together.

Not all children in a group may be ready to graduate at the same time. One child can graduate without the others. The other children can profit by understanding what it takes to graduate and observing the process.

Graduation from the group can be made into a ceremony. Certificates can be made for the parents and the graduating children. All parents and children can meet for the ceremony. The children's therapists, the parents' therapists, and others including other parents, may want to make statements about each person who is graduating. Often the persons graduating want to say something about their experience in treatment. This creates a very warm and congratulatory experience.

Phase 6: After-Group Care

When children and their parents are told they will be graduating, they should be told at the same time about the after-group plan. Since the family members will most likely be in family or group therapy while the children are in group, the family therapy will probably continue beyond the life of the group. In addition, children profit from several postgraduation meetings over a six- to twelve-month period, which can provide an opportunity for the children to renew friendships and check on each other's progress.

Some agencies have parties during the holiday season to which past clients can be invited. This can be a practical, if informal, way to do a longitudinal study of the results of treatment and gives families a welcome opportunity to meet each other again and share their postgroup experiences. Formal longitudinal studies are encouraged in order to assess recidivism rates; the cost of longitudinal studies is often prohibitive and most programs can only estimate recidivism based on new reports of suspected abuse, or referrals back to the program.

While the group was ongoing, therapists encouraged parents to have children participate in community or after-school programs. Families should be encouraged to continue these activities for the child.

Special Issues that Arise in Group Therapy for Children Who Molest

Mandated Treatment

It is important to have a mandate to treatment from some outside agency. The two available systems are protective services or the criminal justice system. The main agency of choice is protective services, because it is their duty to protect children. Protective services may not open a case, however, if the child does not disclose any victimization. If the mandate of protective services in a given state is intrafamilial sexual abuse, they may not open a case if the child who molests is not in the family. It can be argued that although these are children who molest and not victims (at least at the time), they are oftentimes children at high risk in their own homes and children in need of special services. Protective services generally provides more services that may be of benefit to parents and children than probation. If parents do not comply with treatment demands, children can be removed by protective services to a therapeutic setting. If children are prosecuted in the criminal justice system (unlikely for a child under age eleven) or put on informal supervision, services are coordinated with the probation agency.

A mandate to treatment is essential. Children who molest are often difficult to keep in treatment, because it requires their parent's cooperation. After an initial intake interview, the parents may not return with the child for treatment, unless there is an authoritative incentive such as a government agency that requires their participation. The issues the parents need to work on in the parallel group treatment are often very painful for them to face. Many parents have never talked about, moreover come to terms with, the trauma and abuse in their own histories. Some parents are more comfortable just bringing their children to treatment. Even this may be difficult, because their own lack of consistency and follow through makes their performance sporadic. Oftentimes an agency with authority can encourage the parents' cooperation in therapy as a condition to returning children to the home, or avoiding an out-of-home placement.

Coordination of Treatment

A treatment contract is very helpful. Consistency on the part of the therapist in monitoring attendance and treatment compliance, is important. If the parents are not bringing the child to therapy regularly, it is essential that the therapist not let this slip by without addressing it. Because the parents are not consistent, they do not anticipate consistency in treatment staff. Being consistent and following through provides good modeling for the parents. Parents should be warned that they may need to be reported to the agency mandating the treatment, if they do not attend regularly. The contract should be specific so the parents know when they are out of compliance.

If the treatment staff feel that children at school are at risk, contingency plans must be made with the school. Special precautions must be put in place. An initial on-site visit by clinicians and parents with appropriate school personnel, will foster a close working relationship and ensure the greatest safety for other children, and confidentiality for the child. Children should not feel shamed in front of their peers or other teachers. Some children may not be able to be on a school campus until treatment progresses.

Consistent interchanges with the teacher regarding school performance and behavior are valuable. For maximum generalization the teachers, parents, and treatment staff can coordinate some of the goals for children using the same verbal interventions and consequences. If children are in an after-school program or with a baby-sitter, information sharing should occur.

All people who interact regularly with the child are valuable assets to the treatment plan.

Dealing with Victim and Victimizer Issues

Many clinicians struggle with whether to deal with children's victimization or perpetration issues first. It is essential to first work on stopping the molesting behaviors so that other children are not further victimized. It is then possible to deal with the issues simultaneously and throughout the life of the group rather than separate them completely. If children's victimization is worked on first, it is important to ensure that they do not come to believe their perpetration behavior is a direct result of their victimization. This can result in the children feeling they will always molest because they were victimized. Alternatively, children may use victimization as an explanation for perpetration and not take responsibility for it. An example of how to deal with perpetration and victimization simultaneously is in plays. Children can take the victim's role and relate how it feels. Another time children can take the perpetrator's role. This can be in sexual, emotional, or physical victimization and perpetration. Working on both issues simultaneously can provide an opportunity for children to understand each role better. Building empathy for the victim can be a by-product of this approach.

Another example of how to deal with both issues simultaneously is when the group is working on feelings. Children can be encouraged to identify feelings they had when they were being victimized and feelings they had when they were victimizing. The dichotomy between the feelings can be examined. There may be similar feelings such as anger, shame, fear, and anxiety.

It is important to pay attention to the behavior of children in the group in relation to the victim-victimizer dichotomy. Many instances surface in which children are playing out victim and perpetrator roles outside the sexual context. In one group, a child was being victimized by having the ball constantly thrown away from her and being taunted that she couldn't catch it. In another instance, some boys were mercilessly teasing a group member who had a palsied arm. These instances provide powerful opportunities to review the concepts and feelings related to the victim and victimizer roles.

Sexual Behaviors in Group

It is not uncommon for children to exhibit sexual behaviors in the group. A child may rub his penis or leave his pants unzipped; a girl may spread her legs with a dress on; a child may try to rub the therapist's leg or brush against the therapist's genitals; a child may draw sexual scenes on paper or write sexual comments. Sometimes a child attempts to touch another child's genitals. Each occasion must be dealt with directly, openly, and explicitly. The meaning and purpose of the behavior, and the feelings and thoughts that preceded the behavior, are explored. Other children's perceptions of the behavior can be examined. In some instances, the therapists may decide to give consequences to the child for the behavior. Some male children develop erections in group. If this happens and the child begins to manipulate his penis, the therapists can decide whether it is appropriate to mention it. This depends on whether the therapists think the group members can learn something from mentioning the behavior, and if others have focused on the behavior. Otherwise, the behavior is observed, documented, and discussed in an individual session or in group if it persists.

Sometimes the group material stimulates children, and they rush to the bathroom to try to get rid of the feeling in their genital area. At these times, it is generally useful for children to understand any connection between the material that was being discussed and the genital feelings to increase their understanding of what stimulates them. The nature of the stimulation can also be discussed. In some instances, children may go to bathroom to masturbate. It is useful to have a time limit for visits to the bathroom.

Therapists decide when and if it is appropriate for parents-caretakers to be informed about sexual behaviors in group. When this information is shared, children should know about it in advance. It is generally beneficial to have children participate in the conversation.

It may be necessary to develop a behavioral plan with parents-caretakers in order to extinguish certain behaviors both sexual and nonsexual which occur in group. The plan may include the school as well, if pertinent. Children feel more contained if they are not allowed to behave in inappropriate ways in group. If therapists are tolerant of behaviors that would not be tolerated elsewhere, children have difficulty learning proper rules and boundaries. The difference in group is that the therapists do not get angry or shout at children for inappropriate behaviors, but the rules of propriety are not different in different places.

Boundaries

The issue of boundaries pervades much of the work of children's and parents' groups. Most children who molest have not learned about personal space requirements, the right to privacy, or the right to emotional distance and separateness. All these issues need to be raised throughout the life of the group. The group format provides very good opportunities to observe and correct children while they are actively engaged in overstepping others' boundaries. The family session provides opportunities to observe the abrogation of personal boundaries of family members.

Before therapists start to work with children who molest, they need to decide about their own personal space and how they want to handle it. Although many therapists touch and hug children, particularly young children, physical contact is approached with caution. Many of these children attempt to place their faces and bodies against the therapist's body to receive a hug. They may try to bury their face in between the therapist's breasts. Kisses may take the form of the child's tongue licking, or attempts to insert the tongue inside the mouth. Fairly aggressive hugs by these children may occur.

It may be that children can gain more by observing personal space boundaries with the therapist than by receiving hugs. Therapists can decide to teach children how to shake hands as a greeting. If therapists decide to hug the children, the type of hug is important. Sideways hugs can be taught. Once children's preoccupation with sexualizing their interactions decreases, safe, appropriate touching can once again become a more natural process requiring fewer safeguards.

Rules on the use of bathrooms before, during, and after group can teach guidelines about privacy for personal functions. These rules can be shared with parents for use at home. During the time the inappropriate sexual behaviors are occurring, and until children learn how to control their aggressive impulses, it is best for children to avoid being in the toilet area with other children.

When a person projects feelings onto another, they believe the feeling belongs to the other person. Children can understand that sometimes they confuse how another person feels about something with how they feel about it. They can be taught the value of asking someone how they feel, rather than being sure they know. Children can also learn they can have their own opinion and other people can have different opinions. Although emotional boundaries can be difficult concepts, they are important to learn. Many parents project their negative feelings onto their children, and the children in turn do so with other children and with therapists.

Discussing Sex and Sexuality with Children

Children who molest often find it difficult to differentiate between sex and sexuality in general, and sexual victimization. It is helpful to discuss these topics with children in a group format, in which clinicians can reassure the children the discussions will not lead to touching behaviors. A prerequisite for therapists who work with sexualized children and children who molest is the ability to talk openly, clearly, and without anxiety about sex and sexuality. This is not as easy as it may seem because transference and countertransference issues may interfere.

Children who molest have an intensity about sex uncharacteristic of children their age. Because they do not have good boundaries about sexual issues, they are likely to ask therapists about their sexual activities and preferences. Therapists must be prepared for this and decide what responses will be provided. To give the children a model of appropriate boundaries, therapists' personal life should remain private. If a question is not too intrusive, children can be asked what they think the answer might be and what they would think about that answer. Allowing children to be expansive regarding their fantasies about the therapist may be too stimulating, and sometimes frightening for the group and therefore firm limits are required.

Fantasy material is important to understand and should not be lost. Therapists may want to have a session with the child apart from the group, or the child's individual therapist can be asked to address the issue. Careful consideration should be given to a child's fantasies about the therapist. These fantasies often include sexual and highly aggressive material. Therapists must examine, with the help of their cotherapist, any of their behaviors that may elicit these responses from children.

Therapists must use the proper terminology for the genitalia and sexual acts, intermixing this with the children's vocabulary (and that of their families) so there is a clear understanding of what is being discussed. This allows children to feel comfortable and learn the proper vocabulary.

In talking about the touching problem, it is very important to listen carefully to children to understand the meanings they attach to sex and sexuality. Many children perceive sex as a weapon, something that can be used to hurt others and something that can hurt them. Some perceive sex as a tool for getting things such as favors, drugs, attention, or acceptance. Some children think that sex and anger and anxiety are close to the same thing. Some children think sex is bad, others are fascinated with it. Although most children do not speak of sexual pleasure when they talk about their molesting behaviors, some children not only speak of it but have physiological signs of arousal (flushed cheeks, shortened breath, heightened energy and/or discomfort and frustration, and erections). When discussing the molesting behaviors, the therapist must not assume anything about the sexual aspects of it. Each child experiences the behavior differently. The genesis of the behavior and each child's patterns are different. Therapists and children need to understand the behavior as clearly as possible. This understanding is generally very important for parents to know. Questions to ask the child are:

"When you are going to touch another child what feelings do you get? Where do you get feelings in your body? What kind of feelings do you get in your [review all body parts]. Do you like the feelings? Does anything happen to your penis [vagina] at these times? If you could get rid of the feelings would you want to?" These questions can help you discern how sexual or eroticized the feelings are. In my experience, the younger the child, the less frequent are descriptions of arousal as sexually pleasurable.

Discussions about sexual arousal, erections, orgasm, and masturbation are part of the discussions the group will have off and on throughout the course of treatment. As the children grow older during the course of treatment, they relate to these topics differently. The group discussions should be at the appropriate level for the group at that time.

The distinction between sex play and victimizing behavior is very hard for these children to understand and needs as much clarification as possible. The issue of normal sex play is best addressed later in therapy, since some children whose behavior initially feels compulsive may perceive the elements of age-appropriate play as permission to abuse.

Erratic Attendance

Whereas all group therapy programs have difficulty with attendance, groups with children who molest have a high rate of absences. Although programmatic problems may need addressing, a fundamental issue is the reluctance of parents to engage in parallel group treatment because of their own emotional problems and the pain of focusing on problematic aspects of their lives. It may be difficult for parents to focus on children's problems when they are in such pain. They may see coming to group sessions as being only for the child's benefit and be less than enthusiastic about attendance. When parents are erratic, this causes the children to miss their sessions, creating substantial difficulties for children's groups.

Attendance in group is generally not the only time parents have difficulty following through. Parents need continual reassurance about their ability to feel better themselves and help their children. Although parents' groups focus primarily on the children's needs, it is important to address the parents' concerns and fears as well. Clinicians must take care that parents' issues do not overshadow childrens' issues, as this may recapitulate the home environment.

The contracts signed by parents at the beginning of treatment are to help keep parents in therapy. Therapists and parents should have a close working relationship with the person who referred the child to treatment. This encourages parents to keep on track and also provides the family with more support.

Accepting children into treatment without a mandate from an outside agency becomes very difficult, because an authoritative incentive to attend is one of the reasons parents best understand for consistent attendance. Some mental health practitioners refuse to provide treatment without a mandate.

Poor Parental Boundaries versus Sexual Abuse

A challenge in working with parents of children who molest is to determine when parental behaviors are within acceptable limits and when they become abusive. Sexual abuse may involve subtle behaviors, which are more difficult to observe or identify. In one instance, a mother had been told that her two children who were five and six years old must not bathe or sleep together and should not be in any situation in which they were not fully clothed in each other's presence. The children felt more comfortable with these rules. The six-year-old told his therapist in group that his mother had made him bathe with his sister. He said he hated it because he hated to see her vaginal area. It made him feel like hurting her. (He had been forced to have intercourse with her while his father and grandparents took videos.) The mother was approached and said she had forgotten; it was so much easier to have them bathe together. This was clearly neglectful of her children. The therapist reinforced that the mother had to keep clear what to do, and that the children would help remind her. The children replied that they had told her and she had ignored them. This concerned the therapist greatly because the six-year-old, a year earlier, had forced the five-year-old to have sex, and he had been clear that one of the precipitants was his anger when he saw his sister undressed. The therapists became more forceful with the mother about her need to protect her daughter and son. Although she insisted she would protect them, her actions jeopardized the children living together at home. The protective services worker was appraised of the situation.

Several weeks later, as the therapists continued to monitor the bathing, the little boy said he hated to sleep with his mother because it was too crowded. After questioning it became clear that the mother had all three children in bed with her. She was sleeping in the nude. Her explanation was that she felt more comfortable that way. She had been told that none of the children were to sleep together. Is this abusive? What would we think if the parent had been a male who was sleeping nude with the children? Was this mother able to provide an environment for her children in which they could heal?

Is a mother who insists that her eleven-year-old son kiss her on the mouth, even though he does not want to, abusive? What if she also refuses to let him have doors on his bedroom or on the bathroom, and she walks in whenever she wants to without warning? Is it abusive or poor boundaries when a mother tells her six-year-old daughter about her sexual fantasies, her boyfriends, and the types of contraceptives she uses? Is there a difference if the daughter is older, or the child is a boy? What about the parents who allow the child to come into the room when they are engaging in heavy petting or sexual intercourse?

All these situations and many more come up in the treatment of families of children who molest (see Chapter seven). Close attention to the interactions of children and parents is essential, because a great deal of tension and confusion regarding sex comes from the home environment. All therapists who work with the family need to discuss these issues and develop a plan. It is critical that therapists remain clear about their reporting criteria and responsibility and articulate specific recommendations to the protective services worker regarding the safety of the children. If the children's therapy is being sabotaged by parents who do not cooperate in following therapy guidelines, or persist in sexualizing family interactions, the therapist may recommend out-of-home care.

Premature Termination of a Child From Group

Some children at intake appear appropriate for group treatment, but after entering the group cannot profit from this format. This is a difficult situation, because the therapists do not want to make the child feel bad by asking him or her to leave, and yet the work of the other children must not be jeopardized.

Because the group is continually working on the issue of sexualized behaviors, the material itself provides its own source of anxiety. When this is compounded by other problems the child brings, the combination may overwhelm his or her ability to cope effectively. Some children become highly agitated in the group setting and cannot sit in their chairs even for a limited period of time. Receptive language disorders may inhibit a child's ability to learn in a group setting. Children with severe Attention Deficit Disorder may find group settings too distracting. Hyperactive children may find it too difficult to remain seated and attend to the group work.

Therapists should assess the group situation thoroughly to ensure that everything has been done to assist the child to profit from it. Many aspects of the group may need to be strengthened: Placement of children at the group table can be modified, group sessions can be better organized, therapists can provide greater containment of the children, transference and countertransference issues can be analyzed, distracting events in the group process can be minimized, the reinforcement system can be made more compelling, and therapists can be more proactive in calming the group when disruption occurs and in curtailing sexual and aggressive impulses. Many possibilities can be explored regarding the group and its structure before children are considered unable to profit from the setting.

After these elements are assessed and managed, and the child continues to have difficulty, therapists can work with the child individually to help him or her conform to the group expectations. The child can be coached in the group by one of the therapists who sits next to the child to offer more support; the reinforcement system can be augmented. The child can be given time-outs. Another adult can be available to accept the child for a time-out outside the group. Therapists can meet with the child and his or her parents to understand outside precipitants of the behavior.

Many steps should occur before the child is transferred from the group. In this way, it will not be a surprise to the group, the child, or the child's parents. If a transfer is imminent, a farewell should take place in a group session. The possibility can be left open to return to group if the child's behavior improves. There should be no secrets about why the child is leaving. It should be openly discussed in a caring manner in the parents' and children's groups, because both are losing members.

Having the child and parents leave in an open manner, with no secrets and with warning, is an important model for clients to observe. Most families have experienced dramatic and often frightening separations, after which people have disappeared. This way of separating minimizes angry and resentful feelings and does not leave anyone feeling abandoned, confused, distrustful, or suspicious.

Some children may be transferred out of group because they are far more seriously disturbed than the other children. This may not be evident in the behavioral manifestations previously mentioned, but in their pathological behaviors and thinking. If one child has murderous fantasies that include rape and mutilation, and these are mirrored in aggressive and destructive discussions with therapists and other children, a decision may need to be made about the costs and benefits to the child, the other children, and the group. Particularly if this is an outpatient group, and is the only place children would come in contact with this child, it may not be desirable to have this child discussing and playing out these issues. In some cases, the group format provides a platform for the child's exhibitionist pleasure in acting out his or her sexual and aggressive impulses. Therapists may be unable to contain the child, and the group may feel unsafe to others.

Bottom Lines

Although the intent of group work is to develop empathy for the victims, an increased understanding of one's own impulses and desires, and stronger coping skills, it is also helpful to have children understand the possible serious consequences of their behaviors if they were to continue. When this information is brought up, it should not appear threatening or frightening.

If children are living in their natural homes, it is possible they may be removed because of their parents' failure to keep them and others around them safe, and their own inability to curtail their behavior. If they are in a group home, they may be referred to a more restrictive environment.

Most children who molest engage in behaviors that, if they were adults or perhaps even adolescents, would be punishable by incarceration. Although it is rare that a child is adjudicated and sentenced to a juvenile facility, it is possible, and it has happened. There is also a serious threat of venereal disease. AIDS is a possible consequence.

Religion

People's religion is very personal and important, and their beliefs must be respected. In some cases, the parents' religion is a positive force. In some cases, the parents of children who molest have religious beliefs and practices that mitigate against using psychotherapy to its fullest. When this happens, the therapist must respect the religious beliefs but try to come to an understanding with the parents.

One issue that arises is finding the answers to the child's problems in the Bible and not finding the therapist's counsel useful. The therapist should try to work in parallel with the Bible. Another issue is that some persons believe, based on their religion, that masturbation is a sin. Many children who molest masturbate. In some cases, masturbation decreases the inner tension they feel about sexual and aggressive topics. For some children, masturbation decreases the molestation precursors.

When parents insist that children stop masturbating or be punished, the therapist can try to gain the parents' agreement to decrease the masturbation over a period of time. During this period, children can be helped to isolate the behavior to places and times they are not observed by anyone and gradually decrease the amount of time spent masturbating, until it stops altogether.

Some parents who describe themselves as strongly religious shame their children for their sexual behaviors and portray them as sick, dirty, and damned. Parents need to be helped to alter their perceptions. If parents continue to feel children are damned, an agreement should be reached that they will not say this to the child.

Cultural Considerations

Therapists must create opportunities to highlight unique cultural differences among group members. Therapists should learn as much as possible about a family's culture in order to support important family values and strengthen children's sense of cultural identity.

Walking the Tightrope

With children who have severe problems involving sex and sexuality, it is important that they don't view sex as bad. Children who molest have little real experience with sexuality, but are constantly reprimanded for everything that has to do with their genitalia. In this atmosphere, they may feel that sex is bad, dirty, to be hidden and avoided. They must be taught that there is nothing wrong, bad, or dirty about sexual behaviors themselves. When they grow up and feel love for someone approximately their own age, that person will willingly engage with them in sexual behaviors to express their mutual caring.

Information from Home

Once issues in the family are identified as problematic for increasing sexualized behaviors, it is helpful to monitor the home situation. Parents may be doing something that increases children's propensity to act out, in which case children are very likely to tell the therapist in an outspoken fashion that the parents are still breaking the rules. Children are generally interested in having the provoking situations modified.

This situation creates problems for therapists and parents. Parents may resent children and not want to come to group. These situations must be handled carefully and thoughtfully, because the parent must be helped to remain in the parental role and children must not be stimulated to act out sexually. It may be helpful to speak to parents apart from the children so they do not have to watch their parents feeling reprimanded.

Some children, particularly those who are in residential care, may be reticent to speak about their families. It may be difficult to learn much about what the home environment was like. Some of this occurs because children repress memories; other times children have been removed when very young and don't remember. Some families have a very strong rule against saying anything outside the family. Family loyalty frequently keeps children from progressing in treatment, because the harmful as well as the pleasurable aspects of their home life are relegated to silence or flights of fantasy.

If children are living at home and the parents are demanding secrecy about home life, this situation must be carefully assessed. There can be little therapeutic progress if children are always having to screen what they are saying to avoid telling things that parents-caretakers want to hide. The basic tenet of treatment is that sexual abuse occurs in secret, and there must be no more secrets.

Homework

Ideas, skills, and knowledge gained in group should be translated into children's daily life. To this end, children are often given homework assignments. An assignment might be to catch themselves about to do something they know is wrong and stop themselves from doing it. Children can be asked to tell the group about it at the next session. They might also be asked to make a list of all the things that made them think of touching during the week, or to list things that made them mad and what they did with their angry feelings, or tell the group three times when they were proud of themselves during the week.

Parent Conferences

If children are in group therapy with a therapist different from the family and individual therapist, it is important for the group therapists to meet with the parents on a regular basis. Therapists can decide, based on the goals of the meeting, whether the children should be in the session. The time can also be split with the children attending half the session.

Parent conferences often build a bridge between parents and therapists to the benefit of the child. Information is shared before and after group, but the thirty to forty-five-minute parent conference provides a structured time for the therapists to become better acquainted with the parents.

Assessment of Parents and Children During the Therapy Process

The progress of parents and children should be assessed throughout the life of the group. To assess the progress of children, the Child Behavior Checklist (CBCL) and the Child Sexual Behavior Checklist (CSBCL) are helpful (see Appendix B for CSBCL). There are two forms of the CBCL. One is filled out by the parents, and the other is filled out by the teacher. The CSBCL is filled out by the parents. The teacher can also be asked to assess the child using the CSBCL. These measures can be given every six months, and are a good way to determine progress. Parents can be asked to fill out the Adult-Adolescent Parenting Inventory every six months to assess the development of their parenting skills.

Other measures can be used to assess progress in the groups. Specific behavioral goals are helpful for each group member and provide a focus for the therapists. The goals are highly individual. Examples of goals for children are expression of a greater range of feelings, increased ability to make friends, and increased ability to attend to and respond to the material in group. Parental goals can include listening to children when they speak, answering children's questions, giving children positive validation for nonabusive behaviors, decreasing angry outbursts aimed at children, and talking to children about age-appropriate topics. Their progress toward these goals can be assessed at the end of each cycle, and new goals can be set.

Group Supervision of the Group Treatment Program

Supervision is one of the most important aspects of therapy with children who molest. Due to the complexity of the problems of the children and the families, group supervision provides additional input and resources. Attempting to work with multiproblem families alone, or in an individual private practice setting, can be extremely difficult.

Supervision can serve many functions: Training, information sharing about family members; examination of the group process for children and parents and the individual processes of children and parents; planning for future group sessions; assessment of the direction, needs, and structure of the program and participants; assessment of the stresses on therapists; titrating of treatment plans for each client and family; evaluation of case management; discussion of the need for child abuse reporting; discussion of any issues arising between cotherapists; and examination of transference and countertransference issues arising in the groups between therapists or between therapists and the supervisor or between therapists and clients.

If a treatment program runs parallel groups for children who molest and their parents, as well as groups for sibling-victims and siblings of the children who molest, therapists must share information. Group supervision after the treatment groups finish allows all the therapists working with family members to work in coordination. This diminishes the possibility of therapists working at cross purposes with families and increases each therapist's understanding of the dynamics of the family. Cotherapists for each group can also meet outside the large group supervision. Frustration with the slow progress, or at times lack of progress, of these families can be attenuated by the group format.

Summary

Although many treatment modalities are helpful for children who molest, group therapy is the primary treatment of choice. Adjunctive therapies are also important, particularly family therapy. Individual therapy is also very helpful. When treating children who molest, goals are specific and focused on the sexually aggressive behaviors, sexual patterns, any history of abuse, healthy sexual knowledge, values and attitudes, and positive relationships with others.

Specific issues are related to each of the goals. Because children who molest are deficient in most skills, this is an important treatment focus. Structured activities are used in the groups to help the children attain the goals. To develop a structured activity, the clinician selects a goal and a specific issue, and uses one of the therapeutic techniques to develop the activity. Skills can also be a focus of the structured activity.

The group therapy of children who molest occurs in several phases. Initially, the emphasis is on the child becoming a member of the group, then having the group enter the work phase, after which there is an integration and consolidation of the material. In the fourth phase, children begin the process of leaving the group. This ends in the celebration called graduation. The final phase is the after-group care of the child.

There are many special issues in the group treatment of children who molest. Requiring a mandate from a supportive government agency and coordination of services is important in the treatment of children who molest. Talking about sex, victimization and perpetration, bottom lines, religion, boundary issues, and handling the sexual behaviors of the child all provide the clinician with challenges. Erratic attendance, and premature termination of a child from treatment, are issues that need to be addressed with the parents. Homework, parent conferences, and ongoing assessment are valuable aspects of a group treatment program. Group supervision of a group treatment program is advised.

References

Cunningham, C., & MacFarlane, K. (1991). *When children molest children: Group treatment strategies for young sexual abusers*. Orwell, VT: Safer Society Press.

Damon, L., & Waterman, J. (1986). Parallel group treatment of children and their mothers. In K. MacFarlane, J. Waterman, S. Conerly, L. Damon, M. Durfee, S. Long, (Eds.), *Sexual abuse of young children*. New York: Guilford.

Davis, N. (1990). *Once upon a time—Therapeutic stories to heal abused children*. Oxon Hill, MD: Psychological Associates of Oxon Hill.

DiLeo, J. H. (1983). *Interpreting children's drawings*. New York: Brunner Mazel.

Friedrich, W. N. (1990). *Psychotherapy of sexually abused children and their families*. New York: W. W. Norton.

Gardner, R. A. (1971). *Therapeutic communication with children: The mutual storytelling technique*. New York: Jason Aaronson.

Johnson, T. C. (1989). *Human sexuality: Curriculum for parents and children in troubled families*. Los Angeles: Children's Institute International.

Johnson, T. C., & Berry, C. (1989). Children who molest: A treatment program. *Journal of Interpersonal Violence* 4:185–203.

Kaufman, B., & Wohl, A. (1992). *Casualties of childhood: A developmental perspective on sexual abuse using projective drawings*. New York: Brunner Mazel.

Kramer, E. (1971). *Art as therapy with children*. New York: Schocken.

Kwiatkowska, H. (1967). Family art therapy. *Family Process* 6:37–55.

Lane, S. (1991). Special offender populations. In G. D. Ryan and S. L. Lane (Eds.), *Juvenile sexual offending: Causes, consequences, and correction*. Lexington, MA: Lexington.

Lark-Horovitz, B. (1976). *The art of the very young: An indicator of individuality*. Columbus, OH: Charles E. Merrill Publishing.

Mandell, J. G., & Damon, L. (1989). *Group treatment for sexually abused children*. New York: Guilford.

Mills, J. C., & Crowley, R. J. (1986). *Therapeutic metaphors for children and the child within*. New York: Brunner Mazel.

Nickerson, E. T. (1983). Art as a play therapeutic technique. In C. E. Schaefer and K. J. O'Connor (Eds.), *Handbook of play therapy*. New York: Wiley.

Oster, G. D., & Gould, P. (1987). *Using drawings in assessment and therapy*. New York: Brunner Mazel.

Rasmussen, L. A., Burton, J. E., & Christopherson, B. J. (1992). Precursors to offending and the trauma outcome process in sexually reactive children. *Journal of Child Sexual Abuse* 1(1): 33–49.

Wohl, A., & Kaufman, B. (1985). *Silent screams and hidden cries: An interpretation of artwork by children from violent homes.* New York: Brunner Mazel.

12

Family Treatment

Eliana Gil, Ph.D.

The treatment of young children with problematic sexual behaviors (including molesting) must include conjoint family treatment. Children's behavior originates within their family, and the younger the child the stronger the family's influence. Attempts to curtail the behavior must be negotiated within the family system, which has inherently contributed to the emergence and maintenance of the problem behavior.

Family members of children with sexualized or molesting behaviors tend to resist direct therapeutic interventions, asking instead for treatment of the "problem child." Family members seem more responsive to educational directives about how to keep the behavior from escalating and becoming more troublesome.

When clinicians offer services to parents (or caretakers) of sexualized children or children who molest, it is important to work toward the goal of providing family therapy by building a therapeutic alliance with family members. This can be accomplished by empathizing with the family's current concerns, emphasizing the family's strengths, and being sympathetic to the fact that the child's problematic sexual behavior has more than likely been a shock to them. Parents may have discovered the child's behavior from neighbors, teachers, or other persons outside the family, or through direct observation.

In either case, the child's behavior has probably caused embarrassment, alarm, anger, guilt, and other difficult emotions. If the child has molested another child outside of the home, the news of this incident is communicated by either a frightened or angry parent or authority figures such as the police or social workers. The first task of treatment then is to "join with" the parents, demonstrating empathy as well as supportive and clear guidance during this crisis.

When children molest other children, or develop unusual or extreme sexualized behaviors, the presence of these behaviors may signal that the child has either been overtly or covertly abused. The early research indicates that many children who molest, and many children with problematic sexual behaviors, may be children with histories of physical and sexual abuse. It is important, therefore, to assess families using some of the known data about the dynamics that typically prevail in families in which physical and sexual abuse or neglect of children occurs. These dynamics are highlighted later in this chapter.

Joining

Joining is a term that refers to building rapport with families who come into treatment (Minuchin, 1974). Building rapport means making efforts to put the family at ease. Clinicians must convey both a willingness and an ability to be of assistance and demonstrate the expertise to do so. Therapists can decrease the anxiety typical of individuals entering treatment by making empathetic and nonjudgmental statements that encourage the family to share their private thoughts and feelings.

Rapport building is particularly difficult when the family is not seeking help voluntarily but rather is court mandated (Lehmer, 1986) or referred by authorities such as police or protective services. Although some families are referred through court order, others are encouraged to attend to avoid an impending unfavorable outcome. For example, children may be allowed to remain in the home with the stipulation that the family attend therapy and adhere to other specific conditions. Protective services workers may communicate to the family that if they fail to meet certain conditions (e.g., attending therapy, seeking medical attention for the child, taking the child to daycare or school), a petition will be filed with the juvenile court to make the child a dependent of the court, thus giving social services responsibility for the child's placement outside the home.

As described in Chapter eight, the response from authorities charged with investigating cases of children who molest varies greatly. Referrals for evaluation or treatment include situations in which parents seek therapy voluntarily, situations in which protective authorities have imposed therapy as a "condition" to avoid further action, and situations in which the court has mandated that the family obtain therapy. It is unlikely that young children with sexual acting-out behaviors will be removed from the home unless an investigation reveals that children are being victimized or neglected in their own home. If the investigative or protective agency workers believe that the family may be contributing to the child's problematic sexual behaviors, or needs education to learn to give appropriate guidance to or to set limits for the child—and yet the child can safely remain in the family's care—the family may be referred for therapy to address contributing factors. When investigators remain uncertain about the family dynamics, they may rely on therapists to conduct a comprehensive assessment of the parents' ability or willingness to provide the necessary monitoring and guidance to help stop the problematic sexual behaviors.

When working with court-referred or otherwise involuntary clients, clinicians can verbalize their understanding of their situation. "I know how hard it is to do something you don't want to do. I've been in similar situations, and I know how angry and helpless I've felt. You aren't seeking out therapy . . . you probably feel forced or intimidated. I imagine you are in a very difficult and frustrating position. Tell me about it." Mandated parents are not in control of the situation, and anything clinicians can say or do to help them feel more in control is helpful. For example, find areas of choice for them. Allow them to choose when they can come and at what time. If possible, give parents an opportunity to negotiate the method of payment and express your willingness to help process insurance forms. Give them a chance to ask anything they wish and encourage them to give you their version of the story. Often, parents coming into treatment under these circumstances tend to feel that no one cares, and no one listens. The clinician sets a positive and respectful tone by allowing each family member to talk about his or her perceptions and concerns.

If the clinician is of a different ethnic group than the clients, it is likewise important to acknowledge the situation and express a willingness to learn about the client's cultural practices. Clinicians can say, "I'm wondering what it's like for you to be in treatment with a therapist from a different cultural background than your own." Give clients an opportunity to talk about this issue. Many clients belong to minority groups and may have not encountered professionals of their own ethnic group. It is useful for clinicians to acknowledge what they know or don't know about the client's culture. For example, a Caucasian therapist meeting with an Asian family may give his or her understanding of child-rearing practices and then ask the family to provide additional information. In addition, talking about problems with outsiders may be culturally prohibited. As clinicians talk with families of different cultures, they can ask about any hesitancies to reveal information. Several books discuss cross-cultural therapy and they are valuable resources (McGoldrick et al., 1982; Ho, 1987; Sue & Sue, 1990; Ting-Toomey & Korzenny, 1991; Tseng & Hsu, 1991).

Assessment

The first step in formulating a treatment plan is to conduct a comprehensive assessment, beginning in the first session. The clinician encourages family members to give their opinions and perspectives of the specific behaviors of the children that has been deemed problematic.

In the initial sessions, the clinician focuses on the incident in question and the family's reactions to the behavior. It's useful to determine how parents and/or siblings have reacted to the child's problematic sexual behaviors and what corrective measures have already been taken. If parents are seeking therapy voluntarily, the clinician should inquire why therapy is being sought at this juncture. Incidents of concern may include either a range of sexualized behaviors (see Chapter six) or molesting behaviors such as fondling; oral copulation; and digital, oral, or penile penetration. Children may have molested their siblings, extended family members, neighborhood friends, or unknown children. In cases of familial abuse, parents have both offender and victim under the same roof, which further complicates the situation. The clinician must assess the family's responses to the child-victim, the current sibling relationship, safeguards the family has initiated to prevent the recurrence of molesting behaviors, and consequences they imposed on the child who molested. Generally speaking, it is a good prognostic sign if the parents are taking precautions to prevent further incidents of abuse (e.g., by not leaving the children unsupervised, not requiring the child who molests to baby-sit). In addition, it bodes well for the family if parents have acknowledged the inappropriateness of the molesting behavior (as opposed to denying or minimizing), sought help and guidance, and set consequences for the child's inappropriate behavior.

A family assessment tool (See Appendix F) was designed by Gil and Bodmer-Turner at A Step Forward for use in the initial family interviews with parents of adolescent sex offenders. This tool can be used with families of sexualized or molesting children. The interviews are usually conducted with all family members, including the child who precipitates the concern and the child-victim if he or she is a family member. If the child-victim is too young to participate in the family session, or if for other reasons the child-victim's attendance is contraindicated, the child is excused from these initial sessions; many child-victims are in need of, and benefit from, their own individual therapy.

At this early stage in the assessment, some important issues are explored. Is the family in denial about the events? Does the family minimize the problem? Are family members explicitly or inadvertently supporting or encouraging the problematic sexual behaviors? How does the family communicate about sexuality? How do the parents set limits with their children? Are the children behaving appropriately in the session, or do they seem detached, overly compliant, or frightened? Are family members physically and emotionally distant from each other? Do some family members collude against others? Is the affect or emotional tone flat or volatile?

Family fortitude is also assessed. What are the strengths of the family? Is the communication clear? Are the parenting approaches nonpunitive yet firm? Do the children appear affectionate and warm to the parents and vice versa? Are family members able to be spontaneous and can they enjoy themselves, laugh, have fun? Does there seem to be adequate emotional contact and support? What are the family's individual and joint interests and activities?

Once the clinician has conducted the family interviews and has a preliminary sense of the family's reactions and responses to the sexualized or molesting behaviors of the child, as well as the family dynamics, a social/family history is taken.

History taking usually begins with the childhood, adolescence, and young adulthood of each parent, progressing to an account of how the parents met, courted, formed a relationship (which may include marriage), and how they made the decision to have children. A history of each child is then taken, including developmental milestones for each. Any unusual or significant life events are recorded. If the children have endured parental separations, death of parents or significant family members, or other important events, the clinician documents these events and their subsequent impact on family members.

The clinician should obtain individual and collective data about the children's personalities, likes/dislikes, hobbies, TV-watching habits, friends, teachers, pets, and other relevant information. These data assist in formulating a treatment plan for the child and his or her family. Once developmental information is recorded, the clinician places the child's sexual problem within the context of his or her developmental history. Although the primary goal of meeting with the whole family is to gather data both about the problem behavior and the family's response to the behavior so far, the underlying goal is to assess many other family variables, as discussed in the following section.

Structural Issues

Minuchin developed "structural family therapy" in the 1970s after extensive work with underprivileged families (Minuchin et al., 1967), conceptualizing family structures along a continuum of healthy functioning. He postulated that problem behaviors (symptoms) would surface and then be maintained by an underlying dysfunctional structure. Minuchin suggested that clinicians assess the family's organization including the hierarchical structure, functioning of family subsystems (marital, parental, sibling, parent-child), emotional distance or closeness (often represented physically by where people choose to sit), boundaries (the invisible lines that regulate interactions), and the level of flexibility or rigidity in the family. Rigid families often engage in power struggles and untenable conflicts, whereas flexible and dynamic families may weather crises in a healthier and less disruptive way. In families in which there is ongoing or sporadic abuse of any kind, there are varying levels of stress, lack of family cohesion, isolation, secrecy, and feelings of helplessness that affect the nature and persistence of emerging problems. Since there are many unspoken disappointments and frustrations, emotional contact between family members is compromised. Abusive and neglectful families can be characterized by emotional distance; lack of communication; high levels of personal, social, and economic stress; community isolation; power imbalance between spouses or partners; parentification of children; general depression; and a feeling of helplessness arising from the inability to effect change in the family system (Waterman, 1986; Sgroi, 1988; Friedrich, 1990).

Physical abuse can cause crisis orientation—the family's emotional contact is organized around periods of alternating explosiveness and calm, punctuated by the presence of physical abuse. Walker (1979) describes a "cycle of violence" in cases of domestic abuse in which distinct phases of violence exist: "tension building," "explosion," and "honeymoon." These phases of violence can be observed with parents who physically abuse their children. Tension builds, chaos erupts, and a calm (temporary) reunification follows providing emotional closeness. The impact on family members is the presence of inconsistency, chaos, and fragile respite periods. Resultant feelings among family members include terror, shame, guilt, and helplessness—the very feelings that contribute to feelings of low self-esteem, entrapment, isolation, and an unwillingness to interact with others.

In cases in which there is parental neglect, the parents withdraw the necessary attention and nurturing from their children due to their own inability or unwillingness to function as parents (Polansky et al., 1981). Many neglectful parents have histories of severe neglect themselves. In these families, the boundaries are diffuse or disengaged, and it is the lack of emotional and physical contact that underlies family problems. Likewise, when parents psychologically abuse their children, they are either emotionally unavailable or they are critical, punitive, or unresponsive (Garbarino et al., 1987). Extremes in contact between family members, either through enmeshed or disengaged boundaries, result in a range of behavioral or emotional problems in children as well as adults.

Structural Problems

Hierarchy

Healthy or functional families have a clear delineation of power; adults seem able to use their authority to provide guidelines and limits for their children. When a hierarchy is well defined and in place, the adults are clearly in charge, creating a "united front" that enhances the enforcement of necessary rules and regulations.

In families in which one or more children engage in sexually inappropriate, problematic, or molesting behaviors, it is important to explore how well or how poorly the parents are providing clear boundaries, guidelines about sexuality, or appropriate limit-setting with acting-out behaviors.

Marital/Parental Subsystem

Ideally, the adults in a family are willing and able to function as a partnership; decisions are made jointly after clear discussions and negotiation. The adults present a united front because a united front in fact exists. This ability for individuals to work collaboratively and effectively usually happens when the marital relationship is strong, flexible, and cooperative. If conflicts in the partnership or marriage are approached and resolved effectively, these conflict-resolution skills can be applied to the many decisions involved in the parental roles.

Sometimes the adult relationship functions well, and yet parenting tasks seem unmanageable. The individuals may have such different backgrounds and divergent views about child rearing that an impasse in effective communication and decision making can occur. In these families, the conflicts in the parental subsystem can create problems for the marital system, or the marital system may become stronger as a result of feeling greater success. In addition, it is possible for parents to acknowledge the discrepancy between their functioning as marital partners and parents without developing a clear strategy for resolution; the couple simply ignores parenting issues.

Triangulation

Triangulation occurs when a third party (or situation) is thrust upon a relationship between two individuals. Triangulation can be used to diffuse conflict, or to obtain support for a position. For example, two individuals engaged in a heated argument may turn to a third person to diffuse escalation of the conflict. As soon as a third person enters the discussion with a new point of view, or to point out new aspects of the situation, the argument changes in intensity and focus. Likewise, a third person can be brought in for support and alliance. A frustrated individual may look for a vote of confidence from a colleague or friend, hoping to shift the balance of power in his or her favor. "Dexter and I both think that you need to take a different position," is a much stronger argument than "I think . . ."

Many unhealthy patterns of interaction can develop when children are triangulated into arguments between parents. Children can be recruited as allies and involuntarily drafted into a heated exchange between parents. Children can also learn how to inject themselves into the parental dyad, weakening one or the other parent's power hold. It is very common for children who have been told "no" by one parent to approach the other parent with the same request. Children quickly learn which parent is more or less likely to acquiesce to their demands and act accordingly. Unless parents function as a parental team, children will succeed in getting their needs met while pitting one parent against the other. In less functional families, parents triangulate children to meet their own needs. For example, a parent who feels there is insufficient physical affection from his or her partner or spouse, and has failed to resolve this issue directly, may consciously or unconsciously seek out a child to obtain desired increased physical affection. A parent who feels lonely, isolated, or dissatisfied may turn to the child for substitute companionship, restricting the child's normal developmental needs for peer contact and social activity.

Children may develop interesting and complex coping strategies to deal with physical abuse between parents or adult caretakers. Children may try to protect one parent from another by eliciting negative attention; children may learn to "provoke" negative attention, feeling relieved and powerful when they "take" a beating for a hurt and weary parent. A parent may also turn on a child. Some parents who are abused or maltreated feel incapable of standing up for themselves against their perpetrator. They may harbor deep feelings of pain, resentment, and anger, which can find their expression through hostile verbal and physical attacks on their helpless children who cannot fight back.

In incest families, triangulation is at its most obvious. The parent-perpetrator is likely experiencing feelings of isolation, pain, helplessness, low self-esteem, frustration, and anger. These feelings can cause the individual to seek comfort from a dependent and trusting child. The child will certainly try to please, comply, and adapt to parental expectations and requests. The parent-perpetrator relates to the child as a mate rather than a child, perceiving the child capable of providing adult companionship and comfort. The relationship gradually takes on imposed aspects of an adult intimate relationship; intimacy becomes inappropriately sexualized. In sexual abuse situations, the parent places his or her needs in front of the child. The parent who

becomes sexual with his or her child forsakes all the privileges and responsibilities of parenthood, violating the child's trust.

Triangulation can become a habitual problem in families and can
jeopardize parental gratification of the child's developmental needs.

Correlated Issues

Drug and Alcohol Abuse

In many families, drug and alcohol abuse exists alongside physical and
sexual abuse, as well as psychological abuse and neglect. While the statistics
may not yet be exact, several studies have found a correlation. In 1954,
Kaufman and co-workers found that 73 percent of incest fathers were
alcoholic. Cavallin and co-workers (1965) found that 25 percent of fathers
imprisoned for sex with prepubertal daughters were alcoholic: Cavallin
(1965) found that 33 percent of his sample of incestuous fathers were
alcoholic. Ryan et al. (1987) noted that in a study of one thousand adolescent
sex offenders referred for treatment, substance abuse was found in 27 percent
of mothers and 43 percent of fathers. Approximately 40 to 50 percent of
cases I've treated (including physical and sexual abuse, neglect, and emotional abuse) have included parental difficulties with drug use. In familial
child sexual abuse, a parent-perpetrator crosses parental boundaries and
becomes sexual with a child, often using substances to disinhibit the impulse
to molest. In extrafamilial abuse cases, substances may be used to seduce
and disinhibit targeted victims. Perpetrators often befriend young children
by acting as confidantes and peers who provide children with the excitement
of using illicit drugs. Once the children's natural defenses are lowered
through substance use, sexual activity can be introduced and encouraged,
increasing the youngster's interest, arousal, compliance, and participation.

Parents who neglect their children are incapacitated by their use and
abuse of substances. Under the influence of drugs, parents have impaired
judgment and engage in narcissistic tending to their own needs, neglecting
the responsibility to provide adequate care, nurturing, and protection of their
children. In addition, violence may often erupt in families in which drug use
seems to ignite existing frustrations and feelings of despair.

Drug use does not *cause* abusive or neglectful behavior. The parents'
capacity to abuse or neglect already exists, and this preexisting condition,
often kept under control while sober, becomes uncontrollable while under
the influence of drugs. The impulses toward abuse or neglect may have
existed for a long time without expression, and yet the influence of drugs
may contribute to acting-out behaviors. Obviously, drug use is relevant to
family functioning. Even when parents verbalize ongoing or renewed efforts

to minimize or normalize their drug use, clinicians must keep a sharp focus on drug use, refer the parents to specialized treatment programs, and rigorously evaluate child safety. The problems of physical and sexual abuse, or neglect, cannot be put on the sidelines while drug recovery occurs. Conversely, the problem of drug abuse cannot be overlooked or postponed in order to work on parental abuse or neglect. Drug use may well place the children at risk, and should be carefully assessed when considering the family's amenability to therapy and children's need for protection.

History of Violence

In addition to a history of drug use, clinicians should assess the family's history of violent behavior, whether it is violence between the adults (often witnessed by children), violence from parent to child, or violence between siblings. When children develop problematic sexual behaviors, they may have experienced abuse or may have been exposed to violence in the home. Ryan et al. (1987) noted that of one thousand juvenile sex offenders referred for treatment, parental violence was frequently witnessed by the adolescents. A treatment plan must include a clear and ongoing program of violence abatement.

The issue of physical violence cannot be minimized, normalized, and placed on the back burner in order to focus on children's sexual acting-out behaviors. The problems must be addressed simultaneously, and the treatment plan must include ongoing risk assessments of the children with appropriate referrals to complementary recovery programs, such as violence abatement programs and shelters.

In addition to assessing overt physical abuse, many parents have issues with powerlessness, abuse of power, and difficulties with anger management (Thomas, 1991). Fathers who physically and sexually abuse have been found to be domineering (Goodwin et al., 1982), as well as demonstrating a need to control others out of pervasive feelings of inadequacy (Kaufman & Wohl, 1992). Dominance and control issues permeate parent-child interactions in abusive families.

Prior Contact with Authorities

Clinicians should also inquire about the family's prior contacts with authorities, including probation officers, the police, social workers, and mental health professionals. These involvements may be chronic or episodic and may shed light on the family's overall functioning; families may fail to accurately report prior involvements with authorities in an effort to protect themselves and appear in a better light.

Inappropriate Affective Expression (Sexualized Intimacy)

Families may be stymied in their efforts to achieve emotional closeness with each other. They may feel isolated, frustrated, lonely, and inadequate. Family members may be unable to give or receive physical affection or emotional support. Emotional distance and disappointment becomes progressive. Verbal and nonverbal communication decrease in emotionally flat families, and eventually both parents and children feel as if they are coexisting. The longing for intimacy remains elusive.

One way that intimacy is achieved in emotionally barren families is through sexual contact. Individuals who initiate sex are often seeking the feelings of intimacy that can accompany lovemaking. In families with inappropriate boundaries, adults may turn to children to meet their intimacy needs. Groth et al. (1982) note that incest fathers sexualize their nonsexual needs. Gilgun (1988) suggests a "nonnormative" sexual environment in the home. Kaufman and Wohl (1992) state that often in incestuous families fathers are incapable of establishing adult intimate relationships. Intimacy can take overt or covert sexual expression as children are perceived as sexual objects. Given these circumstances, the family dynamics create a climate in which abuse can emerge. Although most of the literature discusses the family dynamics in which parent-child incest occur, these dynamics also occur in families in which one child molests another (see Chapter seven). The end result is that family boundaries are confused and garbled, and children are at high risk for either hands-on sexual abuse, or covert sexual exploitation.

Deviant Arousal Patterns (Thinking and Perception Errors)

As adults turn to children as sexual objects, a series of deviant arousal patterns emerge. Adults develop errors in thinking that affect their perceptions. They become sexually aroused by children and justify their actions by telling themselves that their children are asking for sex, reciprocating equally, enjoying themselves, and so on. Frequently, offenders view children's inability to verbalize "no" as a sign that they desire and reciprocate sexual activity. In addition, if children's bodies respond to manual stimulation and become erect or orgasmic, offenders may view the physiological changes as evidence of the children's cooperation and enjoyment of the sexual abuse.

Parents who become sexually aroused by their children become conditioned to be sexually aroused by other children as well. Arousal can become generalized to other children (siblings or other children), although in some cases the arousal is restricted to one specific child. The literature on child sexual offenders presents a range of offending behavior: some molesters eventually molest all their children, molest only children of specific ages, or may molest only children of one gender. The variations in offender behaviors is vast, and several typologies attempt to conceptualize the offending patterns of adult offenders (Groth, 1978; Knight & Prentky, 1990; Patton, 1991; Finkelhor and Williams, 1992).

One thing is certain. Recent research (Marshall et al., 1990) has challenged the notion that intrafamilial molesters do not molest out of the home, or that molesters who choose a family member to victimize won't select others (in and out of the home).

Acts of Omission/Commission

Not all inappropriate parental behaviors are acts of commission (hands-on contact). Acts of omission occur when parents fail to provide adequate guidance and limits. For example, a child may approach a parent and grab his or her genitals. The parent ignores the behavior and allows the child to fondle him or her. The parent denies wrongdoing on the basis of a passive response ("I never touched her") and the child's initiation of the behavior ("She wanted to do it"). Children need appropriate guidance and limits that will shape necessary social behavior. Finkelhor (1978) found that some families were sex positive and others sex negative. The sex-positive families have a positive attitude toward sexuality and respect boundaries, provide accurate information about sex, positive attitudes about bodies, and show physical affection. Sex-negative families give inaccurate information about sexuality, convey anxiety about sexuality and physical affection, and react in punitive and shaming ways.

Level of Content Focus/Denial

Some parents are sexually preoccupied themselves, and therefore may consciously or unconsciously interject sexual themes and suggestions into most of their interactions with adults and children. Boat (1990) has categorized families erotophobic and erotophilic. Erotophobic families might be punitive and anxious about children's sexual behaviors. Erotophilic parents may be unable to set any appropriate limits or respond to children's request for guidance. These extremes become problematic for the development of healthy sexuality in children. Parents may constantly direct children's attention to sexual matters on television or in print, or may project sexual motives to the children. One parent constantly said, "I know what you're thinking right now. You're probably imagining yourself caressing that beautiful body, or kissing those voluptuous lips." When these parents made love, they told their children what they were going to do and then made loud noises so the children could hear—the door was always ajar, inviting the children to peek. In these cases, parents are focusing their children's attention on sexuality. When confronted with their sexualized behavior, they may remain in denial.

Family of Origin Issues

A wide range of family of origin issues may influence the organization of family hierarchy, roles, boundaries, and interactions. No linear cause and effect is seen between childhood experiences and adult family interactions, and yet early experiences contribute greatly to unconscious reenactments of prior events. Ryan (1991) describes families of juvenile sex offenders as having "manifold problem areas, frequently involving a multigenerational history of interpersonal violence and sexual abuse" (p. 158). Mrazek and Kempe (1981) found that of all the contributing factors mentioned in the literature, the most predictive (of sexual abuse) were likely to be the absence of a strong, satisfying marital bond, and prior incestuous behavior in the histories of parents. Not everyone with a history of childhood abuse repeats the abusive patterns. The contribution of negative childhood experiences can decrease significantly when individuals make efforts to challenge the lessons they learned and make conscious choices to live their adult lives in a different manner. For example, adults raised by alcoholic parents themselves may become alcoholic parents or may make a clear decision to avoid involvement with alcohol and be sober.

Unresolved Traumas

One of the factors that has an impact on adult behavior is the adequate resolution of childhood traumas. Unresolved traumatic material can influence adult functioning. Parents who have ignored, avoided, or forgotten their history of childhood abuse may inadvertently become abusive. One such parent confided her thoughts about hitting her daughter: "I don't know why I hit her. I look at her face, her eyes are red, she's sobbing, and I see myself. I can't seem to stop myself from hitting her, I feel terribly guilty after I do, but when I hold her and comfort her it's as if I'm being comforted also." This parent had a history of physical abuse, which she preferred to avoid, insisting that it no longer affected her life, and that she was too busy to undertake therapy for herself. The unresolved history of abuse became clear and present in her relationship with her daughter.

Another woman who sought therapy did so because she was in a relationship with a man who abused her physically. Reflecting on her boyfriend's abuse, she stated, "One day I'll have the courage to leave him . . . it won't be like it was when I was a child and couldn't leave. I was trapped then, I'm not trapped now." After six months of therapy that focused on her own abuse as a child, she was able to extricate herself from the abusive relationship. In this case, the client's history of abuse had propelled her into accepting an adult relationship that included violence. By unconsciously reenacting the dynamics of victim-victimizer, she created a situation that allowed her an opportunity to change the outcome. In her adult abusive relationship, she found the strength to escape as she wasn't able to escape when she was a child. She went from a position of helpless victim to empowered survivor.

Whether it's a history of violence or sexual abuse, some evidence suggests that these traumatic histories have an impact on current abusive patterns in parents. Lankester and Meyer (1986) found that 64 percent of 153 family members of juvenile sex offenders had a history of either physical or sexual abuse.

Prescribed Gender Roles

In some cases, individuals can feel confined or trapped by the roles assigned to them through gender. The confinement of stereotyped gender roles can lead to unhappiness, frustration, or despair. Adults with gender confusion or dissatisfaction can interact with their children in ways that create childhood gender-identity confusion or concern. For example, a mother of a six-year-old boy often dressed him in dresses and let his hair grow long. The boy was named Francis, which could have been either a girl's or boy's name. When outsiders mistook the boy for a girl, the mother made no efforts to correct their misperception. Francis was referred for treatment because he was constantly drawing pictures of nudes with both sets of genitals, telling sexually explicit stories, and grabbing his friend's genitals whenever he could. Francis's acute distress about his own sexual identity, was caused by his mother's unwillingness to accept him as a male, due to her own views of men as both threatening and powerful.

Cultural and Religious Attitudes or Beliefs

Just as individuals develop thinking and perception errors as attempts to rationalize, minimize, or justify their inappropriate actions, so individuals can refer to cultural or religious attitudes and beliefs to do the same.

Clinicians may over- or underreact to abusive behavior in families, pointing to cultural or religious differences that many believe to be untractable and resistant to change. In addition, clinicians may want to exhibit respect for culture or religion by overlooking abusive interactions in misguided fashion. Clinicians must remember that although definite cultural differences exist in child-rearing, no culture openly condones physical and sexual abuse or neglect of children. Many cultures and religions may support physical discipline, but none support injuring children. Although some cultures in northern Europe are more relaxed about adult sexual contact with preadolescents or adolescents, none presently encourage incest or sexual contact between adults and young children.

When cultural or religious beliefs serve as the foundation for physically or sexually abusive behavior by parents toward children, between children, or between spouses or partners, these beliefs must be confronted and alternatives sought.

Social Stressors: Family Vulnerabilities

Trepper and Barrett (1990) discuss the assessment of "family vulnerabilities" when treating incestuous families. This concept allows clinicians to look at those areas of family functioning that need strengthening and support. All families have vulnerabilities to external stressors such as financial problems, family deaths, unemployment, or catastrophic events (e.g., earthquakes, hurricanes, or floods). Internal stressors also emerge from disappointments, resentments, frustrations, unresolved conflicts, and tensions. Family secrets and exclusionary collusions between family members can also cause family vulnerabilities.

Family Treatment

When children molest other children, the treatment must be multilevel. The behavior of sexualized children or children who molest brings the family into treatment; the initial focus is on the problematic sexual behavior. However, all family members deserve concern and attention. Gelinas (1988) describes an approach she labels "multilaterality," in which the therapist takes into account every family member's needs and interests, lifting up people's sides if they are themselves unable to do so. She says that rather than being the agent of only one person exclusively, perhaps in these cases either the victim or child who molests, the therapist persistently attempts to deal with every family member's needs and rights and acts responsibly toward all members of the family. In summary, Gelinas promotes holding each family member accountable for his or her actions, attending to each member's investments and rights, and balancing these issues among individuals.

When children with sexualized behaviors are evaluated, frequently the treatment of choice is to provide brief therapy for the parents. Often sexualized behaviors are alarming to parents, who seek help in providing appropriate responses. When parents apply behavioral strategies (see Chapter six), the problematic aspects of the child's behavior may decrease and normalize. If the behavior persists or escalates, children may require individual or group treatment. It is not advisable to place children with sexualized behaviors in groups with children who have already molested, since the sexualized children may become overstimulated, and the children who molest may role model inappropriate molesting behaviors. Children who molest require a more aggressive therapy approach, which can include individual, group, and family treatment. The treatment plan for children who molest must consider the contribution of the family dynamics on the child's sexual acting-out (including possible overt or covert sexual abuse). Those who work with adolescent sex offenders have consistently stated the importance of having family members participate in the assessment and treatment (Knopp, 1982; Breer, 1987; Steen and Monnette, 1989; Ross & Loss, 1991; Thomas, 1991). The family's participation in treatment is even more critical with younger children. Younger children are more dependent on their parents and parental influence is greater. In addition, young children are more susceptible to lessons taught by parents or caretakers, since behavior is being shaped during formative years.

A comprehensive assessment reveals familial problems. In particular, family interactions that encourage or permit molesting behaviors on the part of children are identified. Parent's overt or covert sexualized interactions, as well as verbal and nonverbal sexualized communication, are pinpointed and addressed in therapy.

Parents of sexualized children or children who molest enter therapy with varying degrees of enthusiasm. Often, they may seek therapy out of fear and shock about their children's behavior. They may feel angry and resentful, particularly if one of their children has molested another. Parents may bring their children to therapy expecting only the child's participation in therapy. Parents may be very resistant to therapy, and may attend only because they are mandated to do so. A variety of treatment approaches can be used with parents of children who molest, regardless of their initial willingness or unwillingness. However, parental resistance is a factor that must be overcome for treatment to have optimal impact. Resistant parents, as well as parents eager to participate in therapy, more often respond favorably to a group setting with other parents whose children have similar problems. Since parents or caretakers of children who molest usually bring their children to therapy, clinicians can schedule parent's educational and/or therapy groups to coincide. That way children and their parents or caretakers are in parallel therapeutic situations. To engage the family in therapy, and to provide a context for future in-depth work, clinicians begin family treatment by providing psychoeducational groups.

Psychoeducational Groups

The primary intent of psychoeducational groups is to provide clear and specific information about children who molest. A secondary purpose is to allow the parents an opportunity to meet, understand, and support each other. One of the benefits that naturally occurs is that parents feel less stigmatized and more willing to share their thoughts and feelings and learn from peers.

Psychoeducational groups differ from general therapy groups in that they provide a structured approach to communicating information. There is less focus on obtaining insights and processing emotional matters, although these can occur spontaneously. Psychoeducational groups seek to equip parents with information and skills through didactic presentations on issues of child sexual abuse. Psychoeducational groups are most often followed by general therapy groups to help parents process their emotional responses to their children's molesting behaviors, as well as other related issues that may emerge (e.g., general discipline and parental conflicts).

Goals of Psychoeducational Groups

Psychoeducational groups convey information on the following topics, which may be discussed in greater depth in group therapy:

1. Characteristics of children who molest: average age, types of offense, gender of molester and victim, and most common situations (e.g., older siblings, extended family members, neighbors, and school friends)
2. Issues for children who molest: typical areas of difficulty including poor boundaries, impulsivity, prior victimization, aggression, low self-esteem, social isolation
3. Molesting behaviors: fondling, digital penetration, penetration with objects, vaginal and/or anal intercourse, and so on
4. Age-appropriate sexual play between children: what behaviors constitute age-appropriate sexual behaviors between peers

5. Differentiation between normal sex play and sexual abuse: how to differentiate between age-appropriate sexual play and sexual molestation

6. Family dynamics: the dynamics of families in which children molest (In particular, some of the dynamics highlighted in Chapter seven are reviewed.)

7. Appropriate external controls: how parents can help their children by limit-setting, monitoring, and holding children accountable for molesting behaviors

8. Appropriate internal controls: how parents can help their children develop ways of stopping the inappropriate sexual behaviors

The first two or three sessions are introductory and more loosely structured to help parents become familiar with each other and the format while establishing basic trust. Parents are instructed to describe how they first learned of their child's molesting behaviors and what their initial reactions were. In addition, each parent tells how he or she got to therapy and what legal procedures have occurred (CPS investigation, probation, etc.). After the introductory meetings, group sessions focus on the molesting behaviors of children and related issues through structured presentations.

Once the parents of children who molest have completed the psychoeducational group (usually lasting eight to ten weeks), they participate in a group therapy program that runs parallel to their children's group therapy. While the parents conclude the psychoeducational group, children are either evaluated and prepared for or begin individual or group therapy sessions.

Family Service Agency of San Francisco provided parallel groups for parents and children who molest during a two-year specialized project for children who molest (1987–1989). The same issue raised in the children's group was raised in the adult groups, although the style differed. While clinicians provided children with games and playful tasks to convey the lesson, adults simply discussed the selected topic.

The parents' and children's groups lasted one hour and were divided in three parts. The first fifteen minutes was used to review what was done the previous week and to allow an opportunity to "settle down" and prepare for the lesson; a snack was provided for the children. The second part, lasting twenty minutes, provided a structured lesson, discussion, and closure. The two groups converged for the last 15 minutes and parents or caretakers told their children what they learned, and children told their parents what they learned. This last part of the group was particularly useful because the lessons were clarified and reinforced. In addition, the very fact that the material was verbalized and discussed, encouraged and modeled open communication about previously uncomfortable or confusing sexual matters. Johnson discusses group formats in Chapter eleven.

Group Therapy

Parents who attend psychoeducational groups become motivated to pursue additional therapy. Since they have been encouraged to cooperate with treatment, and understand that the educational groups precede group therapy sessions, their resistance is less evident during the transition from educational groups to group therapy. To facilitate parental participation, group therapy is provided in the evening, separate from the children's group therapy. This allows for the fact that the adult's group usually runs longer than the children's group, and encourages the participation of parents or caretakers who may have standard work schedules.

Primary Goals of Group Therapy

Group therapy sessions for parents and caretakers maintain a focus on the molesting behavior of children, and at the same time address the wide range of parental emotions and concerns. The goals of therapy therefore, are categorized in the same manner as the child's therapy with primary (offense-specific) goals and secondary (general) goals.

The primary goals of group therapy include the following:

Parental understanding of their children's unique pattern of molesting. Each parent must develop a clear understanding of the specific circumstances or patterns in his or her child's molesting behaviors. For example, if a child has molested when unsupervised in the school playground, the parent must make sure that school personnel are available to monitor the child during recess and that after-school activities are structured accordingly. If the child is molesting his or her sibling after being reprimanded or feeling frustrated, the parent needs to help the child with pent-up emotions, as well as heighten supervision during these times.

Parental clarity on their participation in providing external controls (i.e., supervision). Parents need to demonstrate an ability and willingness to provide direct supervision of the child. If the parent of a child who molests reports, "I just took my eyes off him and his sister for ten minutes . . . I just had to have a shower," and does not comprehend that this places both the child who molests and the potential child-victim at risk (until the child's behavior is controlled), this parent is contributing to the child's sexual acting-out behavior by failing to provide the necessary supervision (external control). Lane (1991) asserts that "The parent's role in monitoring, reinforcing application of concepts and providing support on an ongoing basis are critical to the child."

Parental clarity on their participation in assisting their children with internal controls (e.g., responding when children ask for assistance as part of their prevention strategies). During the course of treatment, children who molest receive information about what to do when they experience an overwhelming desire to molest. Amazingly enough, young children are quite clear about the urgency they feel to "touch a penis," or "stick my dick in her butt." Children receive a variety of instructions designed to decrease their acting-out, separating the impulse (thought) from the action (behavior). One of those strategies may be to talk about what they are feeling with an adult they trust. The children may therefore approach a parent and want to share their feelings. Parents must take the time to be responsive, listen, and assist the child. Parents will hopefully develop the capacity to recognize and respond to children's verbal and nonverbal cues of distress.

Parental cooperation in identifying and addressing high-risk factors for their children. When parents understand the offense-specific patterns, it is possible to identify risk factors for each child. Children's problems vary, and the risk factors change accordingly. Parents of children who molest must make every effort to decrease risk situations, thereby assisting their child. If a parent knows that the child who molests tends to sequester children in the closet, unsupervised play in the child's room is a risk factor. The parent therefore ensures that the child plays with a friend in clear view of the parent and is not allowed to play in his or her own room with the door closed.

Parental ability to maintain open communication with their children regarding molesting behaviors or situations. As difficult as it may be for parents to discuss issues of sexuality with their children, it is important to maintain a focus on the child's problem. If children do not bring it up (and many learn to do so spontaneously), parents may ask from time to time, "Did you think about your touching problem today?" or "Was your touching problem okay at school today?" In this manner, the child knows that the parent has not forgotten the matter, is willing to talk about it, and can communicate an interest in hearing about potential problems and concerns. On the other hand, the parent must not become a warden who thinks about, suspects, and continuously raises the issue of the child's molesting. Parents should make sure they have obtained clear directives from the clinicians about how often, and under what circumstances, to raise the topic with the child.

Parental understanding of family dynamics that may contribute to a family climate in which abuse can occur. During the assessment phase, the clinician identified family dynamics that may have contributed to the occurrence of molesting behaviors in the child. For example, if the parents were making love with open doors and the children had habitually observed their sexual interactions, this exposure to explicit sexual activity might have taught the children about sex, as well as aroused their interest and curiosity, and possibly, the development of sexualized behaviors (this factor alone is not likely to elicit molesting behaviors in children). Clinicians must address the issue of discreet sexual interaction between the parents so that the children are not exposed to highly explicit and arousing stimuli. The parents can discuss alternative times and places for sexual encounters, in addition to the obvious need for privacy.

Parental cooperation with all aspects of the children's therapy designed to help them stop the offending behavior. Clinicians ask parents to cooperate in very specific ways. Sometimes parents are taught to say specific phrases, and at other times they are asked to respond to the child with behavioral interventions. Parents who are cooperative with the therapy clearly create a climate for prompt resolution of the children's problematic sexual behaviors.

Parental clarity about their thoughts, feelings, and reactions to the child who molests, the child-victim, and other family members. Parents may feel initially shocked, scared, confused, guilty, and worried about their child's sexual acting-out. Parents of children who molest have confided that they feel untrusting, suspicious, and angry at the child who molests, while they feel protective, sympathetic, and sad about the child-victim. These are normal responses and they must be processed and resolved. It does not help children who molest to be neglected or abused by parents, which could further escalate their feelings of unworthiness or stigmatization.

The secondary goals of group therapy include the following:

Processing of self-esteem, a sense of parental adequacy, and feelings of guilt, shame, or confusion. When children molest, their parents can have a range of emotions and may feel in some way responsible for the child's molesting behaviors. Parents may reproach themselves for what they did or failed to do; they may blame each other in an effort to relieve their own guilt.

All of these feelings are normal and expectable, and the clinician must actively facilitate the expression and resolution of these feelings. If parents continue to feel responsible, defective, or helpless, it will impact their ability to provide clear and helpful assistance to their children. Usually, contact with other parents challenges feelings of inadequacy—as camaraderie develops, parents feel better able to glean and accept information from others and develop a strong preventive approach within their family.

Identifying strengths and weaknesses of the family. A family with a child who molests is a family in crisis. Initially, the crisis can feel overwhelming and all-consuming, and the stress level may increase as parents find themselves having to interact with outsiders (CPS workers, probation officers, mental health workers). Families may feel shaken by the child's molesting behaviors, and parents may regard themselves negatively for a period of time. Clinicians must help the family identify their own strengths and provide positive reinforcement for desirable parental responses (e.g., showing interest in their child and cooperating with the treatment plan).

Identifying strengths and weaknesses of the marital unit. If a marriage or partnership exists, clinicians must assist the adults to strengthen their support of each other so they can use those skills to develop a strong and effective parental team.

Processing conflicts in an open and safe way. The child's sexual acting out may be in some way related to the family's aggression. The family may have spoken or unspoken aggression that the child has integrated. All family members should identify chronic or acute conflicts openly and make efforts toward positive resolution.

Decreasing dysfunctional patterns of interaction such as secrecy, collusions among family members, and triangulation. If structural problems exist, the clinician addresses these during group therapy. For example, if parents raise the issue of a fight they were having in which the child became involved, the clinician should identify the process of triangulation and inquire about other patterns of triangulation in the family. After discussing how triangulation develops and how it may be helping or hurting the family, the clinician can demonstrate alternative methods of interacting.

Increasing the use of functional patterns of interaction such as open communication, positive conflict resolution, and identifying, expressing, and negotiating needs. During group therapy, clinicians not only role model, but they also identify and support positive and healthy functioning among group members. In this manner, issues such as open communication and identifying and expressing needs are constantly addressed. Clinicians summarize the issues that arose in each group session and emphasize the resolution or consensus about each issue.

Increasing the ability to anticipate problems and use internal and external resources to cope with stress factors. All families have varying degrees of stress, and yet individuals seldom stop to consider the impact of stress and how to decrease its negative effect. Some stress is positive in that it generates excitement and motivates toward action; some stress does the opposite: it overloads the system and causes a virtual breakdown or shutdown.

Issues around stress management should be highlighted. Parents who manage their stress in more effective ways are better able help their children with their stress.

Recognizing and correcting any and all patterns of interaction that contribute to sexualization of the family environment. This topic tends to be difficult to discuss. Parents often deny any "wrongdoing" that may have contributed to their child's sexual acting-out. And yet some families place undue focus on sexuality and seem to expose their children prematurely to sexual matters (see Chapter seven). These issues are brought up during psychoeducational groups, and discussed in group therapy after parents have had a chance to think them through and develop more familiarity with the group process.

In addition to group therapy, individual therapy may be requested or initiated by the therapist or the family. Some parents request individual therapy sessions to spend more focused times on issues that have surfaced during group. Group cotherapists maintain a resource list so they may refer group members into individual therapy. This approach seems to work better than requiring individual therapy from the beginning. I have found that almost 60 percent of parents who attend psychoeducational groups and group therapy request individual therapy as well.

Group Therapy Format

Group therapy usually lasts two hours, a full hour longer than the children's group. Both parents should attend group therapy even if they no longer live together. Since parents' work schedules may interfere with attending groups during the day, evening groups may have higher attendance. (Children, on the other hand, tend to do best in groups that occur immediately after school and before dinner.)

Since full attendance in parent groups can include between eighteen and twenty adults, cotherapists are indicated; a male and female cotherapy team best reflects the makeup of the group.

Family Therapy

In addition to psychoeducational groups, group therapy, and individual therapy, the family is often helped by engaging in family therapy sessions. During these family sessions, the clinician highlights the lessons taught during individual and group therapy, and engages the family in open discussion about how they now view the problematic sexual behaviors, how they will make efforts to prevent future problems, and what each family member has learned about his or her contribution to the problem. Before termination, the clinician identifies and reinforces positive changes, highlights ongoing concerns, and reiterates the skills that have been practiced in therapy. If one child has molested another child in the family, it is helpful if the child who molested is able to verbalize or communicate an apology (letters are sometimes dictated) to the child victim.

Thomas (1991) lists the following goals in working with families of adolescent sex offenders: (1) identify and interrupt family patterns that allowed or supported the sexual abuse; (2) improve family relationships and maximize family strengths; and (3) provide the information needed for the family's participation in relapse prevention. Thomas states that the ultimate goal of therapy, of course, is to prevent further sexual abuse. Gelinas (1988), in discussing treatment of incest families, measures successful outcome by four criteria: (1) the abuse is terminated and not resumed; (2) there is a healthier family structure; (3) the marital relationship has significantly improved; and (4) the victim is significantly less parentified and self-esteem and assertiveness have increased. Although these goals and termination criteria have been developed in work with similar (but not identical) populations, they are relevant and applicable to working with families of children who molest.

Summary

The parents of children with sexualized behaviors or children who molest seek therapy under a variety of circumstances. Parents of sexualized children may seek guidance in responding to their child's unusual or excessive sexual preoccupation. An evaluation may reveal problematic sexual behaviors that will decrease through teaching parents appropriate behavioral interventions. Sexualized behaviors may reflect underlying emotional concerns including, but not limited to, overt or covert abuse in the backgrounds of the children. If prior victimization is uncovered, the children are likely to be referred for their own treatment.

The parents of children who molest frequently seek therapy during a crisis state in which they've discovered that one of their children has sexually abused another child, either a sibling, extended family member, neighbor, or unknown child. If sibling abuse has occurred, the parents have conflicting emotional responses toward both children. Parents need and deserve an opportunity to process their own thoughts, emotions, and reactions about the molesting behaviors of their child (and possible victimization of another child), and to understand and learn about family dynamics that can contribute to the child's molesting behaviors.

Parents have varying degrees of interest in therapy. They may bring the child for therapy and feel uncomfortable with the requirement that they attend group therapy. Some parents of children who molest are mandated into treatment with their children. Resistance can be decreased by engaging the parents in psychoeducational groups in which they are given information about children who molest, and have an opportunity to meet other parents of children who have engaged in similar sexual acting-out. This has the immediate impact of helping destigmatize children's sexual acting-out behaviors, helping parents understand the importance of helping their children stop sexually aggressive behaviors, as well as providing opportunities for parents to develop supportive relationships with peers.

Educational groups (parallel with children's groups) are followed by group therapy, which allows a deepening of understanding and processing. The primary distinction between psychoeducational groups and group therapy is the provision of didactic presentations in the former and a greater focus on parental insights, expression of emotions, and resolution of conflicts in the latter. Psychoeducational groups focus on the unique molesting patterns of each child, and teach parents a variety of strategies to assist the child in preventing the recurrence of additional molesting; group therapy sessions have a broader focus. Sometimes the topics discussed in groups overlap: parents may spontaneously discuss related but not offense-specific issues in the educational groups; these issues are processed as well as possible and referred for more in-depth discussion in group therapy.

The ultimate goal of therapy is to stop the molesting behaviors of children. To effect these changes, most professionals agree that a combination of individual, group, and family therapy will be helpful. Because children's sexual behaviors emerge in the family, and because young children are greatly influenced by family attitudes and values about sexuality, a comprehensive family assessment must be undertaken to identify patterns that might be contributing to the child's molesting behaviors.

Resources are available for parents of children who molest (Gil, 1986; Kahn, 1990). These can be given to parents to read and can serve as a source of discussion topics for psychoeducational and therapy groups.

References

Boat, B. (1990). Personal communication to Dr. William Friedrich, cited in Friedrich, W. N. *Psychotherapy of sexually abused children and their families*. New York: W. W. Norton.

Breer, W. (1987). *The adolescent molester*. Springfield, IL: Charles C. Thomas.

Cavallin, H. (1966). Incestuous fathers: A clinical report. *American Journal of Psychiatry* 122:1132–1138.

Cavallin, H., Gebhard, P., Gagnon, J., Pomeroy, W., & Christenson, C. (1965). *Sex offenders: An analysis of types*. New York: Harper & Row.

Finkelhor, D. (1978). Psychological culture and family factors in incest and family sexual abuse. *Journal of Marriage and the Family* 4:41–49.

Finkelhor, D., & Meyers Williams, L. (1992). A pioneering new study on incestuous fathers. In Vanderbilt, H., Incest: A chilling report. *Lear's Magazine*, Feb., 60-61.

Friedrich, W. N. (1990). Understanding and treating the family, In W. N. Friedrich, *Psychotherapy of sexually abused children and their families*. New York: W. W. Norton.

Garbarino, J., Guttman, E., & Seeley, J.W. (1987). *The psychologically battered child*. San Francisco: Jossey-Bass.

Gelinas, D. J. (1988). Family therapy: Characteristic family constellation and basic therapeutic stance. In S. M. Sgroi (Ed.), *Vulnerable populations: Volume 1*. Lexington, MA: Lexington.

Gil, E. (1986). *Children who molest: A guide for parents of young sex offenders*. Rockville, MD: Launch Press.

Gilgun, J. (1988). Factors which block the development of sexually abusive behavior in adults abused as children. Paper presented at the National Conference on Male Victims and Offenders. MN.

Goodwin, J., McCarthy, T., & DiVasto, P. (1982). Physical and sexual abuse of the children of adult incest victims. In J. Goodwin (Ed.), *Sexual abuse: Incest victims and their families*. Boston, MA: John Wright, PS.

Groth, N. A. (1978). Patterns of sexual assault against children and adolescents. In S. M. Sgroi, A. W. Burgess, A. N. Groth, & L. L. Holmstron (Eds.), *Sexual assault of children and adolescents*. Lexington, MA: Lexington.

Groth, N. A., Holson, W., & Gary, T. (1982). The child molester: clinical observations. In J. R. Conte & D. A. Shore (Eds.), *Social work and child sexual abuse*. New York: Haworth Press.

Ho, M. K. (1987). *Family therapy with ethnic minorities*. Newbury Park, CA: Sage.

Kahn, T. J. (1990). *PATHWAYS: A guide for parents of youth beginning treatment*. Orwell, VT: Safer Society Press.

Kaufman, B., & Wohl, A. (1992). *Casualties of childhood: A developmental perspective on sexual abuse using projective drawings.* New York: Brunner Mazel.

Kaufman, I., Peck, A., & Tagiuri, L. (1954). The family constellation and overt incestuous relationship between father and daughter. *American Journal of Orthopsychiatry* 24:266–279.

Knight, R., & Prentky, R. (1990). Classifying sexual offenders: The development and corroboration of taxonomic models. In W. Marshall, D. R. Laws & H. Barbaree (Eds.), *Handbook of sexual assault: Issues, theories and treatment of the offender.* New York: Plenum Press.

Knopp, F. H. (1982). *Remedial intervention in adolescent sex offenses: Nine program descriptions.* Orwell, VT: Safer Society Press.

Lane, S. (1991). Special offender populations. In G. D. Ryan & S. L. Lane (Eds.), *Juvenile sexual offending: Causes, consequences, and correction.* Lexington, MA: Lexington.

Lankester, D., & Meyer, B. (1986). Relationship of family structure to sex offense behavior. Paper presentation, National Conference on Juvenile Sexual Offending. MN.

Lehmer, M. (1986). Court ordered therapy: Making it work. *American Journal of Forensic Psychology* 4:(2): 16–24.

Marshall, W., Laws, D. R., & Barbaree, H. (Eds.) (1990). *Handbook of sexual assault: Issues, theories and treatment of the offender.* New York: Plenum Press.

McGoldrick, M., Pearce, J. K., & Giordano, J. (Eds.) (1982). *Ethnicity and family therapy.* New York: Guilford.

Minuchin, S. (1974). *Families and family therapy.* Harvard: University Press.

Minuchin, S. Montalvo, B., Guerney, B., Rosman, B., & Schumer, F. (1967). *Families of the slums.* New York: Basic Books.

Mrazek, P. B., & Kempe, C. H. (Eds.) (1981). *Sexually abused children and their families.* New York: Pergamon Press.

Patton, M. Q. (Ed.) (1991). *Family sexual abuse: Frontline research and evaluation.* Newbury Park, CA: Sage.

Polansky, N., Chalmers, M., Buttenweiser, E., & Williams, D. (1981). *Damaged parents.* Chigago: University of Chicago Press.

Ross, J., & Loss, P. (1991). Assessment of the juvenile offender. In G. D. Ryan & S. L. Lane (Eds.), *Juvenile sexual offending: Causes, consequences and correction.* Lexington, MA: Lexington.

Ryan, G., Davis, J., Miyoshi, T., Wayne, S., & Wilson, K. (1987). Getting at the facts: The first report from the uniform data collection system. *Interchange, National Adolescent Perpetrator Network* 1987: 5–7. Denver, CO: Kempe Center.

Ryan, G. (1991). The juvenile sex offender's family. In G. D. Ryan & S. L. Lane (Eds.), *Juvenile sexual offending: Causes, consequences and correction.* Lexington, MA: Lexington.

Sgroi, S. (1988). Family therapy: Characteristic family constellation and basic therapeutic stance. In S. M. Sgroi, (Ed.), *Vulnerable populations, Volume 1.* Lexington, MA: Lexington.

Steen, C., & Monnette, B. (1989). *Treating adolescent sex offenders in the community.* Springfield, IL: Charles C. Thomas.

Sue, D. W., & Sue, D. (1990). *Counseling the culturally different: Theory and practice.* 2d. ed. New York: Wiley & Sons.

Thomas, J. (1991). The adolescent sex offender's family in treatment. In G. D. Ryan & S. L. Lane (Eds.), *Juvenile sexual offending: Causes, consequences and correction.* Lexington, MA: Lexington.

Ting-Toomey, S., & Korzenny, F. (1991). *Cross-cultural interpersonal communication.* Newbury Park, CA: Sage.

Trepper, T. S., & Barrett, M. J. (1989). *Systemic treatment of incest.* New York: Brunner Mazel.

Tseng, W. S., & Hsu, J. (1991). *Culture and family: Problems and therapy.* New York: Haworth Press.

Walker, L. (1979). *The battered woman syndrome.* New York: Harper & Row.

Waterman, J. (1986). Family dynamics of incest with young children. In K. Mac-Farlane, J. Waterman, S. Conerly, L. Damon, M. Durfee, & S. Long, *Sexual abuse of young children.* New York: Guilford.

13

Out-of-Home Care

Eliana Gil, Ph.D.

Out-of-home placements may be viable options for some children who molest. In particular, if children persist in compulsive and aggressive sexual behaviors that put other children at risk, and when behaviors are resistant to change despite consistent limit-setting by caretakers as well as therapeutic efforts, children may need the type of containment and supervision provided in out-of-home care facilities.

Clinicians may find themselves in positions of having to both recommend and oversee children's placement in extended family homes, a psychiatric children's unit, residential treatment center, foster home, or group home. Clinicians are often asked to provide guidance and consultation regarding children's sexual behavior problems. A recent survey of 110 psychiatric units found that staff members reported great difficulty with children's sexual behaviors, and many inappropriate reactions were documented (Kohan et al., 1987).

Children's residential treatment centers have also expressed concern over the most effective response for children with problematic sexual behaviors. The Thirty-Fourth Annual Meeting of the American Association of Children's Residential Centers highlighted the issue of sexuality in the institutional setting at their 34th annual meeting in October of 1990. Johnson and Aoki (in press) surveyed line-staff in eleven residential treatment centers across the United States, using the Child Sexual Behavior Checklist (see Appendix B). They found that 42 percent of the children who engaged in sexual behaviors were described as having serious or very serious sexual problems. As a result of this survey, policy suggestions and recommendaitons for managing specific sexual behaviors in residential settings were articulated.

Foster parent associations have provided discussion of this topic at recent conferences and several books have presented guidelines for working with sexual behaviors of children in foster care (Ford, 1988; Johnson, 1990a, 1990b; Ryan, 1990; Gil, 1993). Clearly, ongoing dialogue must continue in order to define and implement sensitive and helpful responses to children's problematic sexual behaviors in or out of their home.

Extended Family Members as Alternative Placements

When children who molest have parents who are unable or unwilling to provide necessary supervision, or feel that their children's behavior is beyond parental control, the juvenile court usually seeks and evaluates the possibility of placing children with a qualified and willing relative. When children molest other children, relatives may feel alarmed or confused by the behavior, particularly if they have young children of their own. Relative placements may occur occasionally, and clinicians need to prepare and guide caretakers in order to maximize the possibility of a successful placement.

Children's Psychiatric Unit

Many psychiatric hospitals include a children's unit for the evaluation and/or treatment of acute emotional or behavioral problems in children. These units maintain a multidisciplinary staff (psychiatrists, nurses, social workers, psychologists, milieu therapists) who provide comprehensive services to children and their families including psychological evaluations, education, expressive therapies, and family treatment. Children's behaviors are monitored daily, medications may be dispensed, and therapy relationships are established with individual, group, and family therapists. Case managers are assigned to coordinate services and organize case conferences with professionals providing services to children or their family.

Residential Treatment Center

A residential treatment center is a therapeutic program in which children can remain for a period of years if necessary. The residential program also has numerous professionals who provide comprehensive services to children and their family. Educational programs are almost always included to maintain scholastic continuity.

Foster Family Homes

Foster care is provided by foster parents who are licensed to house a maximum of seven children in most states. Foster parents often receive specialized training and yet training funds are often restricted; the quantity or quality of training varies from state to state.

Group Homes

Group homes are larger than foster homes and are staffed by professionals. Older children are usually referred to group homes, whereas younger children are referred to foster family homes. Group homes, like foster homes, are licensed and supervised by state licensing boards.

Day Treatment Programs

Day treatment programs are specialized therapy programs that children can attend during the day. Children go to foster family homes or their natural families in the evenings. Day treatment programs provide a combination of individualized therapy and educational services to small numbers of children.

Children who molest may be referred to any of the settings listed above, or the home of an extended family if one is suitable and willing to care for the child.

Several problems may surface for children residing in out-of-home care. Clinicians who recommend alternative placements, or who provide ongoing therapy to children in coordination with services they receive in placement, must anticipate the following problem areas and initiate discussions with placement personnel.

Sexual Acting-out at Placement Settings

Public masturbation. Children with sexual acting-out behavior may exhibit compulsive masturbatory behavior in public. Peers may ridicule or avoid these children; staff members may feel uncomfortable with the behavior and may chastise or isolate children who do not stop masturbating.

Caretakers should refrain from making judgments about the masturbatory behavior. Attempts to stop children from open masturbation must be made with respect and without harshness. A number of interventions can be made including giving children manual tasks, distracting children with another activity, encouraging physical exercise, or directing children to masturbate in private.

Most children with sexual acting-out tend to masturbate to assuage difficult emotions, decrease tension, or cope with the intrusiveness of trauma-related memories. In these circumstances, the interventions may work on a temporary basis and must be accompanied by therapeutic exploration into the origin of the symptomatic behavior.

Children of all ages masturbate, although younger children engage in random masturbation, while older children have more specific (orgasm-oriented) masturbatory behavior. When masturbation has a compulsive quality, and appears to be reflective of emotional problems, it is counterproductive to simply make efforts to remove children from the sight of others while they masturbate. The concept of masturbating in private is most effective after the compulsive nature of the masturbatory behavior has been explored in treatment.

Sexual aggression toward others. Children who molest may be overstimulated by being left alone with other children, and if unsupervised may attempt to molest. For this reason, children who molest must be carefully assessed before placement so that a clear plan is developed about the type of supervision required. Treatment staff need to provide constant supervision and address risk factors for each child.

Sexual gestures toward peers. In addition to molesting behaviors, some children may not molest overtly, yet they may exhibit sexually suggestive gesturing toward peers including sexual language, sexual jokes, describing sexual scenarios, or engaging in provocative situations that can escalate (e.g., giving massages, dancing, wrestling). These are normal age-appropriate interactions and encouraged under typical circumstances. When children have problem sexual behaviors, that is, until children's internal controls are effective, they must avoid these behaviors since they may be overstimulating and propel them into crossing sexual boundaries.

Risk Factors

Sleeping arrangements. Children who molest may be unable to sleep in the company of other children, and may in fact be unable to control their impulses in this setting. This issue may be addressed by (1) isolating the child so he or she sleeps alone and (2) making sure the child sleeps with children who are physically and emotionally able to protect themselves from sexual approaches. Isolating children may be impossible in facilities where space is a problem. However, staff may be able to review the particulars of the situation and any problematic patterns. For example, if the child who molests has a pattern of molesting only younger and smaller children, that child may be placed in sleeping quarters with older children who are not at risk. It is important for all children (children who molest and the peers who cohabitate) to understand the decisions being made about sleeping arrangements. When staff openly discuss their decisions about sleeping arrangements, supervision, and so on, it is less likely that children who molest will feel rejected or punished.

Hygiene. Bathroom activities with other children may be high risk for children who molest. Children should be isolated during normal hygiene practices until such time that their molesting behavior is no longer an issue.

Unsupervised peer activities. Children who molest cannot play with other children without adequate supervision. They may have learned ways to isolate others or escape supervision. Children who molest must be given supervision until such time when their molesting behavior is not an issue. Often it is difficult and challenging for extended family members, foster parents, group home or residential treatment center staff, and caretakers to provide this type of rigorous supervision. However, round-the-clock supervision serves as a necessary external control and is a temporary response until the children's molesting behavior is contained.

Relevant Situational Factors

Victims in care. Children who molest are often placed in settings with children who have histories of being victimized. This is a statistically probable situation, since over half of children placed in care settings are there due to abuse and neglect. Children who molest may recognize the signs of children who are vulnerable to exploitation, and they may engage in sexually aggressive behaviors.

If the placement includes children who may be potential victims of children with molesting behaviors, the placement should be reconsidered or the placement personnel must stand ready to provide twenty-four-hour supervision of both the children who molest and their potential victims.

Unresponsive or punitive staff. Children who molest require sensitive and nonpunitive interventions by calm and nonjudgmental staff. If placement staff ignore the sexually aggressive behaviors, or if they punish the children for them wihout needed exploration, their behavior may continue or escalate. Children who are sexually aggressive need sensitive, purposeful, and consistent interventions from caretakers who understand the behavior and respond in a careful way.

Family visits and cooperation. Family cooperation is critical to effective treatment of sexual acting-out behaviors in young children. Parents must remain informed about the treatment plan and necessary interventions. They need to be considered part of the treatment team and given the necessary information and strategies to respond to their children in a consistent way.

If parents minimize their children's sexual acting-out, or if they are unwilling to cooperate with the treatment plan, it may become necessary to supervise family visits and ensure that family treatment is ongoing. Family members can sabotage treatment efforts; engaging the family as team members is pivotal in the children's effective treatment.

Summary

When children who molest are unable or unwilling to change the behaviors when provided with parental supervision and limits, they may need placement in a variety of alternative settings in which they can be carefully monitored and problematic sexual behaviors addressed.

Clinicians can anticipate problems, initiate discussion of potential difficulties with out-of-home care staff, and help develop a coordinated response during their placement.

Several problems may surface when children who molest are placed with extended family members, in foster homes, group homes, residential centers, or psychiatric children's units. These problems have received growing attention from concerned personnel in recent years, and include sexual aggression toward peers, excessive and public masturbation, sexual preoccupation and sexually suggestive behaviors. In addition, a number of risk factors must be addressed in order to minimize the occurrence of molesting behaviors in out-of-home care.

Clinicians can be helpful by recommending alternative care settings when needed, and by anticipating and discussing the sexual behaviors that can become problematic or potentially dangerous to other children in out-of-home care. Personnel in out-of-home care settings will need direction so they can provide the necessary treatment and supervision.

References

Ford, J. M. (1988). *Foster home care of sexually abused children.* Reedsport,OR: Ford.

Gil, E. (1993). *Foster parenting abused children.* (2nd Ed.) Chicago, IL: National Committee on the Prevention of Child Abuse.

Johnson, T. C. (1990a). Important tools for adoptive parents of children with touching problems. In J. McNamara & B. H. McNamara (Eds.), *Adoption and the sexually abused child.* Human Services Development Institute, University of Southern Maine.

Johnson, T. C. (1990b). Children who act out sexually. In J. McNamara & B. H. McNamara (Eds.), *Adoption and the sexually abused child.* Human Services Development Institute, University of Southern Maine.

Johnson, T. C., & Aoki, W. (In press). *Sexual behaviors of latency-aged children in residential care: Residential treatment for children and youth.*

Kohan, M. J., Pothier, P., & Norbeck, J. S. (1987). Hospitalized children with a history of sexual abuse: Incidence and care issues. *American Journal of Orthopsychiatry* 57:258–264.

Proceedings of the American Association of Children's Residential Centers, 34th Annual Meeting, October 1990, AACRC. Washington, DC.

Ryan, G. (1990). Sexual behavior in childhood. In J. McNamara & B. H. McNamara (Eds.), *Adoption and the sexually abused child.* Human Services Development Institute, University of Southern Maine.

14

Transference and Countertransference

Eliana Gil, Ph.D. and Toni Cavanagh Johnson, Ph.D.

Children who molest had disrupted childhoods. They are often filled with negative and harsh images of their parents or abusers, feeling distrust or anger at the adults who hurt them. These children have not internalized positive role models and often identify with the negative, destructive, yet powerful people in their lives, in order to achieve a sense of identity.

When sexualized children or children who molest enter therapy, they approach the therapist with great hesitation projecting their negativity, anger, and distrust verbally and behaviorally. Sexualized children may learn that they are special, or safe, when they are sexual objects for adults. They may, therefore, elicit abusive (familiar) responses from the therapist.

Preliminary data suggest that most children who molest live in dysfunctional or abusive families; 70 percent of children who molest have histories of physical and sexual abuse (Johnson, 1988). Children who are not overtly abused, often live in families where dysfunctional dynamics contribute to the emergence of inappropriate sexual behaviors in children (See Chapter seven). When considering transference and countertransference responses we must, therefore, discuss not only abusing children but abused children as well.

The transference reactions of sexualized children and children who molest, as well as abused children, are described in this chapter. Clinicians must manage both the transference responses of child clients and their own countertransference responses.

Transference

Mazce and Witenberg (1955) define transference as "The distorted perception of the present in terms of the past, whereby the individual attributes to people in his current life the attitudes and emotions of those in his early family constellation."

O'Connor (1991) broadened the conventional use of the word "transference" and defined it as "not only the emotions, thoughts, and behaviors that individuals manifest within the context of the therapeutic relationship but to the treatment related interaction between the child or the therapist and the child's ecosystem. That is, transference on the part of the child also occurs when [he or] she reacts to events within [his or] her ecosystem in a manner consistent with those occurring in the therapy" (p. 273).

Transference is defined as the thoughts, emotions, and behaviors that clients bring into the relationship with the therapist; countertransference is defined as the thoughts, emotions, and behaviors that the therapist brings into the relationship with clients.

O'Connor describes three primary transference responses of children in therapy: therapist as parent figure; therapist as omniscient and all-powerful; and "the child's taking emotions, thoughts, or behaviors out of the playroom and into [his or] her ecosystem rather than into the playroom" (p. 276). Abused and abusing children have these and other transference responses.

Therapist as Parent-Caretaker

Because abused or abusing children have experienced dysfunctional or disturbed interpersonal relationships, they may approach new relationships with a reservoir of unmet needs, as well as a host of fears and anxieties. They may hope for and elicit caretaking responses from therapists, engaging them in positive parent roles. They may verbally or nonverbally request physical affection, validation, guidance, limits, and general nurturing. In play therapy sessions, they may want and ask to be fed, sung to sleep, tucked in, or rocked. They may be unable to use play to compensate through fantasy for deficits or concerns in their own life. For example, severely neglected children may not initially be able to use dolls and play materials to engage in nurturing behaviors such as feeding the doll, rocking the doll to sleep, and so on. As they feel safe and begin to see the clinician as trustworthy and consistent, they may be better able to use play symbolically to express their own sense of deprivation. Neglected children look for maternal or paternal warmth and security, often relating to therapists and other adults in withdrawn and regressed fashion.

Conversely, abused or abusing children may expect and elicit abusive responses. Nonabusive behaviors may elicit acute anxiety: children face interactions that are unfamiliar and therefore frightening. These children may seek to reduce their own tension by becoming "provocative" and eliciting abusive responses. Therapists may suddenly find themselves angry with or resentful of their child clients, and may feel discomfort, guilt, or shame over these emotions. When this happens, children have successfully negotiated a familiar interaction and relieve their anxiety; children who elicit negative affect have taken control of the situation by decreasing the intolerable anxiety of anticipating the predictable assault. The attack is over, things settle down, and tension is reduced. This pattern is the same as the one identified by Walker (1984) regarding the cycle of violence and the victims' efforts to control the timing of the battering.

Therapist as Sexual Object

Children who have been sexually abused in or out of the home may have learned that adults expect sexual responses from them. Finkelhor and Browne (1986) refer to a process "in which a child's sexuality [including both sexual feelings and sexual attitudes] is shaped in a developmentally inappropriate and interpersonally dysfunctional fashion as a result of the sexual abuse" (p. 181). He says that children learn sexual behaviors "as a strategy for manipulating others to get his or her other developmentally appropriate needs met" (p. 181).

Based on learning theory, Finkelhor speculates that children are reinforced for inappropriate behavior and therefore learn that sexuality is a necessary part of a relationship. When children enter therapy, they are the focus of attention from a concerned and interested adult; this focused attention can precipitate learned responses designed to reduce stress or provide feelings of empowerment. One four-year-old sexually abused girl went into her new therapist's office, sat on her lap, and licked her face. The child was not trying to "seduce" her therapist. Instead, she was trying to make herself feel safe the only way she knew how. She was probably also testing the limits: "I will make you feel good so you won't hurt me." Therapists must respond quickly, nonpunitively, and most importantly provide a safe and corrective experience.

Children who molest may view all adults as potential sex offenders. The child who has been sexualized through inappropriate adult sexual attention and behaviors, may fantasize and worry about the circumstances under which the therapist will molest. Children who molest may develop an exaggerated sense of sexual power and may attempt to elicit sexual responses from the therapist in order to feel in control (and subsequently safe).

Therapist as Persecutor

Many children who molest will view therapy (and therefore the therapist) as a type of punishment. Therapists are viewed by children as adults who try to exert control over them. If children have a history of abuse, they will sometimes resist being controlled. Children who view their therapists as persecutors may take longer to develop a positive therapeutic relationship. Clinicians are therefore encouraged to be patient, even-tempered, consistent, and to depersonalize the children's rejections or attacks.

Therapist as Judge

Many abused children can mistakenly (or correctly) assume that therapists have some "power" beyond the therapy hour. In other words, sometimes adult caretakers tell children that therapy will determine a particular outcome. A caretaker might say to the child, "Tell [the therapist] the truth, so the therapist can tell the judge and she'll let you come home to live with me again." Therapists may be making recommendations to the court about children's reunification, custody arrangements, visitation, or readiness to testify in court. Children may therefore view the therapist less as a neutral helper and more as a judge who will decide their fate. Children will obviously restrict their behaviors and verbalize specific things to persuade the "judge" one way or another.

Therapist as Rescuer

Abused children may see therapists as potential rescuers from harmful or painful situations: asking them to come over, sleep over, and take them to their own house. Therapists must constantly manage their countertransference responses to children who are often living in desperate and potentially high-risk situations. This dynamic can be exacerbated when therapists report suspected child abuse to the authorities, and little or no action is taken, either due to children's inability to provide information, or an inability to substantiate the allegation. Therapists can then be seen as the "last resort" to children, who may literally beg them for specific kinds of help.

Therapist as Colluder in Denial

Children who are abused may sometimes deny their own reality in order to protect themselves from emotional pain or to protect their parents. They may repress the abuse, unable to acknowledge or discuss its occurrence. At the same time, they may have a number of symptoms manifesting internal turmoil. Children may tacitly request the therapist's acquiescence in denial and train the therapist to avoid the subject of abuse, never ask about it or mention it in the child's presence. Therapists who avoid these subjects do children a real disservice. Some therapists may feel capable of discussing children's own abuse and yet may be resistant to acknowledge children's abusing behaviors. Therapists may minimize sexually aggressive behaviors describing them as inconsequential or normal sexual play. When therapists ignore, minimize, or otherwise fail to address children's sexualized behaviors, children are not being helped, since the behavior doesn't usually disappear on its own—often escalating into more difficult problems for children and their families.

Clinicians who collude with children's denial are not being helpful to their child clients. This denial must be eventually confronted, whether it is denial about their own past abuse, or denial of their current molesting behaviors. In this way, trauma-related issues can be worked through and the child can express the many emotions that exist as a result of abuse. Denial is a protective shield for children who are hurt; clinicians must challenge the defense gently, not with force. Trying to force children to disclose or provide details may recapitulate the dynamics of abuse. Clinicians need to provide opportunities for children to communicate (through expressive therapies or the use of symbolic play) while becoming trustworthy to the child and making efforts to ensure that the child is living in a safe environment.

Therapist as Focal Point

This dynamic is quite distressing and distracting in the therapy. Children with very little ego cannot tolerate personal attention and "lose themselves" to the therapist by focusing their attention exclusively on the therapist's needs. They emulate the therapist and make overtures of caretaking. They scan the therapist for signs of approval or disapproval and behave accordingly. They can become devastated by any change in the therapy routine, and may become severely distressed and depressed by sudden decreased contact with the therapist. The therapeutic relationship in these cases becomes primary, and children are unable to establish a relationship with anyone other than the therapist. This may encourage feelings of grandiosity in the therapist. Clinicians must constantly define and reinforce the child's own sense of self. In addition, therapists need to encourage children's attachment to other helping adults, remain informed about children's behavior outside the therapy office, and establish and maintain contact with family members or caretakers.

Countertransference Responses

Therapists choose their professions for a variety of reasons including a desire to help others who are injured, a feeling of wanting to improve the social condition, a desire to give back to those less fortunate, a need to be seen as special, and a conscious or unconscious desire to help others in a way they perhaps were not helped themselves. Some therapists choose to become therapists for financial reasons or a desire for respect and status. Others may come from dysfunctional families and may unconsciously seek a profession that focuses them on the resolution of their difficult childhoods. Informal surveys indicate that many therapists who specialize in work with child abuse have a history of childhood abuse. A clinician's own history of childhood abuse can become an important factor in the provision of therapy to abused children and is discussed below.

Sexualized children and children who molest have strong emotions emanating from the interactions with the people who abused them and/or their families. Some therapeutic interactions may not be based in reality and distorted through the transference. When children project irrational feelings onto the therapist, therapists must acknowledge and monitor their reactions and responses. Therapists bring their own histories to the therapy replete with feelings and needs—as they interact with children, it is important to moderate countertransference responses that are designed to meet the therapist's needs, not children's needs. Countertransference includes therapists' reactions to children's transference as well as reactions to the objective or actual person of the child. Therapists must remain objective and purposeful in directing the therapy for the benefit of the children, regardless of their feelings for the children's behavior or personality.

The Frightened Therapist

Abused and abusing children frequently have a great deal of untapped rage. They are capable of expressing this rage verbally and physically, and the intensity of expression can overwhelm the clinician, who might respond with physical or emotional paralysis. This rage may tap into the therapist's past experiences and can make them susceptible to nontherapeutic responses.

Children who express rage trust the therapist to absorb, contain, and direct the rage. Therapists must create an environment of safety and unconditional acceptance and also educate children about the safe release of pent-up emotions.

Clinicians must know and implement techniques for creating safe therapeutic environments for the child's expression of rage, as well as be able to offer alternative modes of expression. Countertransference responses can sabotage the clinician's ability to put knowledge into practice. Clinicians should discuss these issues with supervisors or consultants, develop a repertoire of techniques for helping children express anger safely (see James, 1989), and acknowledge and process their own feelings of fear and anxiety.

The Incompetent Therapist

No one likes to feel incompetent. Feelings of incompetency cause self-doubt, hesitation, feelings of insecurity, lowered self-esteem, and guilt. Clinicians usually prefer to work with problems they know about, understand, and have had an opportunity to learn about through practice.

Abused and abusing children may present a challenge. Their histories are incomprehensible, and they can enter treatment with a range of visible or underlying injuries to their body, mind, emotions, and spirituality. Children can feel hopeless and may either turn to the therapist in despair or expect nothing.

Therapists who feel a lack of competence when treating children who have experienced tremendous suffering must remain grounded and not absorb feelings of hopelessness and futility from either the children or other professionals.

Competency can be achieved through efforts at obtaining added knowledge, consulting with objective outside consultants or supervisors, reading, and maintaining a positive attitude about one's own capacity to be of assistance. Clinicians will feel more competent if they develop a clear theoretical framework with a congruent treatment plan, including measurable objectives, keep good notes on each session with the child, and engage in periodic reviews in which the treatment progress is evaluated. This may allow a professional to gauge feelings of competence by observing measurable progress that otherwise could remain elusive and abstract.

The Aroused or Embarrassed Therapist

The interpersonal behaviors of abused and abusing children can be very unnerving to mental health professionals. In particular, these children may exhibit sexual behaviors that are unusual and quite explicit.

A therapist's typical training does not include much information about processing sexual countertransference responses to children. Therapists usually receive minimal information about possible sexual arousal toward adult or adolescent clients; information or discussion about sexual arousal toward child clients is practically unspeakable.

Many adults, professionals included, find it difficult to discuss sexual issues with children. They may feel embarrassed, uncomfortable with language, or remain uncertain about what specifics children require and how much information should be provided.

Children who are sexually abused may use sophisticated sexual language, offering explicit descriptions of sexual acts. They may exhibit sexual behaviors that are completely foreign to other children. They may attempt to engage the therapist in sexual responses by french kissing, humping the clinician's body, reaching over and touching the therapist's genitals, making attempts at partial or full disrobing, and so on. Clinicians may respond in a variety of ways including punishing the child, asking to see the child with another adult in the room, verbally reprimanding the child, setting up a rewards system when the child does not exhibit these behaviors, and referring the child to another therapist. Some therapists don't know what to do and do nothing, hoping the behavior will eventually subside on its own. This avoidance is countertherapeutic. A psychotherapist who conducted an evaluation of a sexually abused girl remarked in her written report, "She sat masturbating for an hour and a half, looking directly at me, as if wondering what I thought." The child in this example may experience the therapist's passive observation as a recapitulation of abuse. She may have felt that she was sexually gratifying the therapist. The therapist's failure to set limits reinforced the child's anxious and inappropriate sexual behavior.

Therapists who work with sexually abused children who act out sexually in the session must be reflective about the impact of the work and specific countertransference responses. In supervision, therapists have confided their exasperation, concern, feelings of incompetence, as well as their own sexual arousal at the content presented during the session. One therapist who sought consultation had a look of despair as she confided (with a great deal of difficulty) that she would regularly experience sexual arousal during her therapy sessions with a sexually abused boy. On the occasion that precipitated her seeking consultation, she found herself not setting appropriate limits for the child when he kept his hand on her lap a little longer than necessary. The consultant responded to the clinician's concern by discussing the potential for many therapists to experience sexual thoughts or sensations, and the necessity for an open and specific working-through of these sexual responses. The consultant advised that acknowledging these responses, and feeling concern over them, were good prognostic signs; the behavior could become problematic if it went unacknowledged, or if the clinician began to act out in response to her arousal. The consultant offered the clinician an opportunity to process her responses and provided behavioral techniques she could use during the session. A careful follow-up was necessary to ensure that this clinician's need to attend to her own sexual arousal did not inadvertently interfere with her ability to provide adequate and careful services to the child in question or any other sexually abused or abusing child. After discharging her shame and concern in consultation, the therapist felt distinctly focused on the work at hand, and capable of processing her own responses in a speedy manner. If therapists notice that persistent fantasies or intrusive thoughts about sexual activities with children surface as a result of working with sexualized children or children who molest, these factors must be discussed with a supervisor or consultant. These fantasies and thoughts can progress to overt or covert behaviors and must be addressed immediately. If they cannot be quickly resolved, the therapist will need to transfer the child to another therapist.

The Overidentified Therapist

Therapists who work with children who have been victimized must achieve a psychic separation from the child in order to avoid absorbing the child's pain in a way that debilitates the therapist. If clinicians themselves have been victimized, this separation is a greater challenge. The greater the similarity between the child's and the therapist's victimization, the more difficult it may be to separate the experiences. Clinicians who identify too strongly with one particular child may anticipate the child's reactions, feelings, and thoughts and create opportunities for the child to process only those feelings that the therapists have already experienced and processed. For example, if clinicians have been able to identify their own rage toward a perpetrator in the family, they may encourage children to express similar rage and yet fail to provide a climate in which children can express a range of feelings, including sadness, longing, or love for the offender. A therapist who is overidentified with the child may also want to alter the child's experience so it aligns with his or her own. If the therapist ceased all contact with an offender, he or she may unconsciously or consciously facilitate that specific outcome for the child. Therapists can loose touch with the individuality of a child's experience of abuse and relive their own experience through the child.

The Rescuing Therapist

Therapists can lose objectivity when they are overwhelmed with the child's plight, and may develop a compromised ability to guide the family if the boundaries of the therapy are not stable.

Everyone who enters a helping profession does so with the intent of being of assistance; therapists usually harbor a desire to help individuals toward greater self-fulfillment or happier lives. This desire to help can grow out of proportion, compromising therapists' judgment about how to best assist their clients. Inevitably, clinicians who work with children from abusive and dysfunctional homes, perform some parenting activities with the children such as helping to identify needs, build self-esteem, develop impulse control, and encourage expression of emotions. Clinicians may be perceived by the children as the "good and safe parents," particularly when compared with abusive, unsafe, or unrewarding parents. Children may learn to appreciate or crave the validation, respect, and safety that accompany therapy and on occasion may even verbalize, "I wish you were my mommy [or daddy]" or "Can't I come and live with you?" Children experience a qualitative difference of being well regarded and treated warmly and with respect.

Clinicians working with abused children need to consider the treatment of the family in order to begin to get the children's needs met not only in the therapy hour, but in the family system itself. Whether or not the child's therapist provides family therapy is an individual decision. If the child's therapist does not opt to see the family, he or she must take steps to ensure that another professional is able to work with the family to improve parenting skills, discuss discipline, teach appropriate nurturing behaviors, teach parents how to deal with sexualized behaviors, and ensure family safety and integrity .

If therapists overidentify with the "good parent" role and see themselves as capable of rescuing the child from the family situation, these perceptions will hinder their ability to use sound clinical judgment when making recommendations to the court about the potential for family reunification, the need for supervised visits for parents, or the monumental suggestion that parental rights be terminated.

Therapists who overidentify with the rescuer role may believe that they are the only reliable individuals who have the child's best interests in mind, and they may be unable to support or encourage the child's attachment to other adults.

The Helpless Therapist

Working with child abuse is challenging and difficult. Oftentimes therapists are exposed to horrific types of child maltreatment and may provide treatment to children who have had traumatic abuse at the hands of parents or caretakers.

Occasionally, therapists may feel engulfed by feelings of helplessness and hopelessness. They may marvel at the child's survival skills to date and see the potential for long-term damage as a result of traumatic experiences. Therapists may reflect on whether the therapy may be "too little too late," and may grow discouraged about the child's needs.

Therapists need to be cautious when these feelings become abundant. Probably all therapists who work with abused and abusing children have situational and temporary depression as well as feelings of hopelessness for the child's and family's recovery, but if these feelings persist, it's important to get assistance from consultants, supervisors, or other therapists.

Children who are abused usually have increased feelings of vulnerability and a sense of futility (Terr, 1990). They are often unable to look ahead to their futures. Therapists' ability to convey a sense of hope is critical in helping children develop feelings of control and future-directedness.

The Angry Therapist

It is human nature for therapists to feel anger in clinical situations; it would be uncommon and inappropriate for therapists to act out the anger with a client. Instead, clinicians usually acknowledge the anger, explore it, may seek a colleague's opinion, and then discharge the anger safely away from the child. Clinicians choose in advance under what circumstances to role-model safe and appropriate expression of anger with clients.

Child therapists know that anger can surface in the therapy with children, probably because children can engage in many more acting-out behaviors than adults, and can persist in a chosen behavior after a therapist sets limits. Children with abuse backgrounds can develop both aggressive and sexualized behaviors that can test the therapist's patience and endurance.

Therapists may be surprised or alarmed to find that they have developed hostile feelings toward their child clients. Therapists may feel shame and guilt over these emotions.

Certain children may elicit more angry responses than others. For example, women may find themselves viewing aggressive male children as behaving in "typical macho" fashion. Male therapists may find themselves wanting their female clients to "speak up" or "fight back," and may have intolerance for the victim role. Of course some women may have similar disdain for the victim role in female children, and some men may abhor the male children's overidentification with the role of the aggressor. Angry feelings may inadvertently invade the therapists' interactions with child clients, and they may react in an exaggerated manner, raise their voices, become punitive, or express their frustrations through threats to terminate the children's therapy.

The Overcontrolling Therapist

Some therapists fall into the trap of trying to overcontrol all aspects of the child's life, including the parents' involvement in treatment, school choices, tutoring, recreational activities, vacations, and so on.

Therapists need to maintain firm boundaries, keeping a realistic frame of mind about the services they can and cannot provide. Therapists who attempt to overcontrol the family's life will inevitably suffer severe disappointment and frustration.

Therapists need to understand that abused children have had experiences in which they felt powerless and helpless. Children will likely attempt to resolve some of these issues, sometimes overcompensating for past experiences by developing an exaggerated need to control the environment. Therapists must avoid power struggles if at all possible, giving children a sense that they can make decisions and face the consequences of their choices. For example, if children insist on doing something destructive, therapists can help them view the positive and negative consequences of their behavior, asserting the children's power (or control) over their choice. Once children make a choice, therapists can discuss the outcome and enforce whatever specific consequences were outlined. In this way, children may learn that real control lies in choice and develop a way of thinking through the consequences of behavior. Thus therapists avoid efforts to keep children from specific behavior, and children may therefore develop impulse control and feelings of empowerment.

Some children and their parents elicit therapists' desire to control by being unable to exert control over their own lives. Unless therapists remain cognizant of countertransference responses, they may attempt to organize every part of the family's life, overfunctioning for them. Overfunctioning encourages underfunctioning in families who remain dependent on therapists for their survival. Some therapists need to be needed and severely dysfunctional families can exhibit extreme neediness and dependency.

The Victimized Therapist

If a therapist with an abusive background is working with a child victim of abuse or neglect, the therapist may unconsciously infuse the child with the power of the therapist's perpetrator. The child is smaller and weaker than the therapist, and yet the therapist may have fears of being overpowered by the child, particularly the child who has disinhibited acting-out behaviors in the therapy hour. The therapist perceives the child's behavior as reminiscent of, and consistent with, the behaviors of his or her own perpetrator.

If therapists feel victimized (helpless, hopeless, trapped, injured, guilty, ashamed) they may be unable to set appropriate limits or validate or support children's positive behaviors. The therapist is rendered helpless and the therapy is in crisis. Children may feel power and influence over the therapist which is highly countertherapeutic.

Therapists who feel victimized must get immediate assistance to stabilize the therapy. If this is not possible, a transfer must be considered.

Repercussions of Working with Sexually Abused Children

In addition to the countertransference responses that can disrupt or interrupt the flow or progress of treatment, the following aftereffects of this work are worth noting.

Isolation

Friends often discuss their work. When someone works with abused children or children who are molesting other children, friends may become uncomfortable about listening to them describe the kinds of problems faced in providing treatment to abused children. Friends may listen with initial interest, only to leave the conversation with feelings of despair or fear. Eventually, friends may seem disinterested in the therapist, and invitations to social events may decline or stop completely.

People who work with abused or abusing children therefore feel isolated and may find themselves turning to colleagues who share their interests. Although it may be rewarding to talk with co-workers about shared interests, this may limit the therapists' social life and may cause loneliness or depression.

Sex Offenders Are Everywhere

Working with sexualized children and children who molest can be difficult for therapists who have young children. As therapists who are parents become more aware of the extent of abusive behavior toward children in a variety of settings, they may feel overly protective and unable to trust anyone with their children.

Therapists who are exposed to sexual abuse cases on a daily basis may find many people suspect. As children grow older and attend school or participate in sports, the list of suspects can grow, and parents can find themselves mistrusting any adult who shows an interest in their child.

All parents need to be cautious about the real dangers their children can face in the world. At the same time, it is critical to avoid paranoia, which may limit children's opportunities to engage in a wide range of activities. Children can benefit greatly from positive role models, and if everyone is suspect, parents may inadvertently deprive their children of positive and influential contacts with others.

Something Is Wrong with My Child

There is a well-known adage about medical students that as they learn about new diseases, they tend to recognize the symptoms of the new disease in themselves; likewise, as psychology students study psychiatric conditions, they may become aware of their many symptoms and ailments.

Therapists who are exposed to cases of sexual and physical violence on a daily basis may begin to see indicators of abuse in their own children. Normal vaginal redness, bouts of depression, or angry outbursts may panic a parent who is also a therapist by profession. Normal sexual play or aggressive play between siblings may take on alarming dimensions to someone who sees the extremes of these behaviors on a regular basis.

Parents who are also therapists may find it helpful to observe their children's behaviors compared to the behaviors of their peers. It is also useful to engage in conversations with other parents in which children's typical behaviors can be reviewed.

Despair

Therapists working with child abuse may feel despair and pain at the realities of childhood maltreatment. Clinicians may feel that the world "has gone mad," progress is too slow, and support not forthcoming. Catastrophic events like the riots in Los Angeles in 1992 can further accentuate feelings of despair about the prevalence of violence and pain in our culture.

Therapists may find that participating in national or state organizations and channeling their energies through collective activity may decrease feelings of isolation and increase a sense of contributing to the prevention of child abuse in small but specific ways.

Summary

Children can develop a range of transference thoughts, feelings, or behaviors in the therapy relationship. Transference can be used in a positive way, allowing children to process emotions, learn about appropriate interactions, and develop an understanding of attachment, dependency, and trust.

Transference also assists therapists to understand children's previous relationships, including their feelings, behaviors, and physical and emotional relationship to their parents.

Transference has a negative impact when the transferential issues are not addressed by the therapist, or when therapists express negative countertransference responses that can inadvertently stifle the child's development. For example, clinicians who respond to children's need to be rescued by overprotecting and overfunctioning, are not working in the children's best interests.

It is imperative that therapists working with children in general, and abused and abusing children specifically, maintain a constant vigil on the children's transference issues, as well as their own countertransference responses. As Friedrich (1990) states so eloquently, "We learn early how to soothe, comfort, listen, and direct. However, many of us have not had to deal with such phenomena as exploitation, abuse of power, parental alienation, violence, and a precocious introduction to sexuality" (p. 268). Not only are clinicians challenged by this reality, they must also maintain a constant watch on their own responses in order to work in the children's best interests.

Working with abused children is challenging, rewarding, and replete with difficulties. The topic of child abuse elicits many responses from professionals, many of which are based on their own childhood experiences.

In the course of providing therapy, clinicians face transference and countertransference responses. Transference responses in children may include seeing the therapist as rescuer, "good parent," or offender. Therapists may have a range of countertransference responses including fear, incompetency, arousal, overidentification, rescuing, helplessness, anger, overcontrol and victimization. In addition, therapists working with child abuse may feel isolated, in despair, and paranoid about abuse invading their own families.

Therapists must take great care to acknowledge and address transference and countertransference issues so they do not disrupt or delay the progress of therapy. Likewise, therapists who choose this line of work must surround themselves with a support system of peers, stay current with the literature, attend continuing education seminars when possible, seek consultation or supervision as needed, and stay well informed about forthcoming research, treatment strategies, and resources for their clients.

References

Friedrich, W. N. (1990). The person of the therapist. In W. N. Friedrich, *Psychotherapy of sexually abused children and their families*. New York: W. W. Norton.

Finkelhor, D. & Browne, A. (1986). Initial and long term effects: A conceptual framework. In D. H. Finkelhor (Ed.) *A sourcebook on child sexual abuse*. Newbury Park, CA: Sage.

James, B. (1989). *Treating traumatized children*. Lexington, MA: Lexington.

Johnson, T. C. (1988). Child perpetrators—children who molest other children: Preliminary findings. *Child Abuse and Neglect* 12:219-229.

Mazce, T. C., Witenber, E. (1955). *An outline of psychoanalysis*. New York: Modern Library.

O'Connor, K. J. (1991). *The play therapy primer*. New York: Wiley.

Terr, L. (1990). *Too scared to cry*. New York: Harper & Row.

Walker, L. (1984). *The battered woman syndrome*. New York: Springer.

Appendix A

Frequency of Sexual Behaviors and Discriminating Items

(Percentage Endorsement)

No. a	Item (Abbreviated)	Normative Overall	Clinical Overall	T	P
10.	Puts mouth on sex parts	0.1	8.2	4.46	.0001
15.	Asks to engage in sex acts	0.4	11.6	4.29	.0001
7.	Masturbates with object	0.8	11.2	5.45	.0001
17.	Inserts objects in vagina/anus	0.9	11.2	4.34	.0001
9.	Imitates intercourse	1.1	14.1	4.50	.0001
14.	Sexual sounds	1.4	13.1	4.42	.0001
30.	French kisses	2.5	13.1	2.60	.01
28.	Undresses other people	2.6	18.0	6.70	.0001
29.	Asks to watch explicit TV	2.7	15.0	3.23	.0014
19.	Imitates sexual behavior w/dolls	3.2	17.5	3.65	.0003
2.	Wants to be opposite sex	4.9	10.2	3.64	.0003
22.	Talks about sexual acts	5.7	31.6	6.13	.0001
1.	Dresses like opposite sex	5.8	6.8	n.s.	
8.	Touches others' sex parts	6.0	25.7	7.48	.0001
16.	Rubs body against people	6.7	22.3	4.20	.0001
31.	Hugs strange adults	7.3	28.1	4.90	.0001
32.	Shows sex parts to children	8.1	24.8	4.89	.0001
12.	Uses sexual words	8.8	30.6	5.98	.0001
33.	Overly aggressive/overly passive	10.4	35.4	7.17	.0001

No. a	Item (Abbreviated)	Normative Overall	Clinical Overall	T	P
27.	Talks flirtatiously	10.6	15.0	2.11	.04
13.	Pretends to be opposite sex	13.0	13.0	14.1	n.s.
4.	Masturbates with hand	15.3	28.6	4.33	.0001
21.	Looks at nude pictures	15.4	18.4	3.62	.0004
20.	Shows sex parts to adults	16.0	18.0	3.36	.0009
3.	Touches sex parts in public	19.7	21.8	2.94	.0035
34.	Interested in opposite sex	23.0	33.5	4.65	.0001
18.	Tries to look at people undressing	28.5	33.5	2.04	.04
6.	Touches breasts	30.7	30.6	2.76	.0062
26.	Kisses nonfamily children	33.9	29.6	n.s.	
23.	Kisses nonfamily adults	36.2	39.3	n.s.	
25.	Sits with crotch exposed	36.4	36.0	n.s.	
24.	Undresses in front of others	41.2	42.7	n.s.	
11.	Touches sex parts at home	45.8	42.2	3.09	.0022
5.	Scratches crotch	52.2	45.1	n.s.	
35.	Uses opposite sex toys	53.9	29.1	n.s.	

a The preferred order of the items in the scale are identified in this column, e.g., Item No. 1, "Dresses like the opposite sex."

Appendix B

Description of Child Sexual Behavior Checklist (CSBCL)
Revised

This inventory is designed to be used by mental health professionals, child care workers, protective services workers, and other professionals interested in the range of sexual behaviors shown by a child. It provides information useful for evaluation and treatment planning and can be used as a pre- and posttreatment measure. Protective service workers can use it with foster and residential care providers to get an accurate picture of the child's sexual behaviors. It can be used for research on children's sexual behaviors.

The items listed are related to sex and sexuality in children twelve (12) years and younger. They range from natural and healthy childhood sexual exploration to behaviors of children experiencing severe difficulties in the area of sexuality. Although at face value some items may not appear related to sex and sexuality, these behaviors become sexualized in some children.

Part I is a list of over 150 behaviors and should be filled out by an adult who has been in close contact with the child during the previous three months. The time span that is being evaluated can be changed. A long enough period to get a reasonable sample of the child's behaviors should be used. If the person filling out the checklist has known the child for a limited period of time, this period can be assessed with the checklist. If the span of time being represented on the checklist is other than three months, this should be clearly noted on the first page.

Part II is comprised of questions related to the child's background. The answers provide a useful context in which to evaluate the behaviors in Part I.

Part III is designed for use when a child has been engaging in sexual behaviors with other children. The answers, together with parts I and II, provide information helpful for determining the type of intervention necessary to provide for the child.

It was not possible to reproduce this instrument due to its length. To order, contact:

Toni Cavanagh Johnson, Ph.D.
1101 Fremont Ave., Ste. 104
South Pasadena, CA 91030

Appendix C

Child Sexual Behavior Inventory, Version 1

Please circle the number that tells how often your child has shown the following behaviors *recently or in the last six months:*

Never	Less than 1/month	1–3 times/month	At least 1/week
0	1	2	3

1. 0 1 2 3   Dresses like the opposite sex
2. 0 1 2 3   Talks about wanting to be the opposite sex
3. 0 1 2 3   Touches sex (private) parts when in public places
4. 0 1 2 3   Masturbates with hand
5. 0 1 2 3   Scratches anal or crotch area, or both
6. 0 1 2 3   Touches or tries to touch mother's or other women's breast
7. 0 1 2 3   Masturbates with object
8. 0 1 2 3   Touches other people's sex (private) parts
9. 0 1 2 3   Imitates the act of sexual intercourse
10. 0 1 2 3   Puts mouth on another child's or adult's sex parts
11. 0 1 2 3   Touches sex (private) parts when at home
12. 0 1 2 3   Uses words that describe sex acts
13. 0 1 2 3   Pretends to be the opposite sex when playing
14. 0 1 2 3   Makes sexual sounds (sighing, moaning, heavy breathing, etc.)
15. 0 1 2 3   Asks others to engage in sexual acts with him or her
16. 0 1 2 3   Rubs body against people or furniture
17. 0 1 2 3   Inserts or tries to insert objects in vagina or anus
18. 0 1 2 3   Tries to look at people when they are nude or undressing
19. 0 1 2 3   Imitates sexual behavior with dolls or stuffed animals
20. 0 1 2 3   Shows sex (private) parts to adults
21. 0 1 2 3   Tries to view picture of nude or partially dressed people (may include catalogs)
22. 0 1 2 3   Talks about sexual acts
23. 0 1 2 3   Kisses adults not in the family
24. 0 1 2 3   Undresses self in front of others
25. 0 1 2 3   Sits with crotch or underwear exposed
26. 0 1 2 3   Kisses other children not in the family

27. 0   1   2   3   Talks in a flirtatious manner
28. 0   1   2   3   Tries to undress other children or adults against their will
                      (opening pants, shirts, etc.)
29. 0   1   2   3   Asks to view nude or sexually esplicit TV shows (may
                      include video movies or HBO-type shows)
30. 0   1   2   3   When kissing, tries to put toungue in other person's mouth
31. 0   1   2   3   Hugs adults he or she does not know well
32. 0   1   2   3   Shows sex (private) parts to children
33. 0   1   2   3   If a girl, overly aggressive: if a boy, overly passive
34. 0   1   2   3   Seems very interested in the opposite sex
35. 0   1   2   3   If a boy, plays with girls' toys: if a girl, plays with boys' toys
36. 0   1   2   3   Other sexual behaviors (please describe)

A. _____

B. _____

This instrument was developed by Dr. William Friedrich. Permission to reproduce this instrument was provided by Mayo Clinic: Rochester, MN.

Appendix D

Testing of Children with Problematic Sexual Behaviors

Some clinicians prefer to have psychological testing completed before formulating a treatment plan. If the child's sexual behavior problems do not require an emergency response, psychological testing can be requested. A number of diagnostic tests provide valuable information for treatment planning for children with problematic sexual behaviors. Tests that have been found useful are listed below.

Children may have already been tested in school to assess the need for special services. To avoid duplicating standard testing, clinicians should contact the school for results of previous assessments. If children are having school difficulties and school personnel have not provided specialized testing, clinicians can do an initial screening and then help parents encourage the school psychologist to provide testing.

The Weschler Intelligence Scale for Children-III is a standard test used to measure intelligence. Knowing the children's intelligence level is very useful. This test is divided into different areas so the children's strengths and weaknesses across categories can be ascertained. The Kaufman Brief Intelligence Test can also be used to measure intelligence.

The Peabody Picture Vocabulary Test gives a quick assessment of children's receptive vocabulary. This is used as a very rough screening device for children's intelligence level and can be used if the resources to do the Weschler are not available. A low-level score on this test may indicate that children may not be able to participate and profit from group therapy geared toward verbal interactions.

Harter Self Perception Test is a paper and pencil test that children fill out regarding themselves. Depending on age and educational ability, some children need assistance in reading the questions. This provides a measure of children's perception of their worth.

The Child Behavior Checklist (CBCL) is a standardized checklist of childhood behavior problems and social competence. It measures factors that are important to assess about children such as the amount of anxiety, depression, somatic complaints, hyperactivity, aggressiveness, and delinquency that the parent sees in the child. There are six questions regarding children's sexuality on the CBCL. Parents are asked to complete a CBCL for every child in the family. In a two-parent family, both parents are asked to fill out the CBCL separately. Any large discrepancies in the parents' perceptions are carefully discussed with them because these often signal projections interfering with their ability to interact with their children, a scapegoated child, or a severely dysfunctional marital dyad.

Evaluations utilizing this instrument can be done at six-month intervals to provide information on treatment progress.

The Child Behavior Checklist (school version) is a standardized measure similar to the CBCL, which is filled out by children's teachers with norms for age and gender, providing a profile of the children's behavior at school. Evaluations utilizing this instrument can be done at six-month intervals to provide information on treatment progress.

The Roberts Apperception Test (RAT) is a projective test composed of sixteen cards depicting common situations and conflicts in children's lives. Included in the scenes portrayed are situations such as displays of parental disagreement and affection, peer conflicts, observation of nudity, and sibling rivalry. Children tell a story about each picture. The scoring of the RAT allows the clinician to assess perceptions children may have of common interpersonal relationships and provide a general description of children's personality, ability to identify problem situations, and coping styles.

Projective Storytelling Cards are a set of twenty-five projective cards representing a wide array of themes dealing with problematic issues that children have in their lives, especially traumatic events, family and social conflict, and physical and sexual abuse. There are no formal scoring methods, so this does not lend itself to a written assessment; however, the stimulus cards do encourage children to tell meaningful stories that often come directly from their own lives. This can be a valuable way to encourage more reluctant children to begin to speak with the clinician. These cards are very useful in individual or group therapy.

Assessment of the Parents of Children with Problematic Sexual Behaviors

The following instruments gather pertinent data from the parents that is useful for treatment planning:

The Child Abuse Potential Inventory (CAPI) contains 160 items that screen at-risk subjects and is useful in discriminating between abusers and nonabusers. This self-administered inventory measures factors such as distress, rigidity, unhappiness, loneliness, and problems with children, family, and others. A Spanish version is also available.

The Millon is a standardized intake assessment tool that measures personality and characterological disorders. Computerized scoring provides a printed assessment of the subject using a large normative base. A Spanish version is also available.

The FACES III paper and pencil test measures two critical aspects of family functioning, adaptability, and cohesion: testing has shown it to have adequate reliability and validity. A Spanish version is also available.

The Adult/Adolescent Parenting Inventory paper and pencil test gives an assessment of the adults' parenting ability.

Appendix E

Additional Issues Related to the Goals of Group Therapy

GOAL: Decreasing children's molesting behaviors
Daydreams and fantasies
Masturbation fantasies
Persistent thoughts; recurrent thoughts; intrusive thoughts
Impulsive versus compulsive sexual behaviors
Sex play versus sexual abuse; perpetration versus victimization
Sibling rivalry, sibling incest
Legal issues related to perpetration— the bottom line
Children who focus their sexual interest on adults
Power and control versus powerlessness
Assertion versus aggression
Revenge

GOAL: Increasing children's understanding of their unhealthy associations
and beliefs regarding sex and sexuality
Sex equals secrecy; sex equals dirtiness, filth, shame, guilt; sex equals love and
caring
Daydreams and fantasies
Masturbation fantasies; fantasies that precede actions
Betrayal
What is love? How do I know if someone really loves me? How do I know if I
really love someone?
Nurturing: where and how to get it

GOAL: Increasing children's understanding of natural and healthy sexuality
Why are people sexual together? What is the purpose of sex?
Values, attitudes, and feelings related to sex and sexuality
Sexual intercourse is a healthy way to express love between adults
Homophobia
Body image
Pregnancy
Contraception
Sexually transmitted diseases
Anatomy and physiology of sex organs and reproduction

Masturbation
Sexual arousal
Gender identity
Sexual object choice
Gender roles
Homosexuality, bisexuality, heterosexuality
The real meaning of scatological language

GOAL: Increasing children's awareness of their own and family patterns that
    precipitate, sustain, or increase sexually abusive and other nonadaptive be-
    haviors
    Physical battery in the family
    Scatology used by adults and children in the home
    Alcohol and drug abuse
    Role definition in the family; role reversals; parentified children
    Family scapegoats; family favorites
    Sibling rivalry
    Sociopathic tendencies of the family
    How predictable are the consequences of my actions in my family?

GOAL: Understanding and integrating feelings and thoughts associated with
    prior victimization including physical, sexual, and emotional abuse; aban-
    donment; neglect; family breakups; and deaths
    Secrecy
    Nightmares
    Is the world a just place?
    Where do I feel safe? How can I make myself safe? Who makes me feel safe?
    Whose responsibility is abuse?
    Abuse reminders
    PTSD symptoms
    What are my rights and what are the rights of others?
    Dissociation
    Boundaries: emotional, physical, and sexual
    Feelings about offenders
    Feeling damaged

GOAL: Helping children observe and assess their own behavior, be aware of
    the circumstances preceding their behavior, and think of the consequences
    of their behaviors before they act
    When I get in trouble, does it make a difference to anyone? Do I care about
    what others think of my behavior? Do I care how my behavior affects others?
    Responsibility versus blame
    I'm okay, you're okay

How do I make choices? What are the rules I go by?
If I could get away with it, what would I do?

GOAL: Increasing children's ability to observe and appreciate other people's feelings, needs, and rights
Make up a story with a beginning , a middle, and an end about animals who come to the emotional rescue of a baby doe whose mother was eaten by a lion in deepest Africa.
Antisocial and sociopathic behavior
Assertion versus aggression
Moral development

GOAL: Helping children understand their needs and values and develop their own goals and internal resources
Holding multiple contradictory feelings is okay. Loving and hating the same person at the same time happens.
How do others see me?
What am I proud of about me? What do others like about me?
Asking for help is a good idea. Who can I talk to?
What are the positive things about me?
Leader versus follower
Self-esteem; self-respect
Dreams

GOAL: Increasing children's ability to meet their needs in socially appropriate ways
What do I want to change about me? How can I do it? Whose help do I need?
Trusting is okay. Who can I trust?
What is happiness? How do I go about finding it?
Do I want friends? How can I get some?
What are my rights? What are other people's rights?
If someone says no, what do I do ?
How can I know when I am doing something wrong?

GOAL: Increasing children's connectedness to positive others and building internal objects that support future growth
What is it okay to ask for? What can I expect from others? What can others expect from me?
When I get hurt who can make me feel better? Do I know how to soothe myself?
Who do I like the best? Who likes me?

Appendix F

Youthful Offenders' Family Assessment Form

1. Explain what happened that caused the child to be identified as a "sexual offender."
2. How did each family member find out about the sexual offense?
3. How did each family member react?
4. What are each family member's explanations for what occurred?
5. What consequences, if any, were imposed at home on the offender for the sexual offenses?
6. [For sibling incest only] What consequences, if any, were imposed on the siblings of the offender?
7. Which family member is the most concerned about the sexual offense and why?
8. Which family member is the least concerned about the sexual offense and why?
9. Which family member is this child most similar to? Which family member is this child least similar to?
10. What does each family member think should happen to the child?
11. What does each family member think would help the child?
12. Is there any history of sexual abuse in the family, whether it occurred years ago, recently, or was always in doubt? History of physical abuse?
13. Is there any history of alcohol or drug abuse in the family? Have you ever had concerns about your child using alcohol or drugs?
14. Does any family member feel there are important relevant circumstances that must be known in order to help the child?

This Family Assessment Form (developed by Drs. Gil And Bodmer-Turner) is part of a comprehensive Youthful Sex Offender Assessment instrument developed by Dr. Bodmer-Turner. For information, contact:

Dr. Jeffrey Bodmer-Turner
A STEP FORWARD
2827 Concord Blvd.
Concord ,CA 94519

Resources

The following resources were designed for or about children who molest:

Ballester, S. and Pierre, F. (1989). *A matter of control.* Monsterworks Publications, Torrance, CA.

Berliner, L. and Rawlings, L. (1991). A treatment manual: Children with sexual behavior problems. Unpublished monograph, Harborview Sexual Assault Center, Harborview, WA.

Children sexually abusing other children—The last taboo? Summary of the Report ot the Committee of Enquiry into Children and Young People who Sexually Abuse other Children. Policy and Information Department, NCH, 85 Highbury Park, London N5 1UD.

Cunningham, C. and MacFarlane, K. (1991). *When children molest children: Group treatment strategies for young sexual abusers.* Safer Society Press, Orwell: VT.

Gil, E. (1987). *Children who molest: A guide for parents of young sex offenders.* Launch Press, Rockville: MD.

Johnson, T. C. *Let's talk about touching in the faimly.* This is a game designed for children invilved in parent-child or sibling incest, and their non-molesting parents. *Let's talk about touching.* (2nd Ed) A therapeutic game for sexualized children and children who molest. To order: Toni Cavanagh Johnson, Ph. D., 1101 Fremont Avenue, Ste. 104, So. Pasadena, CA   91030 (Cost: $15.00 each + $2.50 s/h).

Johnson, T. C. (1989). *Human sexuality curriculum for parents and children in troubled families.* Children's Institute International, Marshal Resource Library, 711 S. New Hampshire Avenue, L.A., CA 90005.

Johnson, T. C. (1991). Behaviors related to sex and sexuality in preschool children; Behaviors related to sex and sexuality in kindergarten through fourth-grade children. These charts separate children's behaviors into three categories: "Normal range," "Of concern," and "Seek professional help." (Cost: $3.00 for both).

Lane, S. (1990). *Special offender populations*. In G. D. Ryan & S. L. Lane (Eds.), Juvenile Sexual Offending. Lexington, MA: Lexington.

MacFarlane, K. and Cunningham, C. (1988). Steps to healthy touching. Kidsrights, P.O. Box 851, Mount Dora: FL.

Wachtel, A. (1992). *Sexually intrusive children: A review of the literature.* United Way of the Lower Mainland, 4543 Canada Way, Burnaby, BC V5G 4T4, Canada.

The following resources were designed for assessment
and treatment of children and may be useful with children who molest:

Games or Other Tools

Anatomical Drawings. Developed by Dr. Nicholas Groth for use in the investigation and intervention of child sexual abuse. To order: Forensic Mental Health Associates, 7513 Pointview Circle, Orlando, FL. 32836-6335.

Communication Skillbuilders. A set of cards depicting "feelings." To order: Communication skillbuilders, P. O. Box 279, Kalispel, MT 59903.

Projective Storytelling Cards. Developed by Dr. Kent Caruso. To order: Northwest Psychological Publishers, P. O. Box 49458, Redding, CA 96049-4958.

The Talking, Feeling, Doing Game. Developed by Dr. Richard Gardner. To order: Creative Therapeutics, 155 County Road, Cresskill, NJ 07626.

Books and Other Material

Davis, N. (1990). *Once upon a time—Therapeutic stories to heal abused children.* Revised Edition. Psychological Associates of Oxon Hill, Oxon Hill: MD.

De Domenico, G. S. (1988). *Sand tray world play: A comprehensive guide to the use of the sand tray in psychotherapeutic and transformational settings.* To order: Dr. De Domenico, 1946 Clemens Road, Oakland, CA 94602.

Kaufman, B. and Wohl, A. (1992). *Casualties of childhood: A developmental perspective on sexual abuse using projective drawings.* Brunner/Mazel: NY.

Mandel, J. G. and Damon, L. (1989). *Group treatment for sexually abused children.* Guilford Press: NY.

Malchiodi, C. and Peterson, I. R. (1985). *Creative arts modalities with children from violent homes.* Communication Arts Department, Cardinal Stritch College, 6801 North Yates Road, Milwaukee, WI 53217.

Play Therapy Bibliography, compiled by the Center for Play Therapy, University of North Texas, P. O. Box 13857, Denton, TX 76203-3857.

Distributors or Publishers

Creative Therapy Store
  Western Psychological Services
  12031 Wilshire Blvd.
  Los Angeles, CA 90025-1251

Childswork, Childsplay
  Center for Applied Psychology
  P. O. Box 1586
  King of Prussia, PA 19406

Feelings Factory
  5089 St. Mary's Street
  Raleigh, NC 27605

Kidsrights
  P. O. Box 851
  Mt. Dora, FL 27605

Safer Society Press
  RR # 1, Box 24-B
  Orwell, VT 05760

Uniquity
  P. O. Box 6
  Galt, CA 95623

Associations or Organizations

American Professional Society on the Abuse of Children
  332 So. Michigan Avenue, Ste. 1600
  Chicago, IL 60604

Association for Play Therapy
  1350 "M" Street
  Fresno, CA 93721

National Resource Center on Child Sexual Abuse
  106 Lincoln Street
  Huntsville, AL 35801

Interchange, National Adolescent Perpetrator Network.
  c/o Gail Ryan

C. Henry Kempe National Center for the Prevention of Child Abuse
and Neglect
1205 Oneida Street
Denver, CO 80220

Journals

American Journal of Orthopsychiatry
19 West 44th Street
New York, NY 10036

Child Abuse and Neglect: The International Journal
Pergamon Press
660 White Plains Road
Tarrytown, NY 10591-5153

Dissociation: Progress in the dissociative disorders
c/o Bridgeview Institute
3995 South Cobb Drive
Smyrna, GA 30080-6397

Journal of Child Sexual Abuse
Haworth Press
10 Alice Street
Binghamton, NY 13904-9981

Journal of Interpersonal Violence
Sage Publications
2455 Teller Road
Newbury Park, CA 91320

Journal of Traumatic Stress
Plenum Press
233 Spring Street
New York, NY 10013

Videos

Assessment and Treatment of Sexualized Children and Children who Molest: Conversations with Eliana Gil. J. Gary Mitchell Film Company, 1313 Scheibel Lane, Sebastopol, CA 95472 (800) 369-5367. The discussants on this two-tape series include Toni Cavanagh Johnson, Eugene Porter, Karen Cancino and Sharon Marks.

Treatment Outcome Studies Of Sexual Behavior Problems Of Children
(Funded By The National Center On Child Abuse And Neglect)

Children with Sexual Behavior Problems: Assessment and Treatment
Barbara Bonner, Ph.D.
Dept. of Pediatrics, CHO-4N-410
P.O. Box 26901
Oklahoma City, OK   73118
405-271-8858

This is a five-year treatment outcome study (beginning in 1992) in which children are assessed at two sites: the Department of Pediatrics in Oklahoma City, and the Sexual Assault Center in Seattle, Washington (with assistance from Lucy Berliner). The treatment will be conducted over three years at the University of Oklahoma site.

The treatment for children with sexual behavior programs lasts 12 weeks and consists of weekly, hourly group therapy for children 6-8 and 9-11 years of age. The primary caretakers also receive group therapy. Two treatment modalities are utilized: cognitive-behavioral (highly structured and directly focused on the sexual behavior); and dynamic play therapy (relatively unstructured and addressing the inappropriate sexual behavior only when the child brings it up). Children may be referred to other therapists for their own victimization issues. Male and female children attend groups together.

STEP Program
Center for Prevention Services
William D. Pithers, Ph.D.
Alison Stickrod Gray, M.S.
Box 254
Underhill Center, VT 05490-0254
802-899-2824

This grant was awarded to the Vermont Department of Social and Rehabilitation Services and contracted to the Center for Prevention Services, with Dr. Pithers as Principal Investigator and Alison Stickrod Gray as Project Director.

The treatment outcome study will provide treatment to children ages 7-12 across the state of Vermont, in multiple treatment sites. One additional site is out of state.

The program will develop specialized treatment responses for children with problematic sexual behaviors and their caregivers; emprically evaluate the efficacy of specialized interventions for these children and their families; and prepare and disseminate publications and treatment manuals regarding the assessment and treatment of sexually aggressive preadolescents.

Index

Note: Page numbers followed by (t) indicate tables.

C

Caretaker, therapist as, 312–313

Cartoons, in group therapy, 244–245

Child abuse. *See also* Sexual abuse, childhood.

reporting laws for, 133–134

Child Abuse Potential Inventory (CAP), 333

Child Behavior Checklist (CBCL), 332–333

in group therapy, 269

of children who molest, 69–70

Child Dissociative Checklist, 188

Child protective services (CPS), data collection from, 139

investigations by, 126, 128–129, 134–135

gender bias in, 129

referrals by, for family therapy, 276–277

reports required by, 175

response to molestation by, recommendations for, 131–132

treatment mandate from, 257–258

Child Sexual Behavior Checklist (CSBCL), 142

description of, 329

in group therapy, 269

in residential settings, 303

of children who molest, 72–73

Child Sexual Behavior Inventory (CSBI), 8, 142, 330–331

Children, abuse-reactive, behaviors of, 54–55

hypothesis of, 53–54

development of sexuality during, 1–20. *See also* Sexuality, development of.

developmental history of, in evaluation interview, 143–144

eroticized, 57

latency-aged, sexual development in, 25, 26(t)

physical, emotional boundaries of, inadequate parental socialization about, 18

school-age, sexual development in, 24–25, 26(t)

sexual behaviors of. *See also* under Sexual behavior.

range of, 42

sexualized, 91–99

caretaker concerns over, 92

community response to, 121–136

definition of, xiv, 91

excessive masturbation by, 93–95

family dynamics of, 101–120. *See also* Family dynamics.

individual therapy for, 180

inserting objects into genitalia by, 95

interview with, goals of, 154–168

nudity in, 96

peer sexual play in, 96–97

sex abuse history in, 98

sexual knowledge of, 12

sexual language use by, 95–96

sexual preoccupation in, 91–92

hormonal excess in, 3

therapeutic relationship with, 311. *See also* Countertransference; Transference.

treatment of, 129–130

sexually reactive, behaviors of, 54

Children who molest. *See also* Molestation, by children.

sex offenders vs., xv

terminology for, 67

Children's Institute International, 53

Chlamydial infection, sexual transmission of, 35

Chowchilla children, 57

Coercion, by children who molest, 75–76

in problematic sexual behaviors, 49

treatment plan for, 174–175

Cognitive strategies, teaching of, 234–235

Cognitive therapy, for attention deficit disorder, xi

Community response, referral options in, 129–131

to children who molest, 121–129

general suggestions for, 133–134

recommendations regarding, 131–134

Competency, of therapist, 317

Compulsion, in aggressive sexual behaviors, 49

masturbatory, 47

repetition, overstimulated sexuality and, 45

sexual, 195

trauma model and, 58–59

Conditioning, in child sexual abuse, 63

sexual, 102

Conduct disorder, coercive sexual behavior in, 61

in children who molest, xv, 70, 84–85

treatment model for, 179–180

Confidentiality, limits of, in clinical evaluation, 141